Reproductive Health: Advanced Researches

Reproductive Health: Advanced Researches

Editor: Sidney Alvarado

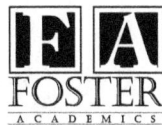

FA

FOSTER
ACADEMICS

www.fosteracademics.com

www.fosteracademics.com

FA FOSTER
ACADEMICS

Cataloging-in-Publication Data

Reproductive health : advanced researches / edited by Sidney Alvarado.
    p. cm.
Includes bibliographical references and index.
ISBN 978-1-63242-804-2
1. Reproductive health. 2. Fertility, Human. 3. Reproductive health--Research.
4. Human reproduction. I. Alvarado, Sidney.
RG133 .R47 2019
618.178--dc23

Foster Academics,
118-35 Queens Blvd., Suite 400,
Forest Hills, NY 11375, USA

ISBN 978-1-63242-804-2 (Hardback)

Contents

Preface

Reproductive health is concerned with the processes and functions of the reproductive system at all stages of life. It is meant to ensure that people enjoy a responsible, satisfying and safer sex life. Access to appropriate health care services related to reproductive medicine, and knowledge of safe, secure, and affordable birth control methods also come under the scope of reproductive health. Some of the common issues associated with reproductive health include adolescent health, contraception, sexually transmitted infection, abortion and female genital mutilation. This book aims to shed light on some of the unexplored aspects of reproductive health and the recent researches in this field. It attempts to understand the multiple branches that fall under the discipline of reproductive health and how such concepts have practical applications. This book aims to equip students, researchers and experts with the advanced topics and upcoming concepts in this area.

Significant researches are present in this book. Intensive efforts have been employed by authors to make this book an outstanding discourse. This book contains the enlightening chapters which have been written on the basis of significant researches done by the experts.

Finally, I would also like to thank all the members involved in this book for being a team and meeting all the deadlines for the submission of their respective works. I would also like to thank my friends and family for being supportive in my efforts.

Editor

Perceptions of counsellors and youth-serving professionals about sexual and reproductive health services for adolescents in Soweto, South Africa

Mamakiri Mulaudzi[1], Busisiwe Nkala Dlamini[1], Jenny Coetzee[1], Kathleen Sikkema[3], Glenda Gray[1,2] and Janan Janine Dietrich[1*]

Abstract

Background: Adolescents in South Africa remain vulnerable to HIV. Therefore, it is crucial to provide accessible adolescent-friendly HIV prevention interventions that are sensitive to their needs. This study aimed to investigate the perceptions of HIV counsellors and other youth-serving professionals about the barriers to providing adolescent youth-friendly sexual and reproductive health services to adolescents in Soweto, South Africa. The study also explored how sexual and reproductive health services in South Africa could be improved to become more accessible to adolescents.

Methods: The research team conducted two focus group discussions with HIV counsellors, and 19 semi-structured interviews with youth-serving professionals from organisations working with adolescents. Audio-recorded data were transcribed verbatim and analysed using thematic analysis.

Results: The results of the study reveal that counsellors were expected to give adolescents HIV counselling and testing (HCT) but felt restricted by what they perceived as inflexible standard operating procedures. Counsellors reported inadequate training to address adolescent psychosocial issues during HCT. Healthcare provider attitudes were perceived as a barrier to adolescents using sexual and reproductive health services. Participants strongly recommended augmenting adolescent sexual and reproductive health services to include counsellors and adolescents in developing age- and context-specific HIV prevention services for adolescents.

Conclusion: Continuous upskilling of HIV counsellors is a critical step in providing adolescent-friendly services. Input from all relevant stakeholders, including counsellors and adolescents, is essential in designing adolescent-friendly services.

Keywords: Adolescent-friendly, Youth-friendly, HIV, Sexual and reproductive health, HIV counselling and testing (HCT), Qualitative

* Correspondence: dietrichj@phru.co.za
[1]Perinatal HIV Research Unit (PHRU), Faculty of Health Sciences, University of the Witwatersrand, Chris Hani Road, Diepkloof, Soweto, Johannesburg 1864, South Africa
Full list of author information is available at the end of the article

Plain English summary

This study reports on the experiences of HIV counsellors and other youth-serving professionals in providing adolescent-friendly sexual and reproductive health services for adolescents in Soweto, South Africa. Information was collected using focus group discussions with HIV counsellors and face-to-face individual interviews with youth-serving professionals from different organisations in Soweto. The study investigated perceptions of HIV counsellors and other youth-serving professionals about the barriers to providing sexual and reproductive health services for adolescents in Soweto and how these services can be improved to become more adolescent-friendly. The results reveal a need to involve key stakeholders in the design and implementation of healthcare services for adolescents. Findings from this study will add to a deeper understanding of the challenges and barriers to providing adolescent-friendly sexual and reproductive health services to adolescents in Soweto, South Africa.

Background

Approximately 7.1% of young South Africans aged 15–24 are infected with HIV, with only 14.3% receiving anti-retroviral (ARV) treatment, the lowest proportion of treatment exposure when compared with other age groups [1]. At an adolescent-friendly HIV counselling and testing (HCT) centre in Soweto, 4% of young people aged 15–24 were HIV infected in 2015 [2]. Prior studies in South Africa have reported high rates of unintended adolescent pregnancies [3, 4]. In 2012, 3.9% of pregnant adolescent girls under 15 years and 19.3% of young women aged 15–24 years, were HIV-positive [5].

Young people in South Africa continue to face barriers when accessing sexual and reproductive health services [6–10]. Commonly cited barriers include lack of confidentiality and privacy, long waiting times (often with adults from the same community), inconvenient operating hours, the remote location of clinics, and a fear of parents finding out about clinic visits [8–10]. Service provider attitudes have been widely reported as hindering adolescents' access to health services, and studies indicate that adolescents tend to avoid health facilities because of the unfriendly, judgmental attitudes of healthcare workers [8, 9]. Researchers found that even after providers received training on how to respond to adolescents seeking sexual and reproductive health services, some remained biased and judgmental [8].

Increased access to and acceptability of sexual and reproductive healthcare among adolescents, achieved through adolescent-friendly services, are a priority for the South African Department of Health (DoH) [9]. Adolescent-friendly services refers to services that are prompt, geographically accessible and welcoming, and that can assure adolescents of confidentiality. These services are staffed with trained personnel to address the sexual and reproductive needs of adolescents [9]. In 1999, the South African DoH, in partnership with loveLife (a sexual health programme for adolescents), established the National Adolescent-Friendly Clinics Initiative (NAFCI). Managed by loveLife between 1999 and 2006, NAFCI was later incorporated into the South African DoH Adolescent and Youth Friendly Services programme [10], an intervention aimed at establishing standards for the provision of adolescent-friendly services in the public health sector [9]. The three key objectives of the NAFCI approach were: to provide high-quality adolescent reproductive and healthcare services and to improve access to health services for adolescents; to establish adolescent-friendly standards and criteria across national healthcare clinics in South Africa; and to equip healthcare workers with appropriate skills for adolescent-friendly service provision [9, 11]. Research on sexual and reproductive health services offered to adolescents rarely addresses service providers' experiences and perceptions. Therefore, this study investigated counsellors' and youth-serving professionals' perceptions of sexual and reproductive health services for adolescents to better understand how services can improve to become adolescent-friendly.

Methods

We conducted a qualitative cross-sectional study to explore the experiences of HIV counsellors and other youth-serving professionals in providing sexual and reproductive health services for adolescents. The aim was to explore barriers to providing adolescent-friendly sexual and reproductive health services.

Study setting

The study was conducted at the Perinatal HIV Research Unit (PHRU), located at Chris Hani Baragwanath Hospital in Soweto, South Africa. Soweto is the most populated black urban area in the city of Johannesburg, Gauteng province, with an estimated population of 2 million people [12].

Study design and participants

A qualitative study was conducted using focus group discussions (FGDs) and semi-structured interviews (SSIs). The FGDs were conducted with HIV counsellors to obtain diverse perspectives in a group setting. As HIV counselling and testing (HCT) is regarded as a non-sensitive topic, the group setting allowed for sharing of work practices and experiences of HCT with adolescents. Participants in the FGDs were purposively selected because they provided HCT services to adolescents, and were recruited from programmes and research sites based in hospitals, clinics and NGOs.

Semi-structured interviews (SSIs) were conducted to obtain specific and in-depth information from professionals working with adolescents. Seven Soweto-based organisations, including research sites and programmes providing services to adolescents, were purposively identified to recruit youth-serving professionals. The SSI participants comprised multidisciplinary team members providing services to both adults and adolescents.

Ethics
Study procedures were approved by the institutional review boards at the University of the Witwatersrand, Johannesburg, South Africa and Duke University, Durham in the United States. Permission for participation was obtained from managers at HCT centres in Soweto. HIV counsellors and youth-serving professionals gave informed consent for participating in the study and for audio-recording the FGDs and SSIs. Anonymity of participants was retained and audio-recordings used participant identity numbers. Participants received a ZAR50 (~ $7) reimbursement for participating in the study.

Data collection
Focus group discussions
Trained facilitators conducted the focus group discussions (FGDs) using a semi-structured interview guide. Each FGD hosted 8–12 participants, comprising HIV counsellors only, and lasted an average of 2 h including refreshment breaks. Interviews were conducted in private rooms at the PHRU. The FGD guide consisted of open-ended questions, with additional probing questions to elicit further information regarding counselling services for adolescents. Discussions elicited information on successful and unsuccessful adolescent sexual and reproductive health service strategies, challenges in adolescent counselling, and recommendations for improving adolescent sexual and reproductive health services.

Semi-structured interviews
Semi-structured interviews (SSIs) comprised youth-serving professionals, including HIV counsellors, who were not part of the FGDs. A trained interviewer administered the semi-structured interview guide, which consisted of open-ended questions with additional probing questions. The interview guide was designed in collaboration with a paediatrician, a psychologist, a nurse, social scientists and social workers, all of whom worked with the adolescent population. The SSI guide was designed to elicit in-depth information about participants' perceptions and beliefs about adolescents' sexual behaviour and HIV risk. In addition, participants were asked for suggestions to improve sexual and reproductive health services for adolescents.

Analysis
The FGDs and SSIs were audio-recorded, transcribed verbatim, translated into English, and entered into Maxqda for data analysis [13]. Transcripts were read by two researchers to facilitate data immersion. Data were first analysed thematically by identifying themes via coded text [14], and the development of themes and codes was data-driven. The primary analyst reviewed the first two transcripts line by line to gain an overall understanding of the data to develop codes, whereafter a second analyst developed a codebook. A meeting including a senior researcher was organised with both analysts to discuss the codebook and to check for consistency. Text from the transcribed data were coded and organised according to themes. Finally, major themes were defined in relation to the aims of the study, to identify key issues regarding perceptions about adolescent sexual and reproductive health services. The researchers arranged a meeting with participants to discuss the findings.

Results
Demographic characteristics of HIV counsellors and other youth-serving professionals
Two mixed gender FGDs (FGD1, $n = 10$; FGD2, $n = 12$) were carried out with 22 HIV counsellors. Two participants were unable to participate because of a scheduling conflict. In total, 10 male and 12 female HIV counsellors, were aged 19–45 years, from similar ethnic and cultural backgrounds (Zulu and Tswana were the two dominant ethnic groups in Soweto) took part. Work experience as counsellors ranged from one to 8 years. All but one participant (with a degree in counselling) had received basic HIV lay counselling training from a variety of organisations.

Semi-structured interviews were conducted with 19 professionals who had an adolescent caseload ($n = 9$ males and 10 females): two counsellors, two doctors, two nurses, three HIV project coordinators, two community outreach officers, two peer educators, two pastors, one teacher, one community liaison officer and two social workers. For inclusion in the study, professionals had to have worked with adolescents in Soweto for at least 1 year. Participants were aged 23–43 and were Tswana- or Zulu-speakers, except for one English-speaking participant. The study staff obtained permission from the organisations to conduct interviews, whereafter candidates were invited to participate. Three teachers and one social worker refused to participate (Table 1).

Key themes identified were: barriers to provision of adolescent-friendly services, and revisiting adolescent sexual and reproductive health services.

Barriers to provision of adolescent-friendly sexual and reproductive health services
Barriers to provision of adolescent-friendly sexual and reproductive health services included provider attitude

Table 1 Demographic characteristics

Participant characteristics	Frequency (n = 41)	Percentage (%)
Gender		
F	22	54
M	19	46
Age (range, years)		
19–25	20	49
26–32	9	22
33–39	9	22
40–46	3	7
Title/Occupation		
Community Liaison Officer	1	2
Doctor	2	5
HIV Counsellor	24	59
Outreach Officer	2	5
Peer Educator	2	5
Professional Nurse	2	5
Project Coordinator	3	7
Social Worker	2	5
Teacher	1	2
Pastor	2	5
Work Experience (range, years)		
1–5	29	71
6–10	10	24
10–15	2	5
Type of Organisation		
Church	2	5
Community centre	2	5
Hospital	5	12
NGO	21	51
Research site	9	22
Schools	2	5

and clinical environment in health care clinics, restrictive standard operating procedures, lack of consultation with relevant stakeholders, and insufficient training in adolescent HCT.

Provider attitude and clinical environment in public health care clinics

Discussions with participants from FGDs and SSIs revealed a critical gap between sexual and reproductive health service provision and adolescent needs. They addressed, primarily, provider attitudes and the clinical environment as barriers to adolescents' access to healthcare. Participants had reservations about integrating adolescent-friendly services into long-established public healthcare clinic settings. HIV counsellors reported that although public clinics were being improved

to provide reproductive health services for adolescents, the clinic environment and the healthcare workers were not adolescent-friendly. 'They [legislators] are busy with the development of a friendly environment for adolescents at the clinics but I doubt that it will work. I am saying this because of the attitude from the clinics, because adolescents don't go to the clinics, really they don't. The environment at the clinics – the health workers, like most of them, they are judgmental; most health workers are not friendly to youth.' (P2 Male counsellor, FGD2)

'A lot of them [adolescents], they know about teenage pregnancies and they have to go to a clinic where it's not teenage friendly and when they get there, they are told they are too young to have sex.' (Male Study Coordinator, SSI 5)

In FGD2, a male counsellor said that 'adolescents don't go to the clinics, really they don't. Why I am saying this? First, the attitude from the clinics- when they need [the] morning after pill, they go to the chemist not at the clinics. Even the condoms they don't fetch them from the clinics, they buy them at the pharmacy.'

Two nurses who participated in the study had different opinions and reported that customer care among clinics and healthcare workers was improving and changes were taking place to accommodate adolescents. One nurse said, 'I see that they enjoy coming here because now it's not like before. Hence we see most of them; they are using the facility especially family planning". (Female nurse, SSI 15).

However, perceptions of provider attitudes towards adolescents appeared to be inconsistent. During an SSI, a nurse stated, 'There are mean nurses but there are good nurses[too]... It's unfortunate that the South African public, it's like every time when they go to the clinic they meet the mean nurses only. They never get to meet the good nurses.' (Female clinical nurse, SSI 4).

Another nurse shared her experience in providing sexual and reproductive health services to female adolescents, stating, 'In this clinic I tell them that you are taking advantage, you are now coming here every day.' (Female nurse, SSI 15).

Restrictive standard operating procedures

Some HIV counsellors who participated in this study worked in organisations that engaged in research on adolescent HIV prevention and treatment. Standard operating procedures (SOPs) may be developed using different counselling models and differ across organisations, but all give instructions to counsellors on how they should conduct their counselling sessions to ensure consistent quality service provision. HIV counsellors, who worked in HIV prevention research for adolescents, reported dissatisfaction with the SOP's guiding counselling procedures. They stated that the inflexibility of SOPs restricted provision of adolescent-friendly services. One of the counsellors said that 'what annoys me the most in counselling is the fact that you are supposed to make this change and yet there is this protocol that says do not [do this] do not [do that].' (P5 female counsellor, FGD2).

Another counsellor maintained that 'this SOP thing that you mustn't be sitting like this or like that, it doesn't matter, but whatever [SOP] law that is set, let it be just a free environment. When you get there, feel free; if you want to put your feet on the table, if it means that person will feel comfortable, let it be, if it's going to make them open ...' (P2 male counsellor, FGD2).

Standard operating procedures included strict behavioural standards to which counsellors were expected to conform, which counsellors perceived as making the environment too rigid and uncomfortable for an adolescent client base. While there was disagreement about how SOPs had to be applied in the counselling session, counsellors recognised that SOPs were merely guidelines. One counsellor stated: 'You have to understand that the manual [SOP] is just there to guide you.' (P3 female counsellor, FGD1).

Similarly, participants in the key informant interviews commented that counsellors should not have to adhere strictly to the counselling manual. One counsellor said: 'I don't entirely believe that everything must be according to what this manual requires...' (male counsellor, SSI 3).

Lack of consultation with stakeholders

Participants from both the FGDs and SSIs raised concern over the lack of consultation with service providers and adolescents in developing SOPs. In their view, while they were expected to provide appropriate counselling services, there was a lack of consultation with the relevant people who knew what was taking place in counselling sessions. For example, one counsellor stated: 'It's one thing for a company to say this is what counsellors might do, but not be in the one-on-one session where counsellors are. It might not always be practical'. (P2 male counsellor, FGD2).

A female counsellor from FGD2 shared her perception regarding the perceived lack of consultation with counsellors when developing adolescent HCT guidelines: 'It is not realistic for me, for directors, to sit and decide what counsellors should say....'

Semi-structured interview participants commented on the lack of consultation with adolescents. A male project manager shared his perception of the lack of consultation with adolescents when developing interventions

for them: 'What we do, we sit in boardroom(s) like this and just think that we know what they [adolescents] are thinking outside there ... It won't have that impact. I need to go down there to these young people on the grassroots level and find out what they want.'

Participants advised that interventions or programmes would not have the desired effect if adolescents were not involved in their design and implementation. They recommended that adolescents be involved in the process of designing or planning from the beginning, including designing HCT programmes:

'... Involve teenagers in the planning and whatever protocols.' (Male peer educator, SSI 6)

'Include teenagers in the programmes. I think that would make a major, major difference.' (P5 female counsellor, FGD2)

A male physician suggested that adolescents provide input about the HIV testing process, regarding how they would like it to be done: 'We can ask kids how they would prefer HIV testing to be done.' (Male physician, SSI 10).

Insufficient training in adolescent HCT

In addition to SOP restrictions in providing adolescent-friendly HCT, participants' perceptions and experiences drew attention to the limited counselling training that they received. Counsellors in this study stated that they had received limited or no training in counselling adolescents. While all counsellors had general HIV/AIDS counselling skills, only a few had received formal training in adolescent development.

'The training that we get is completely directed at how to deal with children. I also got training last year on child participation and even there it deals with how you deal with children.' (P1 male counsellor, FGD1)

While some counsellors had received training specifically geared for adolescent counselling, the length of training was generally brief. This ineffective and low-quality training gave rise to concerns directed at beneficiaries of the services. A male peer educator (SSI participant) suggested that 'the duration for the training must not be too short. It must be longer because we are dealing with the lives of other people; you can't give someone wrong information'.

Although counsellors were expected to provide adolescent-friendly HCT, they had experienced cases that required in-depth counselling knowledge, including rape and psychosocial issues. One counsellor stated, 'We don't only focus on HIV/AIDS ...; we deal with rape, suicide, everything affecting teenagers.' (P5 female counsellor, FGD1).

Despite evidence suggesting the complexities of providing adolescent HCT, accounts suggested that counsellors felt ill-equipped to manage those cases: 'Let's say you are just an HIV counsellor, then they must take you for training on psychosocial counselling. That means if you do happen to pick up, for example, that 'the problem is that they don't love me at home that's why I sleep around' then you can deal with it.' (P5 female counsellor, FGD2).

Other counsellors recognised that adolescence was a unique stage of development, with complex issues that may be challenging for counsellors with limited counselling skills. Counsellors highlighted the need for further training in circumventing or reducing the number of referrals to external organisations. The limited training that many counsellors received resulted in a system of referrals to social workers or other professionals to ensure that clients received support. Some of the counsellors were dissatisfied because they had to refer cases that were perceived to be beyond their counselling level of competence and experience. 'The problem is that they tell you that if you come across this you will have to refer to the social worker and now you have started, your client understands you more and [has] built that trust, but now if you refer him to the social worker, it is going to be different and I am telling [you] he might not come back.' (P2 male counsellor, FGD2).

Revisiting sexual and reproductive health services for adolescents

Participants expressed the need for improvement in adolescent sexual and reproductive health services. They recommended the implementation of healthcare service provision characterised by a prompt, entertaining and welcoming environment that would encourage adolescents to talk freely. They alluded to the need to correct attitudes and provide sexual and reproductive health services at the adolescent's level of understanding, with an innovative approach to HIV information provision. 'The approach is very important, you know, and like creating a very friendly atmosphere where the adolescent can feel safe to say whatever that they want to say.' (Female clinical nurse, SSI 4)

'They really hate waiting ... they hate sitting on those benches for hours. They want something that's quick, if you can get a place where they come in and out.' (P1 Male counsellor, FGD1)

Participants highlighted the need to tailor adolescent health services to be culturally relevant and age specific. A peer educator from the SSIs said that 'when you are talking about adolescents you have to break it in this way: the background, and then the social norms and the communities ... An adolescent from Soweto will be different from an adolescent from the suburbs. You have to know what their values are so that you can understand the adolescent individually.' (Male peer educator, SSI 6).

Participants agreed that effective healthcare services had to be designed to be age- and language-specific, while being delivered at a developmentally appropriate level. 'We need to be able to understand what is their thinking, what are they going through, what makes them tick, what excites them and we bring our interventions at that level.' (Male peer educator, SSI 8).

Participants reported that adolescents were experiencing HIV/AIDS information fatigue, which made it difficult to keep them interested in HIV education programmes. They emphasised that adolescents were well informed about HIV/AIDS and that programmes on HIV education were perceived as boring, hence the call for innovative programmes. 'Most of the youth, they rather do something else than come here and listen to someone talking [about HIV/AIDS]. They will say ... [they] have heard it before; it's boring.' (Female nurse, SSI 15).

Discussion

Our study aimed to capture the experiences of youth-serving professionals and counsellors who work with adolescents, and who experience the systems and challenges that service providers and adolescents encounter in accessing and providing sexual and reproductive health services. Our findings indicate that HIV counsellors were generally prepared to provide adolescent-friendly services to the adolescent client base. However, this enthusiasm was curtailed by their perceptions that HIV counsellors were inadequately trained and were not included in the design of adolescent HCT interventions.

The South Africa government has adopted and initiated training on adolescent HCT based on the WHO and the Centre for Disease Control and Prevention guidelines [15]. Access to HCT in South Africa has increased, with more than 4500 public health clinics across the country providing voluntary counselling and testing and provider-initiated counselling and testing [15]. Access to HCT by adolescents in South Africa increased from 8.7% in 2008 to 51.6% in 2012 among females and from 19.9% in 2008 to 37.3% in 2012 among males [1]. However, due to the burden of HIV in South Africa, HCT remains the responsibility of lay counsellors [16] with limited and generalised skills who, are less confident in providing HCT to adolescents and young key populations [17].

In our study, HIV counsellors considered training on normal adolescent development and management of psychosocial issues, together with practical experience, as essential to enabling counsellors to provide services beyond basic HCT. Although these psychosocial issues were presented during HCT provision, they were beyond the scope of HCT. While the WHO recommendations for additional training to provide adolescent-specific services is echoed by physicians [18, 19] and counsellors [17, 20], addressing psychosocial issues during HCT is beyond the scope of lay HIV counsellors' ability. The notion of HIV counsellors came about as a means of reducing the strain on healthcare workers, in which they would provide pre-and post-test counselling to prepare clients for HIV testing. At the same time, HCT is a critical entry point for other services for adolescents. This paper argues that widening the scope of practice for HIV counsellors would require them to undergo extensive training and education and would require changing the criteria for the selection of HIV counsellors. The training needs reported by counsellors in this study are similar to those reported in previous studies in South Africa [17, 21]. Similarly, Coyle and Soodin [21] found that counsellors identified the need to expand HIV counselling training to include skills to address a range of issues beyond HIV/AIDS, including suicidal ideation, alcoholism and relationship problems [21]. Mwisongo et al. [17], reported that lay counsellors in their study reported a lack of standardised counselling and testing training, and a need for counselling skills for specific groups such as discordant couples, homosexuals, older clients and children.

There appeared to be confusion among participants around the regulatory aspects of the counselling SOP and how it informed the counselling session. In this context, the SOP is a document that outlines procedures to be followed when conducting HCT. The SOP offers essential step-by-step guidelines and is usually developed to facilitate consistency in the application of procedures, reducing the chances of miscommunication and ensuring the safety of the clients or patients [22]. An SOP can serve as a document for counsellors to maintain high quality service provision for adolescents and links with key objective 1 of the National Adolescent-Friendly Clinics Initiative (NAFCI) to provide accessible and acceptable health services for adolescents [9]. Some participants reported being restricted by their SOPs and desired greater leeway to tailor their sessions to individual adolescents. Including essential personnel such as counsellors in the development of SOPs for HCT could address the experiential recommendations of counsellors more adequately. Particularly striking about this finding was that counsellors stated a disconnect between SOPs and providing adolescent-friendly services owing to the restrictive nature of SOPs. To our knowledge, this is a unique finding in our study, but it echoes previous research findings that reported the need to engage all

relevant stakeholders from programme design through to implementation [23, 24]. Engaging counsellors in developing SOPs may enhance understanding of the importance of SOPs and how they can best be implemented to meet the needs of all stakeholders.

According to the South African HCT policy guidelines, adolescents are a unique group and are at increased risk of HIV [15]. As a vulnerable group, adolescents are faced with particular risks for HIV including early sexual debut, unprotected sex, peer pressure, the need to belong, sexual coercion and gender-based violence [15], and HCT services have to be tailored to address adolescent-specific needs. In particular, youth-serving professionals should receive training that provides a sound understanding of adolescent-friendly approaches, adolescent development and appropriate medical, psychosocial and developmental options according to age and maturity [15]. Generally in South Africa, training on HCT is provided by different accredited HCT organisations [17] and rarely focuses on understanding adolescent development. Overall, the findings reveal that sexual and reproductive health services, including HCT, for adolescents in Soweto, South Africa is occurring, but that providers require specific professional training to deliver consistent adolescent-friendly services.

Participants in this study reported that relevant stakeholders, particularly counsellors, were not involved in designing HIV interventions for adolescents, and recommended their involvement in future developments. Study participants recommended further that adolescents, the recipients of the service, should also be included in designing an HIV intervention for adolescents. The *Save the Children* project is a positive example of an adolescent-friendly approach involving adolescents, parents and teachers in improving adolescent-friendly sexual and reproductive health services at pharmacies [25]. In their study, the demand and use of the services increased for both male and female adolescents, with adolescents returning for repeat services. Moreover, training of pharmacists to provide adolescent-friendly services had a positive effect on the pharmacists as well as their service provision. Adolescents were comfortable with the services and experienced less age discrimination from pharmacists.

Another critical idea that emerged in this study was counsellors' lack of confidence in referring adolescents for psychosocial support when required. Although not ascertained in this study, underlying factors such as lack of understanding of the concept of referral [26] and power relations [27] whereby counsellors feel responsible for the life of the adolescent may give rise to counsellors' reluctance to refer adolescents. Other actors may include the lack of evidence for effective referral pathways and comprehensive healthcare service provision. Several studies have shown that adolescents are unlikely to transition to further services at a different location. Moreover, adolescents may be referred to services that are not adolescent-friendly due to limited availability of comprehensive adolescent-friendly healthcare services in South Africa. Adolescents should, ideally, be able to access a variety of services at one clinic. This may decrease the number of cases requiring referral, improve client retention and may be beneficial to adolescent clients. Where comprehensive service provision is impossible, adolescent clients should be referred to services that provide appropriate, and accessible support.

Limitations

The results reflect the experiences and perceptions of the participants, and may not be representative of all HIV counsellors and youth-serving professionals in Soweto. This paper is limited in that it does not include adolescent perspectives. Lastly, FGDs as a qualitative method, have been criticised for facilitating opinions that may be focused on the group norm. Despite the limitations, our study obtained perspectives from relevant contributors about sexual and reproductive health services, including HCT for adolescents in Soweto.

Conclusion

Continuous training and upskilling of lay counsellors and youth-serving professionals is a critical step in providing adolescent-friendly services. Additionally, all relevant stakeholders, particularly counsellors and adolescents, must be involved in designing adolescent-friendly services.

Abbreviations
FGDs: Focus group discussions; HCT: HIV counselling and testing; NAFCI: National Adolescent-Friendly Clinic Initiative; SOPs: Standard operating procedures; SSIs: Semi-structured interviews

Acknowledgements
The authors would like to acknowledge all participants in this study for their willingness to share their working experiences. Special thanks are due to Atholl Kleinhans, Precious Modiba and Sibongile Dladla for their assistance in developing the interview guides. Phindile Maesela is acknowledged for her assistance in facilitating and transcribing the focus group discussions.

Funding
This work was supported by the National Institute of Mental Health (NIM-H) (NIMH -1R21MH083308-01, Glenda Gray and Kathleen Sikkema (PIs), the South African AIDS Vaccine Initiative (SAAVI) and the Canadian Africa Prevention Trials Network (CAPTN). MK has a Thuthuka PhD award from the South African National Research Foundation.

Authors' contributions
GG and KS, as the principal investigators, conceptualised and designed the study. MK and JD were responsible for all aspects of data collection, coding, analysis, and writing of the initial manuscript draft. JC assisted in the interpretation of findings, and revised several sections of the manuscript. JC, BN, GG and KS were also involved in editing the drafts and added significant intellectual content. All authors have read and approved the final version of the manuscript.

Competing interests
The authors declare that they have no competing interests.

Author details
[1]Perinatal HIV Research Unit (PHRU), Faculty of Health Sciences, University of the Witwatersrand, Chris Hani Road, Diepkloof, Soweto, Johannesburg 1864, South Africa. [2]South African Medical Research Council, Cape Town, South Africa. [3]Duke University, Department of Psychology and Neuroscience, Durham, USA.

References
1. Shisana O, Rehle T, Simbayi L, Zuma K, Zungu N, Labadarios D, et al. South African National HIV Prevalence, Incidence and Behaviour Survey, 2012. Cape Town; 2014. http://www.hsrc.ac.za/uploads/pageContent/4565/SABSSM%20IV%20LEO%20final.pdf.
2. Nkala B, Khunwane M, Dietrich J, Otwombe K, Sekoane I, Sonqishe B, et al. Kganya Motsha adolescent Centre: a model for adolescent friendly HIV management and reproductive health for adolescents in Soweto, South Africa. AIDS Care. 2015;27:697–702. https://doi.org/10.1080/09540121.2014.993352.
3. Mchunu G, Peltzer K, Tutshana B, Seutlwadi L. Adolescent pregnancy and associated factors in south African youth. Afr Health Sci. 2012;12:426–34. https://doi.org/10.4314/ahs.v12i4.5.
4. Mothiba TM, Maputle MS. Factors contributing to teenage pregnancy in the Capricorn district of the Limpopo Province. Curationis. 2012;35:1–5. http://curationis.org.za/index.php/curationis/article/view/19/63.
5. Department of Health N. The 2012 National Antenatal Sentinel HIV and Herpes Simplex type-2 prevalence Survey. Pretoria, South Africa; 2014. https://www.health-e.org.za/wp-content/uploads/2014/05/ASHIVHerp_Report2014_22May2014.pdf.
6. Moletsane R. The need for quality sexual and reproductive health education to address barriers to girls ' educational outcomes in South Africa. Brookings; 2014. http://www.brookings.edu/~/media/research/files/papers/2014/12/quality-sexual-reproductive-health-education-south-africa-moletsane/echidnamoletsane2014web.pdf.
7. Frohlich JA, Mkhize N, Dellar RC, Mahlase G, Hons B, Montague CT, et al. Meeting the sexual and reproductive health needs of high-school students in South Africa : experiences from rural KwaZulu-Natal. South African Med J. 2014;104:8–11.
8. Lesedi C, Hoque ME. Youth's perception towards sexual and reproductive health Services at Family Welfare Association Centres in Botswana. J Soc Sci. 2011;28:137–43. https://doi.org/10.1080/09718923.2011.11892938
9. Ashton J, Dickson K, Pleaner M. Evolution of the national adolescent-friendly clinic initiative in South Africa; 2009. http://apps.who.int/iris/bitstream/10665/44154/1/9789241598361_eng.pdf.
10. Beksinska ME, Pillay L, Milford C, Smit JA. The sexual and reproductive health needs of youth in South Africa – history in context. South African Med J. 2014;104:676–8. http://www.samj.org.za/index.php/samj/article/view/8809/6190.
11. Dickson KE, Ashton J, Smith J-M. Does setting adolescent-friendly standards improve the quality of care in clinics? Evidence from South Africa. Int J Qual Health Care. 2007;19:80 9. https://doi.org/10.1093/intqhc/mzl070.
12. Ilgar R, Nazira J. Improving urban and Peri-urban geographical activities in Soweto township, Gauteng for sustainable livelihood. J Basic Appl Sci Res. 2011;1:1386–96. http://www.textroad.com/pdf/JBASR/J.%20Basic.%20Appl.%20Sci.%20Res.,%201(10)1386-1396,%202011.pdf

13. VERBI GmbH. MAXQDA – the art of data analysis. 2014. https://www.maxqda.com/

14. Boyatzis RE. Thematic analysis and code development: transforming qualitative information. Thousand Oaks, CA: Sage Publications Inc; 1998.

15. National Department of Health. HIV counselling and testing (HCT) policy guidelines. 2010. https://aidsfree.usaid.gov/sites/default/files/hts_policy_south-africa.pdf

16. National Department of Health. National HIV Counselling and Testing (HCT). Pretoria; 2010. http://www.genderjustice.org.za/publication/national-hiv-counselling-and-testing-hct-policy-guidelines/

17. Mwisongo A, Mehlomakhulu V, Mohlabane N, Peltzer K, Mthembu J, Van Rooyen H. Evaluation of the HIV lay counselling and testing profession in South Africa. BMC Health Serv Res. 2015;15:278. https://doi.org/10.1186/s12913-015-0940-y.

18. Kershnar R, Hooper C, Gold M, Norwitz ER, Illuzzi JL. Adolescent medicine: attitudes, training, and experience of pediatric, family medicine, and obstetric-gynecology residents. Yale J Biol Med. 2009;82:129–41. https://www.ncbi.nlm.nih.gov/pmc/articles/PMC2794488/pdf/yjbm_82_4_129.pdf

19. Ozer EM, Adams SH, Lustig JL, Millstein SG, Camfield K, El-Diwany S, et al. Can it be done? Implementing adolescent clinical preventive services. Health Serv Res. 2001;36(6 Pt 2):150–65. https://www.ncbi.nlm.nih.gov/pmc/articles/PMC1383612/pdf/16148966.pdf

20. Rachier CO, Gikundi E, Balmer DH, Robson M, Hunt KF, Cohen N. The meaning and challenge of voluntary counselling and testing (VCT) for counsellors–report of the Kenya Association of Professional Counsellors (KAPC) conference for sub-Saharan Africa. SAHARA J. 2004;1:175–81. http://www.tandfonline.com/doi/abs/10.1080/17290376.2004.9724840

21. Coyle A, Soodin M. Training, workload and stress among HIV counsellors. AIDS Care. 1992;4:217–21. https://doi.org/10.1080/09540129208253092.

22. Amare G. Reviewing the values of a standard operating procedure. Ethiop J Health Sci 2012;22:205–208. https://www.ncbi.nlm.nih.gov/pmc/articles/PMC3511899/pdf/EJHS2203-0205.pdf

23. Twine R, Kahn K, Scholtz A, Norris SA. Involvement of stakeholders in determining health priorities of adolescents in rural South Africa. Glob Health Action. 2016;9:1–9. http://umu.diva-portal.org/smash/get/diva2:946131/FULLTEXT01.pdf

24. Villa-Torres L, Svanemyr J. Ensuring youth's right to participation and promotion of youth leadership in the development of sexual and reproductive health policies and programs. J Adolesc Health. 2015;56:S51–7. https://doi.org/10.1016/j.jadohealth.2014.07.022.

25. YouthNet. Creating Youth-Friendly Pharmacies Youth prefer pharmacies for contraceptive services, but training and other efforts are needed to expand youth-friendly pharmacies. Series Number 17. http://www.iywg.org/sites/iywg/files/yl17e.pdf

26. Eskandari M, Abbas Abbaszadeh FB. Barriers of referral system to health care provision in rural societies in iran. J caring Sci. 2013;2:229–36. https://doi.org/10.5681/jcs.2013.028.

27. McDonald J, Jayasuriya R, Harris MF. The influence of power dynamics and trust on multidisciplinary collaboration: a qualitative case study of type 2 diabetes mellitus. BMC Health Serv Res. 2012;12:63. https://doi.org/10.1186/1472-6963-12-63.

Sexual and reproductive health services utilization and associated factors among secondary school students in Nekemte town, Ethiopia

Wakgari Binu[1], Taklu Marama[2*], Mulusew Gerbaba[3] and Melese Sinaga[3]

Abstract

Background: Despite policy actions and strategic efforts made to promote sexual and reproductive health service uptake of youths in Ethiopia, its utilization remains very low and little information was found on the extent to which school youths utilize available reproductive health services in Nekempt town. This study was aimed to assess utilization of Sexual and Reproduactive Health (SRH) services and its associated factors among secondary school students in Nekemte town, Ethiopia.

Method: A school based cross-sectional study design was conducted from April 18 to 22, 2016. Multistage cluster sampling technique was used to select a total of 768 students who attended secondary schools. Sexual and reproductive health services utilization was measured using one item asking whether they had used either of sexual and reproductive health services components during the last one year or not. The data was entered using EpiData Manager with Entry Client and further analysis was done using SPSS version 21 software. Descriptive statistics, cross tabulations, biviarate and multivariate logistic regression analyses were used. All variables were set by p-values less than 0.05 and reported by Adjusted Odds Ratio with its 95%CI.

Result: Out of the 768 study subjects, 739 participants underwent all the study components giving response rate of 96%. About 157 (21.2%) school youths reported that they utilized SRH services. On multivariable logistic regression analysis after adjusting for other variable, discussion with health workers (AOR 3.0, 95%CI [1.7–5.2]), previous history of perceived Sexually transmitted infections (STIs) symptoms (AOR 2.6, 95%CI [1.2–5.5]), being ever sexually experienced (AOR 5.9, 95%CI [3.4–10.2]) and exposure to information from school teachers (AOR 0.36, 95%CI [0.2–0.6]) were found to be independent determinants of sexual and reproductive services utilization among secondary school youths. Inconvenient times, lack of privacy, religion, culture, and parent prohibition were barriers to SRH service uptake cited by the school youths.

Conclusions: The overall utilization of sexual and reproductive services was low among school youths in the town. Discussion with health workers, history of perceived STIs symptoms, sexual experience and information were the association factors of sexual and reproductive service utilization among secondary school youths.

* Correspondence: mtaklu2002@gmail.com
[2]Department of Midwifery, College of Health Sciences and Medicine, Wolaita Sodo University, Wolaita Sodo, Ethiopia
Full list of author information is available at the end of the article

Plain English summary

Even if policy actions and strategic efforts made to promote sexual and reproductive health service uptake of youths in Ethiopia, few literatures showed its utilization remains very low. So, this study was aimed to assess utilization of Sexual and reproductive Health (SRH) services and its associated factors among secondary school students in Nekemte town, Ethiopia.

Students' utilized as well as utilizing Sexual and reproductive Health services before and during April 18th to 22nd, 2016 are included in the study. Among 12 above grade 9 schools, two government and 2 non-government schools were selected using lottery methods. For this study, a total of 768 students were needed. To have these, students from each grade and sections were randomly selected from their attendance lists. On the day of data collection the randomly selected students were told to remain in their classes. Sexual and Reproductive Health services utilization was measured if the students utilized one of the six given components. To keep data quality first data was entered to EpiData Manager and exported to SPSS version 21 software to have the required output. The result was described in table and figures, and cross tabulated. Bivariate logistic regression model was used to see association between utilization and other factors.

In this study, only 157 (21.2%) of students reported their utilization of Sexual and Reproduction Health services. Students who discussed with health workers, perceived history of Sexually transmitted infections (STIs) symptoms previously, experienced sex ever and exposed to information from school teachers were found to be better utilized Sexual and Reproductive Health services.

When summarized, the overall utilization of SRH services was low among school youths in the town.

Background

There were 1.8 billion young people aged 10–24 years among which 1.2 billion youth aged 15–24 years globally in 2015, accounting for one out of every six people worldwide in which Africa comprises 19% (above 226 million) of the global youth population [1]. Young people make up the greatest proportion of the population in sub-Saharan Africa, with more than one-third of the population 10–24 ages [2], and 33.8% of the total population in Ethiopia is between the age of 10–24 [3].

Since the International Conference on Population and Development Key Informant Interview held in Cairo in 1994, governments have pledged to improve the SRH of adolescents by providing access to comprehensive, appropriate information and education and youth friendly health services. Most regions of the world however, still fall short of these commitments, especially for unmarried young people [4].

Even though the comprehensive knowledge of HIV and other Reproductive Health (RH) problems is increasing around the world, many young people do not have the information or means to protect themselves from these problems [5]. Many health problems are contributed by adolescents and young people worldwide: 8.7 million abortions undergone, 41% of new HIV infection, high rate of early marriage and STIs, and high proportion of stillbirth and newborn deaths [6].

In Africa, 430,000 young people are infected with HIV per year; 2.6 million young people are living with HIV; teenage pregnancy rates still remain high and maternal mortality is among the leading causes of death for adolescent girls in this region [7]. Studies done in Ethiopia also show that there was 42.1% sexual risk behavior [8], 19% of youths reported having had premarital sexual intercourse with the mean age of 16.48 years at the first sexual intercourse [9], self-reported STIs prevalence was 19.5% [10] and abortion rate was also 65 per 1000 women [11].

Concerning the utilization of SRH services, it is not enough as expected from the efforts tried in Ethiopia. The SRH services utilization has great variation, 21.5% in Hadya [12] to 96.1%in Harar [13], that refers different factors are affecting the utilization differently in different part of the country. The SRH services utilization is high in areas where youth friendly services are available and accessible at community level [13]. It is evidenced that high school students were visiting SRH services to receive SRH information, for counseling service, to obtain a condom, for treatment of STI, for postabortion care [14] while others were not using SRH services because of inconvenience service hour, feel fear to be seen by others, too long waiting hours, providers are judgmental and unfriendly, feel embracement at seeking RH services [15]. Even, the utilizationof SRH services among secondary school students is not well explored in the country and the existing studies do not show enough information about the SRH situation of secondary school students, resulting in the absence of sustainable school based intervention for secondary chool students. So, additional study that assesses the magnitude and factors affecting SRH service utilization is very crucial to improve SRH service utilization of secondary school young people in the study area in the way that reduce morbidities and disabilities related to sexual and reproductive health.

Methods

Institution based cross-sectional study design was conducted in Nekemte town, East Wallaga zone, Western Ethiopia from April 18th to 22nd, 2016. Nekemte Town is situated 331 km from Addis Ababa city. The town covers an area of 5480 ha. According to data from

Central Statistics Agency Branch in the town, the total population of the town is projected to be 97,289 and young people in the town is estimated to be 37,796 (male = 19,626, female = 18,170) in 2016 [16].

According to the information from Nekemte Town Education Office, the total number of young people enrolled to secondary school (grade 9–12) in 2015/16 was 11,428 (male = 5539, female = 5867) students in seven government secondary schools 9771(85.5%) and five nonegovernment (two Non-Governmental Organizations (NGO) and three Private) secondary schools 1657(14.5%). The government schools are free of charge for educational purposes. From the estimated total population of young people, only 30.24% (28.22% of male and 32.29% of female) of young people were attending schools. The data from Nekemte Town Health Office showed that the town has one general hospital, two government health centers, one higher and twelve medium private clinics, twelve NGO health facilities that are serving the society. From these health facilities, one government health centre and two NGO clinics were delivering SRH services and youth friendly services separately which is free of charge.

All secondary school students enrolled in the year 2015/2016 in the town were the source population and all the students in randomly selected secondary schools were the study population. Sample size was calculated using single population proportion formula by taking the proportion (p) of SRH services utilization by school youths to be 32% taken from the study conducted in Bahir Dar Town (19) [17] with the conservative assumptions in order to get enough sample size that would allow the study to look into various aspects of school youths. The assumptions of 95% confidence level (level of significance, $z_\alpha = 1.96$), 5% margin of error, design effect of 2.0 and 15% non-response were used to determine the sample size. Accordingly, the total sample size was 768.

Concerning Sampling Techniques, Multistage cluster sampling technique was used in order to select a representative sample of students. Four schools (two from government ant two from non-government) were selected randomily. Samples were selected from government and non-government schools proportional to their size of the student population. The total sample was allocated to each grade from grade 9 to 12 proportionate to their student population size; Then four (2 government and 2 non-government) schools were selected using simple random sampling to recruit the allocated subjects for each grade. From each grade, sections were selected randomly and finally the study subjects were selected by using lottery method in SPSS using their attendance lists in the respective schools. On the day of data collection the randomly selected students were told to remain in their classes.

The dependent variable in this study was whether a participant had utilized SRH services within the last 12 months anywhere whether in government or private health institutions. This was measured through the dichotomous response (yes or no). The positive response was further validated with questions on the type of SRH services utilized. This included information and counseling on SRH issues, family planning, voluntary testing and counseling on HIV, abortion care, maternal and child care, testing and treatment of STIs. A positive ("yes") response to any one of these services was regarded as service utilization. The questionnaire was developed by collecting and adopting after customizing into the study context from various literatures [18–20].

The quality of data were assured by translating questionnaires from English to Afan Oromo then back to English by another expert using properly designed and pretested questionnaire. The data was collected by two Diploma Nurses and supervised by 1 BSc Nurse who were trained for two days. The pretest was done on 5 % of the sample size in Gimbi secondary school, a 100 km Town from Nekemte and some modifications such as skipping pattern and sequence sections in the questionnaire were made. To maintain confidentiality, each participant took a single sparsely arranged seat and the participant put the questionnaire on separate table arranged at corner of the room.

The questionnaires were designed by using Epidata manger and entry-client. Regarding data analysis and management, all returned questionnaires were checked for completeness and consistency manually. Thereafter, data was coded, entered into EPI-data entry client 2.0.8. 56 and exported to Statistical Package for the Social Sciences (SPSS) version 21. Frequencies and percentages were used to summarize descriptive statistics. Bivariate logistic regression analysis was done by entering variables that were found to affect SRH utilization. Variables with the p-value of less than or equal to 0.25 were entered into multivariate logistic regression. Those variables statistically significant at p-value less than 0.05 in multivariate logistic regression analysis were found to be taken as statistically significant. Adjusted odds ratio with the confidence level of 95% was considered to assess the strength of the association between dependent and independent variables.

Some phrases are Operationed as follows:
Attitude
Respondents has favorable attitude if they score equal or above mean score (66.48) of the total 24 attitude questions with 1–5 likert scale points.

Knowledge of SRH services
First knowledge about the SRH services was assessed by asking participants whether they were aware of SRH service components or not. Then SRH knowledge was assessed

through 8-item scale on knowledge of SRH service components and the sum of scores ranging from one (minimum) to eight (maximum) for subjects were used in the analysis.

SRH services utilization

This was measured through the dichotomous response (yes or no) by asking whether a participant had utilized one or more of SRH service components within the last 12 months. The positive response was further validated with questions on the type of SRH services utilized. A positive ("yes") response to any one of these services was regarded as service utilization.

Results

Out of the total of 768 study participants, 739 of students took part in the survey giving a response rate of 96.0%. Out of these, 349(47.2%) were males, 665 (90.0%) and 74(10.0%) falls under the age group of 15–19 and 20–24 years respectively with the mean age of 17.3(SD = ±1.7); 25(3.4%) and 136(18.4%) were single and in relationship respectively. Majority of them 925(97.4%) were Oromo by ethnic group, and protestant 525(55.5%) followers. Regarding their current educational status, h 82.9% and 17.1% of them were attending government and private schools respectively. The result also shows that the fathers 666(91.1%) and mothers 573(77.5%) of respondents were formally educated and 291(39.4%) of fathers and 220(29.8%) of mothers were employed. Majority of the students 486(65.8%) were living with their family (Table 1).

Knowledge, attitudes towards SRH services and sexual practices

Three hundred fifteen (42.6%) and 30 (4.1%) of the respondents know at least one and eight SRH service components respectively. Six hundred eighty six of participants have an information on SRH services and 564 (76.3%) of participants were aware of at least one health facility where SRH services could be delivered. Government health facilities, private health facilities, NGO health facilities and traditional facilities were SRH services delivery points as cited by 509(68.9%), 286(38.7%), 187(25.3%) and 50(6.8%) of the respondents respectively. Majority of the respondents (72.7%) have involved in the available school clubs and 400 (54.3%) had discussed on SRH issues with friends followed by health workers 163 (22.1%). 387(52.4%) of respondents had favorable attitude towards the SRH services. A total of 140 (18.9%) of respondents had ever experienced sexual intercourse and 101 (13.7%) of respondents had sexual contact within the last 12 months. The mean age at first sexual contact of respondents was 15.14 (SD = ±2.98) years. This study also showed that 70 (69.3%) of the sexually active respondents were male and 16 (15.8%) of them had more than one sexual partners (Table 2).

Table 1 Socio-demographic, community and family characteristics of secondary school students in Nekemte Town, Ethiopia, April 18–22, 2016

Socio-demographic characteristics		Frequencies	Percentage
Age	15–19	665	90.0
	20–24	74	10.0
Sex	Male	349	47.2
	Female	390	52.8
Marital status	Married	25	3.4
	In a love relationship	136	18.4
	Single	578	76.0
Ethnicity	Oromo	719	97.3
	Others	20	2.7
Religion	Protestant	405	54.8
	Orthodox	155	21.0
	Wakefata	140	18.9
	Muslim	28	3.8
	Others***	11	1.4
Educational status	Grade 9	297	40.2
	Grade 10	173	23.4
	Grade 11	134	18.1
	Grade 12	135	18.3
School type	Government	613	82.9
	Private	126	17.1
Pocket money in ETB	No money	224	30.3
	1–500	450	60.9
	> 500	65	8.8
Mother's education	No formal education	166	22.5
	Formal education	573	77.5
Father's education	No formal education	73	9.9
	Formal education	666	91.1
Mother's occupation	Unemployed	519	70.2
	Employed	220	29.8
Father's occupation	Unemployed	448	60.6
	Employed	291	39.4
Living arrangement	Living with family	486	65.8
	Not living with family	253	34.1
Family residence	Urban	534	72.3
	Rural	205	27.7

Others = Amhara, Guraghe, Tigrie Others*** = Adventist, Catholic, Jhoba

Respondents answered media 333(45.1%), teachers 305(41.3%), health workers 271(36.7%), friends 198(26.8%) as their potential sources of information for SRH services (Fig. 1).

Utilization of SRH services

This study result showed that 157(21.2%) of overall study subjects had received at least one component of

Table 2 Knowledge, Attitudes towards SRH services and Sexual practices among secondary school youths in Nekemte Town, 2016

SRH services and sexual related		Frequencies	Percentage
Awareness of SRH services(n = 739)	Yes	686	92.8
	No	53	7.2
Awareness of Health facilities(n = 687)	Yes	564	76.3
	No	123	16.6
Source of information on SRH services (Multiple Response)	Parent talk	116	12.2
	Friends	198	26.8
	Relatives	60	8.1
	Health workers	271	36.7
	School teachers	305	41.3
	School clubs	149	20.2
	Medias	333	45.1
	Printed materials	154	20.8
Participated in school clubs	Yes	537	72.7
	No	202	27.3
Discussion on SRH topics with (Multiple Response)	Mother	88	11.3
	Father	32	4.3
	Brother/sister	66	9
	Friends	400	54.3
	Health workers	163	22.1
	Relatives	34	4.6
Awareness of health facilities where to get SRH services (Multiple Response)	Government	509	68.9
	Private	286	37.8
	Non-government	187	25.3
	Traditional	50	6.8
Sexually ever experienced	Yes	140	18.9
	No	599	81.1
Currently sexually active	Yes	101	13.7
	No	638	86.3
Currently sexually active	Male	70	69.3
	Female	31	29.7
Partners for sexually actives	Only one	85	84.2
	More than one	16	15.8
Attitude towards SRH services use(n = 737)	Unfavorable	350	47.5
	Favorable	387	52.5

the SRH services in the last twelve months. Majority of the participants 116(54.8%) reported government health facilities from where they received SRH services followed by NGO health facilities 46(29.3%) (Table 3).

The most frequently utilized SRH services was Volunteer Test and Counseling 93(59.2%) followed by information and counseling on SRH issues 80(51%) and condom service 46(29.3%). The result also showed 27(26.7) of the sexually active respondents had utilized family planning methods in the last twelve month (Fig. 2).

In this study, 582(78.8%) of the study participants did not use SRH services in the last twelve months. The most frequently reported reasons for not utilizing SRH services, are not encountering any problem 249(42.8%) ,and believing that the services were not necessary 135 (23.2%) majorly (Fig. 3).

Factors associated with utilization of SRH services
During bivariate analysis, being in 20–24 age (COR 2.36, 95%CI [1.34 to 4.16]), being married (COR 2.69, 95%CI [1.14 to 6.34]), history STIs (COR 4.41, 95%CI [2.46 to 7.91]),

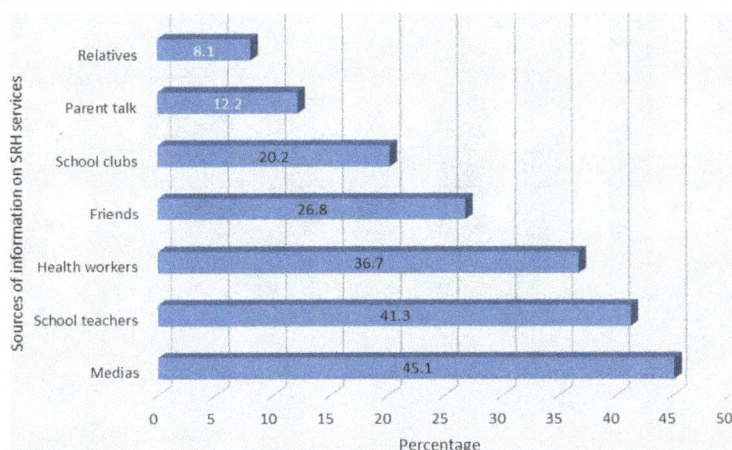

Fig. 1 Sources of information on SRH services for secondary school youths in Nekemte Town, April 18-22, 2016

having ever sexual contact (COR 7.51, 95%CI [4.87 to 11.6]), and having favorable attitude towards SRH services (COR 1.46, 95%CI [1.01 to 2.13]), heard SRH information from school teachers (COR 0.4, 95%CI [0.27, 0.59]) discussing on SRH issues with friends (COR 0.46, 95%CI [0.3, 0.72]), discussing on SRH issues with health care workers (COR 2.78, 95%CI [1.8, 4.3]) and attending non-government schools (COR 0.46, 95%CI [0.27–0.79]) were found to be associated with SRH services utilization (Table 4).

After controlling the effects of confounding, multivariate logistic regression analysis showed that the likelihood of SRH service utilization among secondary school was about 3 times (AOR = 3, 95%CI [1.72 to 5.24]) higher among respondents who discussed SRH issues with health workers than their counterparts. Students who had heard SRH issues from their school teachers were 64% (AOR = 0.36, 95%CI [0.21 to 0.61]) less likely to utilize SRHS than those who had not heard SRH related

Table 3 SRH service utilization and reasons don't use the services by secondary school youths in Nekemte Town, April 18–22, 2016

Characteristics		Frequency	Percentage
Utilized at least one SRH service (n = 739)	No	582	78.8
	Yes	157	21.2
SRH services utilized in the last 12 months (*n* = 157)			
Information and counseling on SRH issues		80	51
Family planning services		34	21.7
Pregnancy test		15	9.6
Pregnancy care		7	4.5
Abortion care services		5	3.2
Condom services		46	29.3
STIs treatment services		28	17.8
Voluntary testing and counseling for HIV		93	59.2
Sexually actives utilized FP methods (*n* = 101)	Yes	27	26.7
	No	74	74.3
Facilities where SRH services received (n = 157)			
Government		86	54.8
Private		35	22.3
Non-government		46	29.3
Traditional		6	3.8

N.B. System missed values were excluded from analysis, some observations may exceed 100% due to multiple options and others may be less than 100% due to missed values

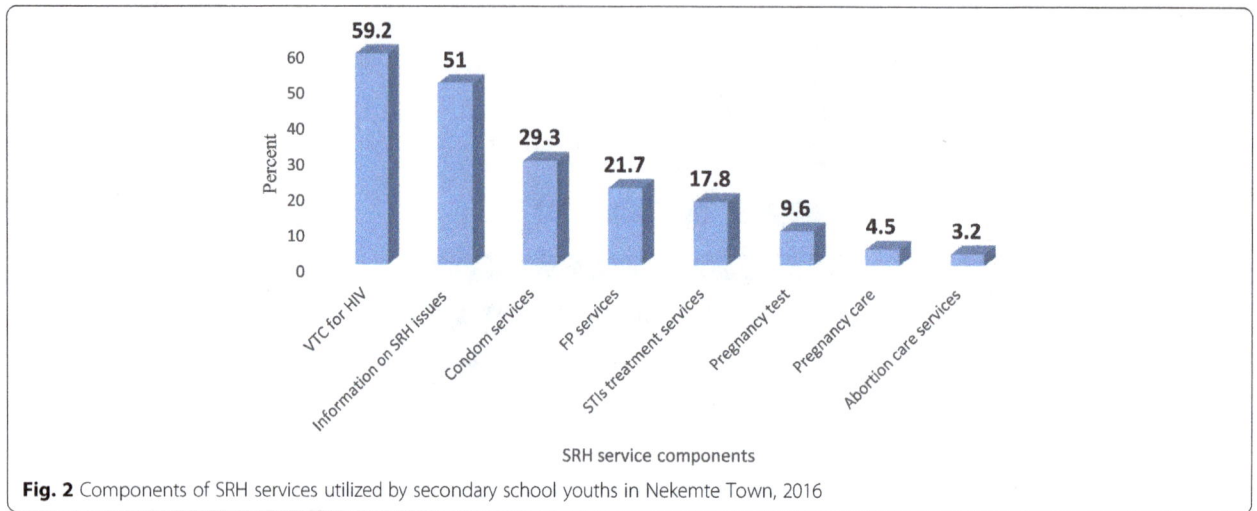

Fig. 2 Components of SRH services utilized by secondary school youths in Nekemte Town, 2016

issues from their school teacher. The odds of SRH service utilization was about 6 times [AOR = 5.87, 95%CI [3.38 to 10.19]] higher among respondents who ever had sexual contact than their counterparts. Respondents who had history of perceived STIs symptoms were 2.6 times (AOR 2.61, 95%CI [1.24 to 5.49]) more likely to utilize the SRH services.

Discussion

The overall utilization of SRH among school youths was 21.2% (95% CI[18.3–24.0]). It is similar with the cross-sectional study conducted in Mekele Town and East Gojjam zone [21, 22]. However, this finding was less than findings from Harar Town, Bahir Dar Town and Hadiya zone [12, 15, 23]. The possible reason for the discrepancy might be due to respondent characteristics,

socio-demographic backgrounds and time reference used in the definition of SRH service utilization [24].

Around 13.7% of the students (9.5% male) were found to be sexually active within the last 12 month. Even though it seems low percentage of respondents, sexual behavior may have been masked because of the socio-cultural context, where sexual intercourse out of marriage is taboo.This result was consistent with another study from Mekele and Nepali [22, 25]. But this percentage is lower than studies in Bahir Dar and Hadiya [17, 26]. The difference might be due to socio-cultural background in which early marriage is encouraged in the two areas. In addition, the number of sexually active male students is greater than of female student. This might indicate that male are having sex with out of school females. The mean age at first sexual contact of respondents was 15.14 indicating early initiation of sexual

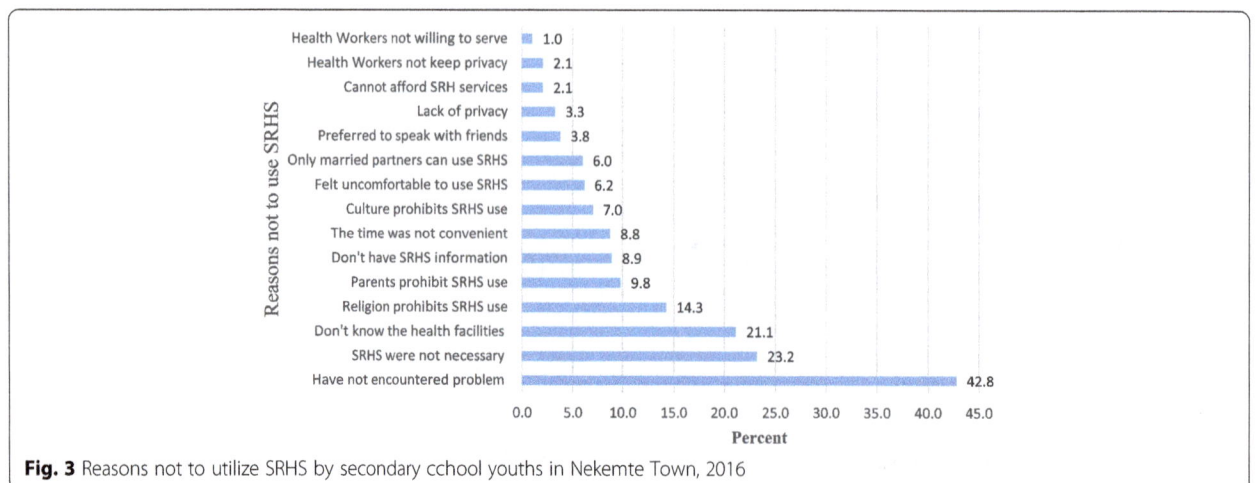

Fig. 3 Reasons not to utilize SRHS by secondary cchool youths in Nekemte Town, 2016

Table 4 Bivaraite and Multivariate logistic regression analysis of factors associated with SRH services utilization among secondary school students, Nekemte, April 18–22, 2016

Variables		SRH service utilization		COR (95%CI)	COR (95%CI)
		Yes (%)	No (%)		
Age					
15–19		132(84.1)	374(92.6)	1	1
20–24		25(15.9)	30(7.4)	2.36 (1.34–4.16)*	1.15(0.51-2.57)
Marital status					
Married		11(7.0)	11(2.7)	2.69(1.14–6.34)*	1.9(0.58-6.48)
Single		146(93.0)	393(97.3)	1	1
School type					
Government		139(88.5)	315(78.0)	1	1
Non-government		18(11.5)	89(220)	0.46(0.27–0.79)*	0.56(0.26-1.20)
Discussion on SRH					
With friends	Yes	76(60.3)	239(76.6)	0.46(0.3–0.72)*	0.73(0.39-1.37)
	No	50(39.7)	73(23.4)	1	1
With health workers	Yes	59(46.8)	75(24.0)	2.78(1.8–4.3)*	3(1.72-5.24)***
	No	67(53.2)	237(76.0)	1	1
Sources of SRH services					
School teachers	Yes	47(29.9)	209(51.7)	0.4(0.27–0.59)*	0.36(0.21-0.61)***
	No	110(70.1)	195(48.3)	1	1
History of STIs	Yes	33(24.3)	22(6.8)	4.41(2.46–7.91)*	2.61(1.24-5.49)**
	No	103(75.7)	303(93.2)	1	1
Sexually ever experienced	Yes	79(50.3)	48(11.9)	7.51(4.87–11.6)*	5.87(3.38-10.19)***
	No	78(49.7)	356(88.1)	1	1
Attitude for SRH services					
Unfavorable attitude		62(39.7)	198(49.1)	1	1
Favorable attitude		94(60.3)	205(50.9)	1.46(1.01–2.13)*	1.21(0.69-2.10)

*significant at bivatiat e ** significant at multivariate, $p < 0.05$ *** significant at multivariate, $p < 0.001$

intercourse. Sixteen (15.8%) of sexually active respondents had multiple sexual partner that may pose them for risky sexual behavior and these are important indicators of exposure to risk of pregnancy and STI during adolescence. This finding was in line with the study conducted in Mekele Town [22].

Majority of sexually active respondents 62(61.4%) had received at least one component of the SRH services in the last twelve months. This finding goes in line with the finding from Hadiya zone [14]. The possible justification of this may be sexually active respondents were more exposed for SRH problems so that they were concerned about their sexual and reproductive healths than sexually inactive respondents.

The commonly utilized SRH service component was voluntary testing and counseling service (59.2%) which is almost similar with the findings of studies done in Goba Town and Gondar Town [27, 28]. Information and counseling on SRH issues, condom services and STIs

services were also commonly recieved by 51.0%, 29.3% and 17.8% of the SRH services seekers respectively. This finding somewhat goes in line with the finding in Mekele Town [22]. Family planning service was utilized by 26. 7% of the sexually active respondents which was similar to the findig from Nepali [25, 29] but less than findings in Gondar Town and Goba Town [27, 28]. The possible explanation for this difference might be due to more implimentation opportunities at the community than at school level and information gap among school youths of the study area as more government and non-government facilities are designed and implementing at community level.

The findings of this study indicated that school youths used various health facilities in which government health facilities most frequently cited (50.9%) followed by NGO health facilities similar to those previous studies conducted in Bahir Dar [17]. The possible explanation for this could be the services in governmental and NGO health institutions were given either free of charge or with a minimal payment.

This study also showed that a small proportion (3.8%) of the participants used traditional health service that goes in line with Bahir Dar and East Gojjam study [17, 21]. Even if this proportion seems insignificant, it needs a special concern because unless it is confirmed by health experts traditional treatments may pose health risks to individuals.

For the successfulness of the YSRH program appropriate and relevant information about SRH should be delivered to youths. In this study, Medias (45.1%), teachers (41.3%) and health workers (36.7%) were found to be the main source of information about SRH services which was in line with the finding from Mekele [22].

The result of this study showed that majority of the respondents had not utilized SRH services diferrent reasons. Absence of SRH problems for a moment and the service was not necessary for the moment were most commonly cited reasons not to use SRH services. Religion, cultural and parent prohibition, inconvenience service hour and lack of privacy at delivery point were also barriers to SRH services utilization. This finding was consistent with the findings of East Gojjam, Bahir Dar and Mtwara Tanzania [17, 21, 30]. This implies that there is a need of tackling the barriers by dealing with the community leaders, religious leaders, families and health service systems.

In this study, discussion with health workers, previous history of perceived STIs symptoms, being ever sexually experienced and exposure to information from school teachers were found to be independent determinants of SRH services utilization among school youths.

This study revealed that discussion of the service with health care workers had a significant association with SRH service utilization. This can be justified by the fact that discussion of services with people allows youths to create more opportunities to exchange information, experiences, and build comprehensive knowledge about SRH. It can also create opportunities to deal with adolescent problems associated with SRH service utilization so that health professionals might be the source of accurate information for youths which help them for appropriate decision making in health services seeking behavior.

School youths who had encountered at least one of STIs symptom were more likely to utilize SRH services than who did not encounter the problem. And also individuals who had ever sexual contact were more likely to utilize SRH services than abstainers. This finding goes in line with study conducted in Hadiya, Nepali and Bahir Dar [12, 15, 29] This might be explained as youths were more concerned about their health when they encounter SRH problems that triggered them to use SRH services

and youths who engaged in sexual intercourse were more vulnerable to SRH problems that might increase the need for SRH services utilization. This implies that youths need an access to a wide range of health information and services as well as health professional support to engage in healthy and safe behavior.

The students who had heard SRH related issues from their school teachers seemed to be 64% less likely to utilize SRH service than students who had not heard from school teachers in contrary to the fact that school teachers were the main sources of information for SRH. The justification of this finding is not simple and difficult to hypothesize that information leads to less SRH service utilization. In fact school teachers may strictly disseminate information that early sexual initiation can lead to risk of unwanted pregnancy and STIs. Therefore, before formulating hypotheses about information from school teachers, additional studies using qualitative designs are needed to dig out the deeper meaning and to identify type of information delivered by school teachers.

Limitation

Since this study examines personal and sensitive issues, obtaining honest responses among adolescent students might have been difficult. Therefore this data might have prone to respondent bias. The quantitative study design did not allow for probing into certain areas which needed further qualitative description. Finally, the study was conducted in schools of only one town, which means the findings may not be generalizable to the overall Ethiopian adolescent and youth population, who are socio-economically, linguistically, and ethnically diverse. In addition factors at community (e.g. parental attitude and control over the children) and health system are needed to be included in the future researches.

Conclusion

This study had showed that low proportion of the school youths visited different health facilities to utilize SRH services in the last 12 months. The most frequently utilized SRH service component was voluntary testing and counseling service followed by information and counseling on SRH issues. Media was the potential source of information on SRH services for school youths followed by teachers and health workers. Discussion with health workers, previous history of perceived STIs symptoms, being ever sexually experienced and exposure to information from school teachers were found to be independent determinants of SRH services utilization among school youths.

Abbreviations
NGOs: Non-Governmental Organizations; RH: Reproductive Health; SPSS: Statistical Package for the Social Sciences; SRH: Sexual and Reproductive Health; SRHS: Sexual and Reproductive Health Services

Acknowledgements

We would like to pass our thanks to Jimma University with its respective College of Health sciences, Department of Population and Family Health. Our thanks also go to the school teachers who devoted their time from the busy schedule during data collection, all the study participants for giving us their busy time of study and who had took part in the survey, data collection facilitation and supervisions.

Funding

Sponsored by Jimma University.

Authors' contributions

These authors contributed equally to this work. All authors of this paper have read and approved the final version before submission.

Ethics approval and consent to participate

Ethical clearance was obtained from Jimma University, Collage of Health Sciences ethical review committee. Then letter of permission was written from the Oromia Regional Health Bureau to Nekemte Town Health and Education Offices. Cooperation letter was taken to each selected School Directors of the randomly selected schools from which the data is to be collected. Verbal informed consent was obtained from the selected individuals after objective of the study was communicated in detail. The respondents were assured that they have the right to be involved or not in the study, and that their non-involvement will not affect them in any way. Participants were not requested for name or any identifier on the questionnaire.

Competing interests

The authors declare that they have no competing interests.

Author details

[1]Department of Midwifery, Arba Minch College of Health Sciences, Arba Minch, Ethiopia. [2]Department of Midwifery, College of Health Sciences and Medicine, Wolaita Sodo University, Wolaita Sodo, Ethiopia. [3]Department of Population and Family Health, College of public Health and Medical Sciences, Jimma University, Jimma, Ethiopia.

References

1. United Nations Development of Economic and Social Association, *Youth population trends and sustainable development*. 2015.
2. United Nations Population Fund, *Status Report on Adolescents and Young People In Sub-Saharan Africa; Opportunities and Challenges*. 2012: 7 Naivasha Road, Sunninghill, Johannesburg, 2157 South Africa.
3. Central Statistical Agency of Ethiopia, *Ethiopia Mini Demographic and Health Survey*. 2014: Addis Ababa.
4. Siegrid Tautz *The Youth to Youth Initiative: an assessment of results in Ethiopia and Kenya*. 2011.
5. Population Reference Bureau, *The World's Youth*. 2013.
6. United Nations, Framework of actions for the follow-up to the Programme of action of the international conference on population and development beyond. 2014.
7. United Nations Education Social and Culture Organization, *One Year in Review | 2013–2014 Eastern And Southern; The Eastern and Southern Africa (ESA) Commitment,*. 2014.
8. Abebe M, Tsion A, Netsanet F. Living with parents and risky sexual behaviors among preparatory school students in Jimma zone, south West Ethiopia. African Halth Sci. 2013;13(2):498–506.

9. Bogale A, Seme A. Premarital sexual practices and its predictors among in-school youths of shendi town, west Gojjam zone, north western Ethiopia. BIOMED Cent Reprod Heal. 2014;11(1):1–9.
10. Yohannes B, Gelibo T, and T. M, Prevalence and Associated Factors of Sexually Transmitted Infections among Students of Wolaita Sodo University, Southern Ethiopia.. Int J Sci Technol Res, 2013. 2(2): p. 86–94.
11. Gelaye, A.A., KNT, and TM, Magnitude and risk factors of abortion among regular female students in Wolaita Sodo University, Ethiopia BMC Womens Health, 2014. 14(50): p. 1–9.
12. Cherie, N., G. Tura, and N. Teklehaymanot, Reproductive health needs and service utilization among youths in West Badewacho Woreda, Hadiya. 7(April): p. 145–153.
13. Harar Bulletin of Health Sciences Extracts Number 4. Youth-friendly health services utilization and factors in Harar, Ethiopia Aboma Motuma. In: 4; January 2012.
14. Bilal, S.M., et al., *Sexual & Reproductive Healthcare Utilization of Sexual and Reproductive Health Services in Ethiopia-Does it affect sexual activity among high school students ?* Sexual & Reproductive Healthcare. 6(1): p. 14–18.
15. Abebe, M. and W. Awoke, *Utilization of Youth Reproductive Health Services and Associated Factors among High School Students in Bahir Dar, Amhara Regional State.* (May): p. 69–75.
16. International, C.S.A.E.a.I., Ethiopia Demographic and Health Survey 2011. 2012, Central statistical agency and ICF international: Addis Ababa, Ethiopia and Calverton, Maryland, USA. p. 450.
17. Abebe M, Awoke W. Utilization of youth reproductive health services and associated factors among high school students in Bahir Dar, Amhara regional state. Open J Epidemiol. 2014;4:69–75.
18. Hynes, M., Et al., Reproductive Health Assessment Toolkit for Conflict-Affected Women. 2007: Atlanta, GA.
19. J., C., Illustrative Questionnaire for Interview Surveys with Young People.
20. Control, C.O.D., Reproductive health assessment questionnaire for conflict-affected WomenCDC. 2011.
21. Abajobir AA, Seme A. Reproductive health knowledge and services utilization among rural adolescents in east Gojjam zone, Ethiopia : a community-based cross-sectional study. BMC Health Serv Res. 2014;14(1):1–11.
22. Bilal SM, et al. Sexual & Reproductive Healthcare Utilization of sexual and reproductive health Services in Ethiopia – does it affect sexual activity among high school students ? Sex Reprod Healthc Elsevier BV. 2015;6(1):14–8.
23. Malarcher S, Social determinants of sexual and reproductive health. 2010: Geneva Swizerland;.
24. Motuma A, Youth-friendly Health Services Utilization and Factors in Harar, Ethiopia. Harar Bull Heal Sci., 2012. 4(5.).
25. Bam K, et al. Perceived sexual and reproductive health needs and service utilization among higher secondary school students in urban Nepal. Am J Public Heal Res. 2015;3(2):36–45.
26. Cherie N, Tura G, Teklehaymanot N. Reproductive health needs and service utilization among youths in west Badewacho Woreda, Hadiya zone, Ethiopia. J Public Heal Epidemiol. 2015;7(4):145–53.
27. Feleke SA, et al. Reproductive health service utilization and associated factors among adolescents (15 – 19 years old) in Gondar town, northwest. BMC Health Serv Res. 2013;13(1):1.
28. Gebreselassie B, et al., Assessment of Reproductive Health Service Utilization and Associated Factors Among Adolescents (15–19 Years Old) in Goba Town, Southeast Ethiopia. 2015. 3(4): p. 203–212.
29. Bam, K., et al., Perceived Sexual and Reproductive Health Needs and Service Utilization among Higher Secondary School Students in Urban Nepal. 3(2): p. 36–45.
30. Mbeba RM, et al. Barriers to sexual reproductive health services and rights among young people in Mtwara district, Tanzania : a qualitative study. Pan Afr Med J. 2012;13(1):1–6.

3

HIV status disclosure to male partners among rural Nigerian women along the prevention of mother-to-child transmission of HIV cascade

Angela Odiachi[1], Salome Erekaha[2], Llewellyn J. Cornelius[3], Christopher Isah[2], Habib O. Ramadhani[4], Laura Rapoport[5] and Nadia A. Sam-Agudu[2,4*]

Abstract

Background: HIV status disclosure to male partners is important for optimal outcomes in the prevention of mother-to-child transmission of HIV (PMTCT). Depending on timing of HIV diagnosis or pregnancy status, readiness to disclose and disclosure rates may differ among HIV-positive women. We sought to determine rates, patterns, and experiences of disclosure among Nigerian women along the PMTCT cascade.

Methods: HIV-positive women in rural North-Central Nigeria were purposively recruited according to their PMTCT cascade status: pregnant-newly HIV-diagnosed, pregnant-in care, postpartum, and lost-to-follow-up (LTFU). Participants were surveyed to determine rates of disclosure to male partners and others; in-depth interviews evaluated disclosure patterns and experiences. Tests of association were applied to quantitative data. Qualitative data were manually analysed by theme and content using the constant comparative method in a Grounded Theory approach.

Results: We interviewed 100 women; 69% were 21–30 years old, and 86% were married. There were 25, 26, 28 and 21 women in the newly-diagnosed, in-care, postpartum, and LTFU groups, respectively. Approximately 81% of all participants reported disclosing to anyone; however, family members were typically disclosed to first. Ultimately, more women had disclosed to male partners (85%) than to family members (55%). Rates of disclosure to anyone varied between groups: newly-diagnosed and LTFU women had the lowest (56%) and highest (100%) rates, respectively ($p = 0.001$). However, family ($p = 0.402$) and male partner ($p = 0.218$) disclosure rates were similar between cascade groups. Across all cascade groups, fear of divorce and intimate partner violence deterred women from disclosing to male partners. However, participants reported that with assistance from healthcare workers, disclosure and post-disclosure experiences were mostly positive.

(Continued on next page)

* Correspondence: nsamagudu@ihvnigeria.org
[2]International Research Center of Excellence, Institute of Human Virology
Nigeria, Abuja, Nigeria
[4]Institute of Human Virology, University of Maryland School of Medicine,
Baltimore, USA
Full list of author information is available at the end of the article

(Continued from previous page)

Conclusion: In our study cohort, although disclosure to male partners was overall higher, family members appeared more approachable for initial disclosure. Across cascade groups, male partners were ultimately disclosed to at rates > 75%, with no significant inter-group differences. Fear appears to be a major reason for non-disclosure or delayed disclosure by women to male partners. Augmentation of healthcare workers' skills and involvement can mediate gender power differentials, minimize fear and shorten time to male partner disclosure among women living with HIV, regardless of their PMTCT cascade status.

Keywords: HIV, Disclosure, PMTCT, Serodiscordance, Male partner, Nigeria

Plain English summary

For women living with HIV, disclosure to male partners is important in preventing HIV transmission to infants and staying healthy on treatment. Gender inequality plays a key role in low rates of disclosure by women to male partners. In addition, HIV disclosure rates may differ depending on whether the woman was recently or previously diagnosed, or whether she is pregnant or has delivered. We interviewed 100 women living with HIV in rural North-Central Nigeria to evaluate their disclosure history and experiences. The women were pregnant and newly or previously HIV-diagnosed, breastfeeding, or had dropped out of HIV care.

Most women (81%) reported disclosing to anyone; with more disclosing to male partners than relatives (85% versus 55%). However, family members were typically disclosed to, first. Also, newly-diagnosed and out-of-HIV-care women were least and most likely, respectively, to disclose to anyone. Male partner disclosure rates were similar across groups. Women who disclosed to male partners did so to motivate them to test for HIV and to keep open, honest couples' communication. Women across all groups reported avoiding male partner disclosure due to fear of divorce and violence. However, when healthcare workers were involved, disclosure experiences were mostly positive.

Our results show that family members were more approachable than male partners for initial disclosure, and that healthcare workers can, and have been instrumental in improving male partner disclosure experiences among HIV-positive women. Therefore, healthcare workers should be trained and proactively involved in helping HIV-positive women to disclose to male partners.

Background

In 2016, there were an estimated 3.2 million people living with HIV in Nigeria, at a prevalence rate of 2.9% in the general population [1]. Unprotected heterosexual sexual intercourse remains the main mode of HIV transmission in Nigeria [2]. Latest available data show HIV prevalence at 3.5% in adult females versus 3.3% in males;

and 3.6% and 3.2% in rural versus urban areas, respectively [2]. In 2016, only 34% of Nigeria's large HIV-positive population were estimated to know their HIV status, and only 30% of those diagnosed received antiretroviral therapy (ART) [1]. Linkage to treatment is important for HIV prevention, because once an HIV-positive client is initiated and is compliant on a suppressive ART regimen, the risk of onward transmission drops significantly [3]. Thus, knowledge of HIV status through massive scale-up of HIV testing, and subsequent linkage to suppressive treatment is critical to containing the HIV epidemic.

Besides personal knowledge of HIV status, disclosure of such status by people living with HIV to others – family, friends, sexual partners – is important for HIV prevention, including the prevention of mother-to-child transmission of HIV (PMTCT) [4]. Disclosure facilitates treatment uptake, drug adherence and retention in care for people living with HIV, including pregnant women [4–10]. For this population, disclosure is important for dual prevention of HIV transmission to sexual partners and for PMTCT, through promoting male partner HIV testing, the adoption of safer sex practices, and partner support for PMTCT service uptake [11, 12].

The PMTCT cascade is a multistep continuum of care package to be completed by HIV-positive mother-exposed infant pairs, and includes maternal HIV testing and treatment, antenatal and delivery care, early infant diagnosis, postnatal services, and linkage to long-term HIV care and support [13]. Women who have disclosed have higher rates of antenatal care (ANC) uptake, facility delivery, and PMTCT ART use compared to women who have not [7]. Non-disclosure has been reported as a predictor of PMTCT cascade dropout [14], while women who disclosed to their partners were up to five times more likely to access and be retained in PMTCT care [15].

Despite the benefits, disclosure rates in PMTCT are widely disparate, particularly in sub-Saharan Africa. Among pregnant and post-partum African women living with HIV, disclosure rates to any person range between 5% and 97% (pooled estimate 67%), and to male partners, 30 to 93% (pooled estimate 64%) [16]. Gender inequities often rooted in socio-cultural factors play a key role in low rates of HIV status disclosure to male partners among women living with HIV [17]. Reasons for male partner non-disclosure among these women include fear of abandonment with the resultant loss of emotional, material and financial support [17–22]; emotional abuse, including name-calling, accusations of infidelity and exposing the family to HIV [19, 20, 22], and sex deprivation [23, 24]. Stigma as well as perceived or enacted discrimination - from male partners and/or the community at large-have also been reported [19, 25]. In extreme cases, women do not disclose for fear of physical violence and other forms of intimate partner violence [17, 19, 26, 27].

As a result of HIV testing in pregnancy, women are often diagnosed before their male partners-regardless of who was infected first-and assume the added burden and responsibility of disclosure [25, 26]. Such gendered asymmetrical disclosure – where only one partner discloses - affects women disproportionately and negatively, as the partner who tests positive first is considered the unfaithful partner and "cause" of the infection, even though the male sexual partner may already be infected [22, 26]. Among HIV-positive women, the first choice of whom to disclose to is often not their male sexual partner(s); rather, where disclosure occurs, it is usually first to a trusted family member who is expected to provide social support [21]. Disclosure to a male partner may occur later or not at all [28, 29]. Despite pre-disclosure fears, many women who disclose report surprisingly positive reactions and support from family and male partners [6, 12, 15, 17, 21, 22, 30, 31]. Nonetheless, negative consequences have also been reported [6, 12, 15, 17, 18, 21, 26, 27].

The reasons for (non)-disclosure and therefore disclosure rates may differ depending on where a woman may be in her PMTCT or HIV treatment journey. Studies in Nigeria have reported HIV disclosure rates from women to male partners between 23.0% and 75.6% in often urban ART clinics [24, 32–34]; and 90.4% among pregnant women [27]. However there is little differentiated data on rates of disclosure among women at different points along the PMTCT cascade, particularly in programmatically challenging rural areas.

Nigeria is an especially important target for scale-up of impactful strategies in maternal and child health and PMTCT. The country has large gaps, especially in rural settings, including low rates of skilled ANC uptake in rural (46.5%) vs urban (86.0%) areas; and facility delivery for only 21.9% of rural, versus 61.7% of urban women [35]. PMTCT gaps include low maternal ART coverage and poor early infant diagnosis uptake of only 30% and 9%, respectively [36]. Studies discussed above highlight

the need for evidence to inform robust socio-behavioral interventions targeting key issues like non-disclosure, to augment biomedical PMTCT strategies in Nigeria and similar settings. This study sought to determine the rates, patterns and experiences of disclosure, primarily to male partners, among women at different stages of the PMTCT cascade in rural Nigeria.

Methods
Study design and setting
This cross-sectional, concurrent mixed-methods study was conducted between July and November 2013, and was nested in the MoMent Nigeria PMTCT implementation research project [37]. The study reported here was designed to understand the rates and context of disclosure (or lack thereof) among women living with HIV. The focus on differences along the PMTCT cascade prompted the study to target core PMTCT consumers (women), and not their male partners. The study was conducted in two high HIV-burden states of Nasarawa and the Federal Capital Territory, with 8.1% and 7.5% general population seroprevalence rates, respectively [2]. Both study states are contiguously located in North-Central Nigeria. The study sites comprised 14 primary healthcare centers and two secondary-level facilities located in rural communities participating in the prospective MoMent study [37]. At the time of the study, all sites were implementing World Health Organization (WHO) Option B regimens per national guidelines, including initiation of maternal ART regardless of CD4 count at booking, and infant breastfeeding concurrent with maternal ART [38].

Study participants and recruitment
Eligible women were HIV-positive, ≥ 18 years old, who were receiving or had previously received PMTCT services at the study sites. Participants were recruited in four groups according to their position along the PMTCT cascade at the time of the study:

- Pregnant, newly HIV-diagnosed (within 7 days), not yet on ART (*"newly-diagnosed women"*)
- Pregnant, on ART, in PMTCT care ("*ANC women*")
- Post-partum (up to three months), breastfeeding, on ART, in care ("*postpartum women*")
- Previously in PMTCT care, lost to follow-up (LTFU), not on ART ("*LTFU women*"). LTFU women were defined as those who had not completed a facility visit in three or more consecutive months.

Women who had not been formally enrolled in PMTCT care and did not have medical records at the recruiting study sites were excluded. We targeted a sample size of 100 participants along the PMTCT cascade, based on recruitment capacity estimations derived from enrollments for women living with HIV at the study sites.

Healthcare workers at study sites identified eligible women during routine clinic visits and contacted LTFU women identified from facility service registers by phone. Thereafter, all interested women were approached by study staff for written informed consent. Self-reported HIV status from participants was cross-checked with medical records at each study facility. To ensure that recruitment calls did not put women at risk of confidentiality breaches, all recruitment calls were made by healthcare workers who only provided details about the call if it was answered by the verified potential study participant; otherwise, a cryptic message or excuse was given by the caller. Those who were not reached by phone, especially those LTFU, were tracked with the assistance of Mentor Mothers (women living with HIV serving as peer counselors at study facilities).

Data collection and analyses

A three-section semi-structured interview guide was used to simultaneously collect quantitative and qualitative data. The first section of the guide collected information on participant socio-demographics (including age, religion, marital status and parity). The second section collected disclosure data (including whether patient had disclosed their status, to whom, and in what order), and data on knowledge of male partner HIV status. The third section collected qualitative information that explored each participant's "lived experience" with disclosure as a woman living with HIV. The key question posed to participants was, "Is there anyone who knows you have HIV?" This was followed by other questions to determine the process, and reasons for disclosure or non-disclosure. The guide was pilot-tested among 10 women and then updated and finalized before implementation.

Two trained study staff fluent in English and the dominant Hausa local language conducted each face-to-face interview in either language, using the semi-structured interview guide. While one study staff interviewed, the other observed and took notes. All interviews were audio-taped, and took place in private rooms at study sites or other designated locations by participant request. Each interview lasted 45 min to one hour. Healthcare workers at study sites neither participated in, nor observed the study sessions. Both English and Hausa audio-taped interviews were transcribed (and where relevant, translated) verbatim in English.

Quantitative data analysis

Participants' socio-demographic and disclosure data (including disclosure status and knowledge of male partner

HIV status) were first analysed with descriptive statistics. This was followed by tests for associations between the independent categorical variable "PMTCT cascade group," and dependent categorical variables, including "disclosure to male partners/others" and "knowledge of partner HIV status" using Fisher's Exact test. Statistical Package for Social Sciences version 16.0 for Windows was used for analysis, and statistical significance was set at $p \leq 0.05$.

Qualitative data analysis

All interview transcripts and field notes were analysed manually by theme and content using the constant comparative method in a Grounded Theory approach [39]. In this approach, inductive methodology is used to systematically generate theory from the data collected. Qualitative analysis was performed by a panel of eight trained and/or experienced researchers including SE, CI, LR, NASA, and an experienced Social Scientist (LJC). We selected a series of code words-the initial code word being "disclosure"-to develop themes and sub-themes from the qualitative data. This led to an iterative content analysis of the transcripts to examine the overall conceptual issues that emerged.

During this process, each researcher independently used the code list to hand-code assigned transcripts by reviewing and summarizing each line, phrase and paragraph to identify key themes. This was followed by group review, triangulation, and content analysis by iteration until a final consensus on patterns and categorizations was achieved. The research team that facilitated the in-depth interviews was maintained for completing transcription as well as conducting the qualitative analysis. AO additionally independently analyzed the transcripts and coded data based on identified themes from the interview guide, and compared these to themes identified by the paired researchers.

Results

A total of 100 women were recruited in the four targeted PMTCT cascade groups: 25 newly-diagnosed, 26 in ANC, 28 postpartum, and 21 LTFU women (Table 1). Overall, 69% (69/100) study participants were between 21 and 30 years old, and 88.0% (88/100) had at least primary school education. The majority (86%, 86/100) of participants were married. Recruited participants had similar characteristics across all four cascade groups except for marital status: women in the LTFU group were more likely to be single, compared to the other 3 groups (Table 1). We collected data for both quantitative and qualitative analyses from all 100 women.

Table 1 Respondents' socio-demographic characteristics

Characteristic	Newly- diagnosed $N = 25$ n (%)	ANC $N = 26$ n (%)	Postpartum $N = 28$ n (%)	Lost to follow-up $N = 21$ n (%)	P value*	Total $N = 100$ n (%)
Age, years						
< 21	4 (16.0)	0 (0.0)	0 (0.0)	3 (13.6)	0.327	7 (7.0)
21–30	18 (72.0)	16 (61.5)	22 (78.6)	13 (59.1)		69 (69.0)
31–40	3 (12.0)	10 (38.5)	6 (21.4)	5 (27.3)		24 (24.0)
Religious affiliation						
Christian	16 (66.7)	18 (69.2)	25 (92.6)	16 (76.2)	1.000	75 (76.5)
Muslim	8 (33.0)	8 (30.8)	2 (7.4)	5 (23.8)		23 (23.5)
No response	1	0	1	0		2
Marital status						
Single[a]	0 (0.0)	3 (11.5)	3 (10.7)	8 (38.1)	0.001	14 (14.0)
Married	25 (100.0)	23 (88.5)	25 (89.3)	13 (61.9)		86 (86.0)
Number of living children						
None	7 (28.0)	7 (27.0)	1 (3.7)	4 (20.0)	0.058	19 (19.5)
1–2	9 (36.0)	13 (50.0)	19 (70.4)	5 (25.0)		46 (46.9)
3–4	7 (28.0)	5 (19.2)	6 (22.2)	8 (40.0)		26 (26.5)
≥ 5	2 (8.0)	1 (3.8)	1 (3.7)	3 (15.0)		7 (7.1)
No response	0	0	1	1		2

Newly-diagnosed: women pregnant and newly HIV-diagnosed within last 7 days
ANC: women pregnant and in antenatal care
Postpartum: Breastfeeding women within 3 months of delivery
Lost-to follow-up: women who had not attended a clinic visit in 3 or more consecutive months
*Fisher's Exact test
[a]Includes single, widowed and divorced women

Table 2 Disclosure by women living with HIV along the PMTCT cascade

Disclosure status	Newly-diagnosed $N = 25$ n (%)	ANC $N = 26$ n (%)	Postpartum $N = 28$ n (%)	Lost to follow-up $N = 21$ n (%)	Total $N = 100$ n (%)	P value[a]
Disclosed to anyone						
Yes	14 (56.0)	21 (84.0)	24 (85.7)	21 (100.0)	80 (80.8)	0.001
No	11 (44.0)	4 (16.0)	4 (14.3)	0 (0.0)	19	
No response	0	1	0	0	(19.2) 1	
Disclosed to family[b]	$N = 14$	$N = 21$	$N = 24$	$N = 21$	$N = 80$	
Yes	5 (35.7)	12 (63.2)	12 (52.2)	13 (61.9)	42 (54.5)	0.402
No	9 (64.3)	7 (36.8)	11 (47.8)	8 (38.1)	35	
No response	0	2	1	0	(45.5) 3	
Disclosed to male partner[b]	$N = 14$	$N = 21$	$N = 24$	$N = 21$	$N = 80$	
Yes	13 (92.9)	17 (81.0)	18 (75.0)	20 (95.2)	68 (85.0)	0.218
No	1 (7.1)	4 (19.0)	6 (25.0)	1 (4.8)	12 (15.0)	
No response	0	0	0	0	0	

Newly-diagnosed: women pregnant and newly HIV-diagnosed within last 7 days
ANC: women pregnant and in antenatal care
Postpartum: Breastfeeding women within 3 months of delivery
Lost-to follow-up: women who had not attended a clinic visit in 3 or more consecutive months
[a]Fisher's exact test
[b]Participants responding "No" to "Disclosed to anyone" have been removed from denominator

Results from quantitative data analysis

Rates of HIV status disclosure among participants

Participants were asked about disclosure of their HIV-positive serostatus to male partners or first-order family members (parents and/or siblings). Approximately 81% of participants reported disclosing to anyone; of these, more had disclosed to their male partner than to family members (85.0% vs 54.5%) (Table 2). At 100%, LTFU women had the highest rates of disclosure to anyone. Newly-diagnosed women had the lowest disclosure rates to anyone or family, while postpartum women had the lowest disclosure rates to male partners. Interestingly, while newly-diagnosed women had the lowest disclosure rates to anyone, they had comparable or higher male partner disclosure rates compared to the other cascade groups. Analysis showed significantly different disclosure rates to anyone across the four groups ($p = 0.001$); however there were no significant differences in disclosure rates to family members ($p = 0.402$) or male partners ($p = 0.218$) (Table 2). Similarly, when compared across pregnant (newly-diagnosed + ANC) and non-pregnant (postpartum + LTFU) women, disclosure rates to anyone were lower among pregnant women (56% for newly-diagnosed women and 84% among ANC women), and were significantly different ($p = 0.0007$) compared to non-pregnant women; but not for disclosure to family ($p = 0.653$) or male partners ($p = 1.000$).

Participants' knowledge of male partners' HIV status

Approximately 67% (54/81) of respondents knew their partner's HIV status, while one-third did not (Table 3). There were significant differences in knowledge of male partner's HIV status across the four groups ($p = 0.004$). The newly-diagnosed group had the lowest proportion of women who knew their partner's status, while the LTFU group had the highest. Among 54 women who knew their partner's status, 30 reported he was HIV-negative, indicating an overall serodiscordance rate of 56%.

Results from qualitative data analysis

Figure 1 displays the core themes that emerged from qualitative data analysis.

Effect of fear on disclosure pattern and experience

One consistent theme that emerged in the qualitative analysis was descriptions of worry and stress experienced by participants, either as they considered disclosing, or as a result of disclosure, particularly with respect to male partners. Digging deeper into the data, we found that fear of marital conflict – in the form of intimate partner violence, or divorce – were important factors during the disclosure process across all four groups:: "*I have not even told my husband, because I don't want to lose my marriage. He is a very difficult person*"- Newly-diagnosed woman. "*Of course he will divorce me since the disease is a license to death*"-Newly-diagnosed woman. "*I feared that telling him would cause a fight*"-LTFU woman. "*I am scared of him beating me and divorcing me at the end*"-Postpartum woman. Some women mentioned being afraid, but failed to explain why, even after probing: "*No, I'm just afraid; I do not know how to tell him*"-Postpartum woman. "*I just feel like not telling him... I know I will tell him, but not now...Yes, he needs to know but it is something you take gradually*"-Postpartum woman.

Nearly 20% of study participants had not disclosed to anyone (Table 2), among whom were women who expressed no intention to disclose their status to male partners and/or others, largely due to uncertainty about the nature of ensuing reactions and/or stigma. "*I haven't told anyone because nobody in my family has experienced anything like this and this is a big shock to me, hearing that I have HIV*"-ANC woman. "*If I tell* [anyone], *I do not know what the outcome will be*"-Newly-diagnosed woman. "*Some people believe that HIV is only from promiscuous people*"-ANC woman.

The fear of marital conflict influenced not only whether women disclosed at all, or whom they disclosed to, but also the timing and pattern of disclosure. While

Table 3 Knowledge of Male Partner's HIV status among Women Living with HIV

Partner's HIV Status	Newly-diagnosed	ANC	Postpartum	Lost to follow-up	Total	P value[a]
	$N = 25$	$N = 26$	$N = 28$	$N = 21$	$N = 100$	
	n (%)	n (%)	n (%)	n (%)	n (%)	
Positive	4 (19.1)	8 (38.1)	5 (21.7)	7 (43.8)	24 (29.6)	
Negative	2 (9.5)	7 (33.3)	14 (60.9)	7 (43.8)	30 (37.0)	
Unknown	15 (71.4)	6 (28.6)	4 (17.4)	2 (12.4)	27 (33.4)	0.004
No response	4	5	5	5	19	

Newly-diagnosed: women pregnant and newly HIV-diagnosed within last 7 days
ANC: women pregnant and in antenatal care
Postpartum: Breastfeeding women within 3 months of delivery
Lost-to follow-up: women who had not attended a clinic visit in 3 or more consecutive months
[a]Fisher's Exact test

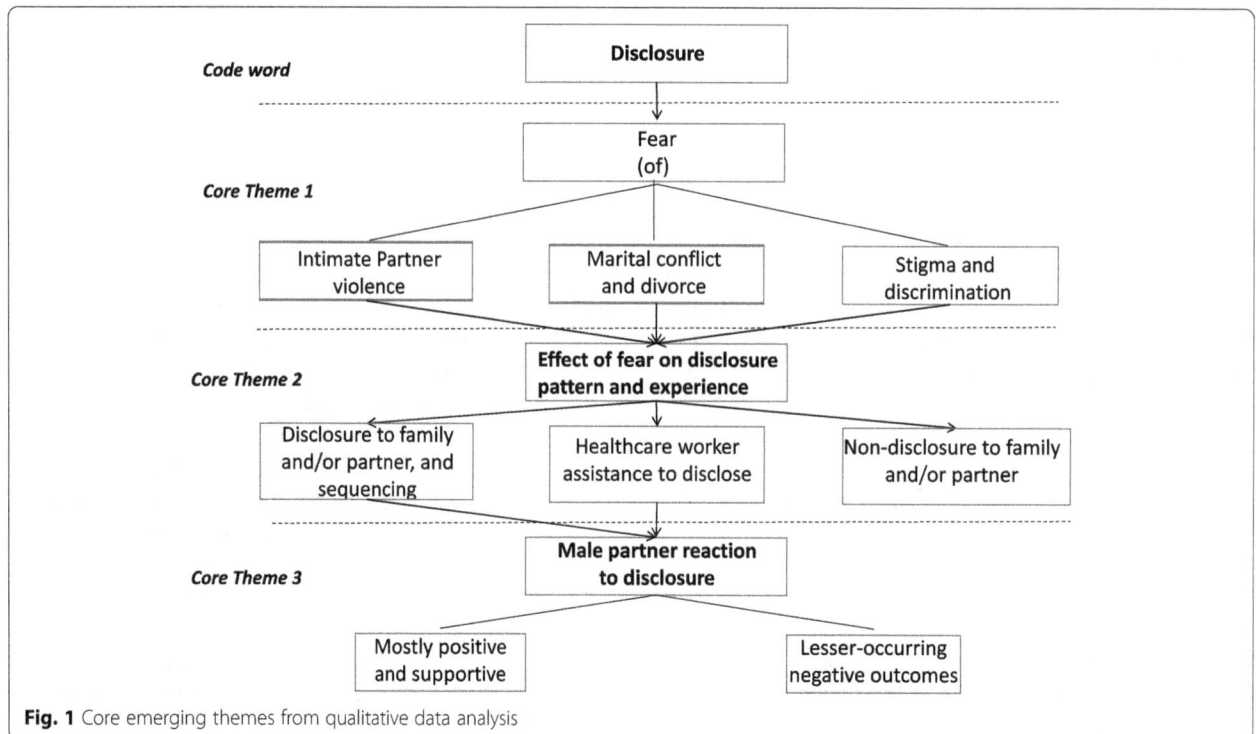

Fig. 1 Core emerging themes from qualitative data analysis

most women who disclosed, disclosed immediately or within days to others, they found it most difficult to disclose to male partners. One respondent stated: *"Only my sister knows. When they told me then I was sad. So I just went straight to her house to tell her...When I told her she was equally sad... I didn't tell him* [husband]*"*-ANC woman, partner status unknown. *"I called her* [sister] *after I have been told about the diagnosis in the hospital. She later found time to talk with me and encourage me about living with it...[But] he* [husband] *is not aware yet"* -Postpartum woman. *"I spoke with her* [friend] *after getting my diagnosis from the hospital. I explained everything to her since I cannot tell my husband. But truly, I am afraid of telling him because it is not something that is easy to disclose"* - Postpartum woman, partner status unknown.

Based on this fear, some women disclosed to only family, and not partners. However, women who first disclosed to male partners were sometimes asked by the latter to refrain from disclosing to anyone else, including family members: *"He begged me not to tell even my family; that we should keep it a secret between the two of us"* -ANC woman, partner HIV-negative. Such partners' requests may be as a result of pride, or fear of stigma "by association," prompting the men to want to protect their families, and their integrity and status in the home and/ or community.

Our quantitative analysis showed that nearly half (42%) of newly-diagnosed women had not disclosed to anyone (Table 2), but most stated that they planned to

disclose to their male partners: *"I plan to tell my husband very soon." "I will tell him when I reach home."* Given the immediacy of the HIV-positive diagnosis (seven days or less), there was less data from newly-diagnosed women on disclosure and post-disclosure experiences, especially involving male partners.

Besides fear, some women did not disclose to their male partner due to mistrust, anger and suspicion that he was responsible for their HIV-positive status through infidelity: *"[I have not told him] because I think that he is the one that gave HIV to me, because he doesn't stay at home"*- Postpartum woman. Yet other women withheld their status from partners due to prior refusal to have himself tested. *"I asked him to go and test, but he refused to go"* -Postpartum woman. In these cases, one could postulate that the women were trying to prevent disclosure asymmetry – not wanting to disclose when they did not know their partner's status: *"I didn't tell him immediately, I brought him here for his own test also, so we found out together that we were both positive"* -Postpartum woman. However, reasons for non-disclosure to family were not due to fear, but more to protect family from stress or HIV-related stigma. *"I did not disclose my status to my mother because she is sick and I knew if I told her she would be thinking as if I will die tomorrow"* -ANC woman, partner HIV-negative.

Women who did disclose to male partners did so mainly to maintain honest communication, they did not trust anyone else, and/or wanted to motivate their partner to test for HIV. *"I told him because I cannot live a life of secrecy*" -ANC woman, partner HIV-negative. "*There is no one I can inform about my status except my husband*" -Newly-diagnosed woman. "*I decided to tell him so that he could get tested, so we will know if we are both infected*" -Postpartum woman, partner HIV-negative. "*I told my husband and sister because I encouraged them to go and know their status*" -ANC woman, partner HIV-negative.

The strategic role and influence of healthcare workers in disclosure to male partners

For women who found it especially difficult to disclose to male partners, healthcare workers played a key role in facilitating disclosure and in convincing male partners to test for HIV. "*The day I was told my diagnosis, the nurse asked if she could help me disclose it to my husband, then I said she should go ahead. He was briefed about my HIV diagnosis, and then I spoke to him and asked him to come for the same HIV test too. He didn't refuse it. He was tested too and found out he is HIV-positive*" – Newly-diagnosed woman. "*I didn't tell him, it was the nurses that told him because I told them that if I should disclose it to him, he may not handle the issue well and I may lose my marriage, so they called him and disclosed everything to him*"-Postpartum woman. "*Initially the matron asked me if I would tell him myself and I said yes, but I couldn't do it. She then asked me to tell him to come to clinic. He met with the matron, they discussed my result, he took it in good faith and he was also advised to go for his own test*" -Newly-diagnosed woman.

In some cases, the health care worker was a co-strategist in the disclosure process: "*You know when I came here, the nurses spoke to me and tried to explain that it is important we let our partners know about it. So I told him, when I went for antenatal the previous day, that I saw a woman crying because they told her she had HIV. So he said, 'How would she be crying?' So that now gave me the courage to open up...you don't just say it outright because it is awkward. So I was just looking for a way*" -ANC woman.

Non-disclosure to female partners among HIV-positive male partners

Non-disclosure also seemed to cut both ways, as some participants reported that their male partners were already diagnosed HIV-positive and on treatment but did not disclose to their female partners until prompted by a sentinel event: "*I called him when they told me I was positive. So he came here* [clinic] *and he told us that he is already positive too, and he has been receiving his medication.*"-ANC woman. "*He was the first to be diagnosed; he did not tell me. He had tuberculosis, so we went to the hospital where he tested HIV positive. But when we came out of the hospital, instead of him to tell*

me, he did not. I confronted him and asked him why he did not tell me when he was diagnosed with HIV." -LTFU woman. In some cases women disclosed to their male partners without asking them to disclose theirs: "*I don't know his status. He didn't disclose it to me, but he knows my status. I wasn't bothered about asking him. I know he did it* [HIV test]." -Newly-diagnosed woman. "*I just told him. He told me it is not something we should discuss at that moment. But I don't know his status*"-Newly-diagnosed woman.

Male partner reaction to disclosure

For majority of the women who disclosed to male partners, partner reactions were often more positive and supportive than expected– with the men continuing to provide emotional, material and financial support, despite the initial shock from disclosure. "*I thought he would take it harsh on me. But he has been very caring since I told him that I'm positive and he reminds me when it is time to take my drugs*" -ANC woman, partner HIV-negative. "*From that day* [of disclosure] *he started loving me better. But he asked me not to talk about HIV anymore since we love each other. And he still supports me*" -Postpartum woman, partner HIV-negative. "*When I went home with the news that day, I was so disturbed. So he noticed and tried to find out what was wrong with me. I couldn't really pronounce it... He perceived that something was wrong, and he knew that I went to the hospital for some tests. So he asked if I was confirmed positive, and I said yes. He told me not to feel anxious about it, not to cry and that I should go and take the drugs.*" ANC woman, partner HIV-negative.

Very few women who disclosed to male partners reported experiencing the negative consequences feared by many women in the first place, including neglect and separation that could potentially impact on PMTCT outcomes: "*I was sick so he brought me to the clinic. That's how he knew my status. So as we were going home he told me he could not live with me anymore. He then sent me away to my father's house. I was there for four months. He came back six days after I delivered...He refused to give me money for transport to come for my drugs here* [clinic]... *That's why I was not taking the drugs*" -LTFU woman, partner HIV-negative. "*Since I disclosed to him, he only gives me some money for food and even if I ask him for any other thing, he won't listen. Before now, he wasn't behaving like this*" -LTFU woman, partner's status unknown.

Discussion

Among our study population of women living with HIV in rural North-Central Nigeria, we found overall disclosure rates to anyone to be relatively high, at 81%. Male partner disclosure reported by our study participants was also relatively high at 85%, compared to 23.0%, 86.5% and 90.4% reported in previous studies among women in South-West Nigeria [9, 24, 27]. Across similar African settings, male partner disclosure rates among HIV-positive women ranged between 44% in Kenya to 93% in Zimbabwe [7, 40]. Similar to our findings, a larger proportion of African women living with HIV ultimately disclose to their male partners than to others [7, 15, 21, 41], although our findings suggest, similar to other studies [21], that family members were often the first to be disclosed to.

Fear of divorce, interpersonal/domestic violence, neglect or other forms of psychological abuse deterred women from immediately disclosing to their male partners. However, with time and encouragement, especially from healthcare workers, women in our study population disclosed with surprisingly, largely positive results, as reported elsewhere in Africa [18, 22], even in situations where male partners were reportedly HIV-negative. Among our study cohort, reasons for male partner disclosure included feelings of obligation and to encourage partner HIV testing, as reported from studies in other African countries [15, 28]. For some women, disclosure to anyone occurred on the same day or shortly after diagnosis, as reported in other Nigerian [42] and African studies [18, 29]. Similar to findings in other studies [6, 21, 43], women who did not disclose a positive HIV status to family members were seeking to protect them.

In our study, newly-diagnosed women had significantly lower disclosure rates to anyone or family, compared to women in the other cascade groups who had previously established care ($p = 0.001$). Newly-diagnosed women also had the lowest rate of knowledge of partner serostatus ($p = 0.004$). This is understandable considering that these women were newly-diagnosed and may not have had enough time to process and share their diagnosis with anyone, or seek to know partner's HIV status. This finding is similar to disclosure data for the ART cascade that shows that newly-diagnosed patients had significantly lower disclosure rates than those in established care [5]. Postpartum and breastfeeding women in care, on the other hand, had the lowest disclosure rates to male partners. The reason for this is not clear from our study. However, Brou et al. [12] suggest that breastfeeding status correlates with partner disclosure by HIV-positive women; with women who choose exclusive formula feeding disclosing at a higher rate than those who choose to breastfeed. We were not able to explore disclosure rates in the context of infant feeding practices, as our study objectives did not include in-depth evaluation of infant feeding practices across all four cascade groups.

Pregnant women (newly diagnosed + ANC) had significantly lower disclosure to anyone than non-pregnant women (postpartum + LTFU) ($p = 0.0007$). Again, one likely explanation could be that non-pregnant women may have known their status for a longer duration. However, we were not able to accurately establish when previously-diagnosed women were diagnosed, as many women in our small rural community study setting did not enrol at the facility where they were first HIV-diagnosed: They often presented at multiple other facilities as "testing-naive" patients. Additionally, when asked, they were often unsure of the exact day or month of testing. This phenomenon was noted in the MoMent prospective study as well [44]. We are therefore limited in explaining if, or how time of HIV testing, and infant feeding practice influenced disclosure across the PMTCT cascade. Further research is needed on these aspects. There were no observed differences across the cascade groups with respect to male partner or family disclosure. However, our small sample size may have precluded the discovery of potential differences in our quantitative results.

Addressing the lack of, or delayed disclosure among couples is important for our study population and the larger HIV community in our study setting because of the relatively high reported HIV serodiscordance rate of nearly 56%, and unknown partner HIV status of 33%. Among our cascade groups, newly-diagnosed and ANC women were less likely to know their partner's status, compared to postpartum and LTFU women, and this difference was statistically significant. Previous Nigerian studies reported a similar serodiscordance rate for North-Central Nigeria of 51.9% [23] and lower rate of 38.5% for South-East Nigeria [45]. Proportions of HIV-positive women with unknown male partner status of 62.4% and 85% have been reported from studies in North-Central and South-East Nigeria, respectively [24, 45], which are much higher than for our study. Studies in similar sub-Saharan African settings have reported serodiscordance rates between 22.9% and 39% [15, 46, 47], and unknown male partner status between 32.7% and 80% among women living with HIV [11, 15, 48, 49]. Since we could not establish time of HIV diagnosis for our cascade groups, it is not possible to determine how and if this played a role in the observed differences in serodiscordance, and knowledge of partner status. For serodiscordant couples, early partner testing, notification and treatment can avert seroconversion in the HIV-negative partner [23].

Similar to previous findings [15, 43] our study highlights that healthcare workers play key motivating and supporting roles in disclosure among women living with HIV, especially to male partners, and actively facilitate partner HIV testing. Pre-existing and longstanding gender inequities in our study communities and similar settings have necessitated women needing more support (including to overcome fear) in order to disclose HIV-positive status to male partners. Intimate partner violence, inequitable laws and harmful traditional practices, including limited decision-making for women, reinforce unequal power dynamics between men and women [50]. Healthcare workers can, and have mediated these power dynamics by increasing their involvement in disclosure, especially by women to male partners. By supporting couples counselling and education on testing and treatment, healthcare workers play a crucial authoritative role in minimizing negative partner reactions for women who have accepted testing and tested positive. This is especially important, as studies show that men living with HIV whose wives know their seropositive status are often less likely to be violent or react negatively to news of female partner's seropositivity; thus, stressing the need for mutual HIV testing and disclosure [20, 26]. Couple testing and disclosure will also lessen the burden on the partner, which in the PMTCT context is the woman, who would otherwise test first and/or positive [51, 52].

As much as healthcare workers in our study setting assisted in disclosure, they and mentor mothers could only provide counselling and psychosocial support: they were not trained to provide professional mental health services. As such, professional mental services were not available to our study participants, especially newly-diagnosed women. Mental health services, if available, are often very expensive and located at large and/or tertiary centers located in urban areas at great traveling distance from rural communities. Thus, the study team could not refer participants for these services. Furthermore, such mental health referrals are not included in routine PMTCT care at the study facilities.

While no respondent in our study reported experiencing physical violence from their male partner as a result of disclosure, fear of such intimate partner violence as well as emotional/financial neglect and divorce/separation were expressed by women across cascade groups as reasons for non-disclosure. Therefore, prevention and management of marital conflict and intimate partner violence in the context of HIV disclosure remain important issues to address in PMTCT programming.

Surprisingly, male partner disclosure rates were no different among LTFU women compared to other cascade groups in our study. This is contrary to previous findings where nondisclosure has been reported as a correlate of PMTCT cascade dropout among women living with HIV [14] [53]; however, the disclosure evaluated in these studies were to anyone and not specifically disaggregated for disclosure to male partners or other individuals. Larger, and more robust studies are needed to examine the relationship between male partner-specific disclosure rates among women in and out of care along the PMTCT cascade.

Study limitations
This study was conducted in rural Nigeria with a purposive sample, therefore study findings may not be generalizable to all HIV-positive women in the study communities, nor to urban settings in Nigeria or elsewhere. There was also significant missing data for knowledge of male partner status: 19 of 100 women did not respond to this question. Analysis was therefore based on the remaining 81 who did. Furthermore, as explained earlier, we were unable to collect reliable data for all study participants on specific initial date of HIV diagnosis. Thus, we could not evaluate if timing of diagnosis was a correlate of overall disclosure rates, and rates between cascade groups. Socio-economic status and male partner socio-demographic data could also not be evaluated vis-à-vis disclosure rates, since we did not collect these data. Disclosure and male partner HIV-status was as reported by participants; it was not possible to verify this information and as such may not reflect reality. Lastly, limitations in cascade-based recruitment (especially for the two post-partum groups) in our rural study settings resulted in a relatively small sample size for each cascade group; this limited robust statistical comparisons between and within groups.

Conclusions
With support from healthcare workers and irrespective of cascade status, male partner disclosure was ultimately achieved with largely positive results for the majority of women in our study. Thus, strategies to increase healthcare worker skills and active involvement are likely to yield high rates of successful male partner disclosure in rural communities - a strategy that is especially important where there are high rates of serodiscordance. Concurrent strategies to enable healthcare workers make successful contact with male partners, either at the facility or in the community, will also be needed to facilitate the disclosure process for women at any stage of the PMTCT cascade. Comprehensive healthcare worker-supported interventions that target male partner disclosure in particular and context-specific women's empowerment in general are important to maximize outcomes in communities with high HIV burdens and low PMTCT performance. Lastly, while mental health and gender-based violence programs are limited in Nigeria and similar settings, the need is well-demonstrated [50], and it is important to establish these services in conjunction with PMTCT program scale-up.

Abbreviations
ANC: Antenatal care; ART: Antiretroviral therapy; HIV: Human immunodeficiency virus; LTFU: Lost to follow-up; PMTCT: Prevention of mother-to-child transmission of HIV

Acknowledgements
The authors would like to thank all the women who volunteered to participate in this study and shared their experiences. We also appreciate the efforts of research staff who assisted with data collection and transcription. Lastly, we thank the funders: World Health Organization, Global Affairs Canada, and the Fogarty AIDS International Training and Research Program for providing financial support for this study.

Funding
The MoMent Nigeria study was funded by the World Health Organization through an award for the Integrating and Scaling up PMTCT through Implementation Research (INSPIRE) initiative from Global Affairs Canada. Additional funding was provided by Fogarty AIDS International Training and Research Program grant number 5D43TW001041.

Authors' contributions
AO performed quantitative and qualitative analysis, drafted the manuscript and conducted final review. SE collected data, performed quantitative and qualitative analysis and contributed to manuscript development and final review. LJC designed the study, performed qualitative analysis and contributed to manuscript development and final review. CI performed quantitative and qualitative analysis and contributed to manuscript development and final review. HOR performed quantitative analysis and contributed to manuscript development and final review. LR collected data, performed qualitative analysis and contributed to manuscript development and final review. NASA conceptualized and designed the study, performed qualitative analysis and contributed to manuscript development and final review as well as provided overall supervision for the study. All authors read and approved the final manuscript.

Competing interests
The authors declare that they have no competing interests.

Author details
[1]Abuja, Nigeria. [2]International Research Center of Excellence, Institute of Human Virology Nigeria, Abuja, Nigeria. [3]School of Social Work and College of Public Health, University of Georgia Athens, Athens, USA. [4]Institute of Human Virology, University of Maryland School of Medicine, Baltimore, USA. [5]Harvard T. H. Chan School of Public Health, Boston, USA.

References
1. UNAIDS. UNAIDS Data 2017. Geneva: Joint United Nations Programme on HIV/AIDS; 2017.
2. CHAI Nigeria. SMS printer program report. 2012.
3. WHO. Programmatic Update. Antiretroviral treatment as prevention (TASP) of HIV and TB. Geneva: World Health Organisation; 2012.
4. Hodgson I, Plummer ML, Konopka SN, Colvin CJ, Jonas E, Albertini J, et al. A systematic review of individual and contextual factors affecting ART initiation, adherence, and retention for HIV-infected pregnant and postpartum women. PLoS One. 2014;9(11):e111421.
5. Ostermann J, Pence B, Whetten K, Yao J, Itemba D, Maro V, et al. HIV serostatus disclosure in the treatment cascade: evidence from northern Tanzania. AIDS Care. 2015;27(Suppl 1):59–64.
6. Winchester MS, McGrath JW, Kaawa-Mafigiri D, Namutiibwa F, Ssendegye G, Nalwoga A, et al. Early HIV disclosure and nondisclosure among men and women on antiretroviral treatment in Uganda. AIDS Care. 2013;25(10):1253–8.
7. Spangler SA, Onono M, Bukusi EA, Cohen CR, Turan JM. HIV-positive status disclosure and use of essential PMTCT and maternal health services in rural Kenya. J Acquir Immune Defic Syndr. 2014;67(Suppl 4):S235–42.
8. Falang KD, Akubaka P, Jimam NS. Patient factors impacting antiretroviral drug adherence in a Nigerian tertiary hospital. J Pharmacol Pharmacother. 2012;3(2):138–42.
9. Ekama SO, Herbertson EC, Addeh EJ, Gab-Okafor CV, Onwujekwe DI, Tayo F, et al. Pattern and determinants of antiretroviral drug adherence among Nigerian pregnant women. J Pregnancy. 2012;2012:851810.
10. Charurat M, Oyegunle M, Benjamin R, Habib A, Eze E, Ele P, et al. Patient retention and adherence to antiretrovirals in a large antiretroviral therapy program in Nigeria: a longitudinal analysis for risk factors. PLoS One. 2010;5(5):e10584.
11. Peltzer K, Jones D, Weiss SM, Villar-Loubet O, Shikwane E. Sexual risk, serostatus and intimate partner violence among couples during pregnancy in rural South Africa. AIDS Behav. 2013;17(2):508–16.
12. Brou H, Djohan G, Becquet R, Allou G, Ekouevi DK, Viho I, et al. When do HIV-infected women disclose their HIV status to their male partner and why? A study in a PMTCT programme, Abidjan. PLoS Med. 2007;4(12):e342.
13. Stringer EM, Chi BH, Chintu N, Creek TL, Ekouevi DK, Coetzee D, et al. Monitoring effectiveness of programmes to prevent mother-to-child HIV transmission in lower-income countries. Bull World Health Organ. 2008;86(1):57–62.
14. Woldesenbet S, Jackson D, Lombard C, Dinh TH, Puren A, Sherman G, et al. Missed opportunities along the prevention of mother-to-child transmission services Cascade in South Africa: uptake, determinants, and attributable risk (the SAPMTCTE). PLoS One. 2015;10(7):e0132425.
15. Sendo EG, Cherie A, Erku TA. Disclosure experience to partner and its effect on intention to utilize prevention of mother to child transmission service among HIV positive pregnant women attending antenatal care in Addis Ababa, Ethiopia. BMC Public Health. 2013;13:765.
16. Tam M, Amzel A, Phelps BR. Disclosure of HIV serostatus among pregnant and postpartum women in sub-Saharan Africa: a systematic review. AIDS Care. 2015;27(4):436–50.
17. Medley A, Garcia-Moreno C, McGill S, Maman S. Rates, barriers and outcomes of HIV serostatus disclosure among women in developing countries: implications for prevention of mother-to-child transmission programmes. Bull World Health Organ. 2004;82(4):299–307.
18. Kiula ES, Damian DJ, Msuya SE. Predictors of HIV serostatus disclosure to partners among HIV-positive pregnant women in Morogoro, Tanzania. BMC Public Health. 2013;13:433.
19. Alemayehu M, Aregay A, Kalayu A, Yebyo H. HIV disclosure to sexual partner and associated factors among women attending ART clinic at Mekelle hospital, northern Ethiopia. BMC Public Health. 2014;14:746.
20. Colombini M, James C, Ndwiga C, Mayhew SH. The risks of partner violence following HIV status disclosure, and health service responses: narratives of women attending reproductive health services in Kenya. J Int AIDS Soc. 2016;19(1):20766.
21. Visser MJ, Neufeld S, de Villiers A, Makin JD, Forsyth BW. To tell or not to tell: south African women's disclosure of HIV status during pregnancy. AIDS Care. 2008;20(9):1138–45.
22. Rujumba J, Neema S, Byamugisha R, Tylleskar T, Tumwine JK, Heggenhougen HK. "Telling my husband I have HIV is too heavy to come out of my mouth": pregnant women's disclosure experiences and support needs following antenatal HIV testing in eastern Uganda. J Int AIDS Soc. 2012;15(2):17429.
23. Onovo AA, Nta IE, Onah AA, Okolo CA, Aliyu A, Dakum P, et al. Partner HIV serostatus disclosure and determinants of serodiscordance among prevention of mother to child transmission clients in Nigeria. BMC Public Health. 2015;15:827.
24. Adekanle DA, Olowookere SA, Adewole AD, Adeleke NA, Abioye-Kuteyi EA, Ijadunola MY. Sexual experiences of married HIV positive women in Osogbo, southwest Nigeria: role of inappropriate status disclosure. BMC Womens Health. 2015;15:6.
25. Crankshaw TL, Voce A, King RL, Giddy J, Sheon NM, Butler LM. Double disclosure bind: complexities of communicating an HIV diagnosis in the context of unintended pregnancy in Durban, South Africa. AIDS Behav. 2014;18(Suppl 1):S53–9.
26. Mulrenan C, Colombini M, Howard N, Kikuvi J, Mayhew SH. Exploring risk of experiencing intimate partner violence after HIV infection: a qualitative study among women with HIV attending postnatal services in Swaziland. BMJ Open. 2015;5(5):e006907.
27. Ezechi OC, Gab-Okafor C, Onwujekwe DI, Adu RA, Amadi E, Herbertson E. Intimate partner violence and correlates in pregnant HIV positive Nigerians. Arch Gynecol Obstet. 2009;280(5):745–52.

28. Maman S, van Rooyen H, Groves AK. HIV status disclosure to families for social support in South Africa (NIMH project accept/HPTN 043). AIDS Care. 2014;26(2):226–32.

29. Abdool Karim Q, Dellar RC, Bearnot B, Werner L, Frohlich JA, Kharsany AB, et al. HIV-positive status disclosure in patients in care in rural South Africa: implications for scaling up treatment and prevention interventions. AIDS Behav. 2015;19(2):322–9.

30. Ogoina D, Ikuabe P, Ebuenyi I, Harry T, Inatimi O, Chukwueke O. Types and predictors of partner reactions to HIV status disclosure among HIV-infected adult Nigerians in a tertiary hospital in the Niger Delta. Afr Health Sci. 2015; 15(1):10–8.

31. Atuyambe LM, Ssegujja E, Ssali S, Tumwine C, Nekesa N, Nannungi A, et al. HIV/AIDS status disclosure increases support, behavioural change and, HIV prevention in the long term: a case for an Urban Clinic, Kampala, Uganda. BMC Health Serv Res. 2014;14:276.

32. Titilope AA, Adediran A, Umeh C, Akinbami A, Unigwe O, Akanmu AS. Psychosocial Impact Psychosocial Impact Of disclosure of HIV Serostatus in heterosexual relationship at the Lagos University teaching hospital, Nigeria. Nigerian Med J. 2011;52(1):55–9.

33. Ebuenyi ID, Ogoina D, Ikuabe PO, Harry TC, Inatimi O, Chukwueke OU. Prevalence Pattern and Determinants of disclosure of HIV status in an anti retroviral therapy Clinic in the Niger Delta Region of Nigeria. African J Infect Dis. 2014;8(2):27–30.

34. Adebayo AM, Ilesanmi OS, Omotoso BA, Ayodeji OO, Kareem AO, Alele FO. Disclosure To sexual partner and condom use among HIV positive clients attending ART clinic at a tertiary health facility in south West Nigeria. Pan Afric Med J. 2014;18:245.

35. International Nal. Nigeria Demographic and Health Survey 2013. Abuja, Nigeria, and Rockville, Maryland: National Population Commission (NPC) [Nigeria] and ICF International; 2014.

36. UNAIDS. On the fast track to an AIDS-free generation: the incredible journey of the global plan towards the elimination of new HIV infections among children by 2015 and keeping their mothers alive joint. Geneva: United Nations Programme on HIV/AIDS; 2016.

37. Sam-Agudu NA, Cornelius LJ, Okundaye JN, Adeyemi OA, Isah HO, Wiwa OM, et al. The impact of mentor mother programs on PMTCT service uptake and retention-in-Care at Primary Health Care Facilities in Nigeria: a prospective cohort study (MoMent Nigeria). J Acquir Immune Defic Syndr. 2014;67(Suppl 2):S132–8.

38. Federal Ministry of Health Nigeria. National Guidelines for Prevention of Mother-to-Child Transmission of HIV. Abuja: Federal Ministry of Health Nigeria; 2010.

39. Glaser BG, & Strauss, Anselm L.. The discovery of grounded theory: Strategies for qualitative research: Transaction Publishers; 2009.

40. Shamu S, Zarowsky C, Shefer T, Temmerman M, Abrahams N. Intimate partner violence after disclosure of HIV test results among pregnant women in Harare, Zimbabwe. PLoS One. 2014;9(10):e109447.

41. Patel R, Ratner J, Gore-Felton C, Kadzirange G, Woelk G, Katzenstein D. HIV disclosure patterns, predictors, and psychosocial correlates among HIV positive women in Zimbabwe. AIDS Care. 2012;24(3):358–68.

42. Amoran OE. Predictors of disclosure of sero-status to sexual partners among people living with HIV/AIDS in Ogun state, Nigeria. Niger J Clin Pract. 2012; 15(4):385–90.

43. Madiba S, Letsoalo R. HIV Disclosure to partners and family among women enrolled in prevention of mother to child transmission of HIV program: implications for infant feeding in poor resourced communities in South Africa. Glob J Health Sci. 2013;5(4):1–13.

44. Sam-Agudu NA, Ramadhani HO, Isah C, Anaba U, Erekaha S, Fan-Osuala C, et al. The impact of structured mentor mother programs on 6-month postpartum retention and viral suppression among HIV-positive women in rural Nigeria: a prospective paired cohort study. J Acquir Immune Defic Syndr. 2017;75(Suppl 2):S173–S81.

45. Lawani LO, Onyebuchi AK, Iyoke CA. Dual Method use for protection of pregnancy and disease prevention among HIV-infected women in south East Nigeria. BMC Womens Health. 2014;14(1):39.

46. Feyissa TR, Melka AS. Demand for modern family planning among married women living with HIV in western Ethiopia. PLoS One. 2014;9(11):e113008.

47. Kaida A, Matthews LT, Kanters S, Kabakyenga J, Muzoora C, Mocello AR, et al. Incidence and predictors of pregnancy among a cohort of HIV-positive women initiating antiretroviral therapy in Mbarara, Uganda. PLoS One. 2013;8(5):e63411.

48. Matthews LT, Smit JA, Moore L, Milford C, Greener R, Mosery FN, et al. Periconception HIV risk behavior among men and women reporting HIV-Serodiscordant partners in KwaZulu-Natal, South Africa. AIDS Behav. 2015;19(12):2291–303.

49. Matthews LT, Moore L, Crankshaw TL, Milford C, Mosery FN, Greener R, et al. South Africans with recent pregnancy rarely know partner's HIV serostatus: implications for serodiscordant couples interventions. BMC Public Health. 2014;14:843.

50. AVERT. Gender Inequality and HIV. 2017. https://www.avert.org/professionals/social-issues/gender-inequality. Accessed 27 Jan 2018.

51. Ateka GK. HIV status disclosure and partner discordance: a public health dilemma. Public Health. 2006;120(6):493–6.

52. Roxby AC, Matemo D, Drake AL, Kinuthia J, John-Stewart GC, Ongecha-Owuor F, et al. Pregnant women and disclosure to sexual partners after testing HIV-1-seropositive during antenatal care. AIDS Patient Care STDs. 2013;27(1):33–7.

53. Watson-Jones D, Balira R, Ross DA, Weiss HA, Mabey D. Missed opportunities: poor linkage into ongoing care for HIV-positive pregnant women in Mwanza, Tanzania. PLoS One. 2012;7(7):e40091.

4

Improved prediction of gestational hypertension by inclusion of placental growth factor and pregnancy associated plasma protein-a in a sample of Ghanaian women

Edward Antwi[1,2]* , Kerstin Klipstein-Grobusch[1,4], Joyce L. Browne[1], Peter C. Schielen[5], Kwadwo A. Koram[3], Irene A. Agyepong[2] and Diederick E. Grobbee[1]

Abstract

Background: We assessed whether adding the biomarkers Pregnancy Associated Plasma Protein-A (PAPP-A) and Placental Growth Factor (PlGF) to maternal clinical characteristics improved the prediction of a previously developed model for gestational hypertension in a cohort of Ghanaian pregnant women.

Methods: This study was nested in a prospective cohort of 1010 pregnant women attending antenatal clinics in two public hospitals in Accra, Ghana. Pregnant women who were normotensive, at a gestational age at recruitment of between 8 and 13 weeks and provided a blood sample for biomarker analysis were eligible for inclusion. From serum, biomarkers PAPP-A and PlGF concentrations were measured by the AutoDELFIA immunoassay method and multiple of the median (MoM) values corrected for gestational age (PAPP-A and PlGF) and maternal weight (PAPP-A) were calculated. To obtain prediction models, these biomarkers were included with clinical predictors maternal weight, height, diastolic blood pressure, a previous history of gestational hypertension, history of hypertension in parents and parity in a logistic regression to obtain prediction models. The Area Under the Receiver Operating Characteristic Curve (AUC) was used to assess the predictive ability of the models.

Results: Three hundred and seventy three women participated in this study. The area under the curve (AUC) of the model with only maternal clinical characteristics was 0.75 (0.64–0.86) and 0.89(0.73–1.00) for multiparous and primigravid women respectively. The AUCs after inclusion of both PAPP-A and PlGF were 0.82 (0.74–0.89) and 0.95 (0.87–1.00) for multiparous and primigravid women respectively.

Conclusion: Adding the biomarkers PAPP-A and PlGF to maternal characteristics to a prediction model for gestational hypertension in a cohort of Ghanaian pregnant women improved predictive ability. Further research using larger sample sizes in similar settings to validate these findings is recommended.

Keywords: Prediction model, Gestational hypertension, Biomarkers, Hypertensive disorders of pregnancy

* Correspondence: ed_antwi@yahoo.com
[1]Julius Global Health, Julius Center for Health Sciences and Primary Care, University Medical Center Utrecht, Utrecht University, Utrecht, the Netherlands
[2]Ghana Health Service, P.M.B, Ministries, Accra, Greater Accra, Ghana
Full list of author information is available at the end of the article

Plain English summary

Gestational hypertension and preeclampsia affect between 5 to 10% of all pregnancies and can result in complications in the mother and the fetus. Early prediction of pregnant women at risk of these conditions will lead to better monitoring and appropriate management. This study was conducted in antenatal clinic settings in Ghana to investigate whether adding two biomarkers, placental growth factor and pregnancy associated plasma protein A, to a previously developed prediction model based on maternal clinical characteristics improved the performance of the model.

Logistic regression was used to derive a prediction model. Adding biomarkers to a previously validated prediction model improved the performance of the model for gestational hypertension.

We recommend further research using larger sample sizes in similar settings to validate our findings.

Background

Hypertensive disorders of pregnancy (HDP) are leading causes of maternal morbidity and mortality globally and affect about 5 to 10% of all pregnancies [1, 2]. The burden of these conditions is greatest in low and middle income countries (LMICs) [3, 4]. Early identification of pregnant women at risk of developing these conditions result in better monitoring and management to minimize complications to the mother and the fetus. Prediction models have been used to identify women at high risk of HDPs, particularly preeclampsia [3–6]. In addition, prevention interventions could be started such as calcium and aspirin supplementation that have been shown to reduce the risk of HDPs, particularly preeclampsia [7–12]. For example, in the ASPRE (Combined Multimarker Screening and Randomized Patient Treatment with Aspirin for Evidence-Based Preeclampsia Prevention) trial with risk selection based on screening, a reduction in the incidence of preterm preeclampsia in the aspirin arm by 62% was observed [12].

PAPP-A is a protease that is involved in the local release of insulin-like growth factors. Low first trimester levels of PAPP-A is associated with hypertensive disorders of pregnancy [13–15]. Placental growth factor (PIGF) is an angiogenic factor and low concentrations have been observed in pregnant women who develop preeclampsia. Suboptimal secretion of PlGF between 8 to 14 weeks gestation as a result of placental dysfunction has been associated with disorders such as preeclampsia, intrauterine growth restriction, small-for-gestational age and still births [16].

The aim of this study was to assess whether the addition of the biomarkers, placental growth factor (PIGF) and pregnancy-associated protein A (PAPP-A) to a previously developed prediction model [17] based on maternal clinical characteristics (diastolic blood pressure, family history of hypertension in parents, history of gestational hypertension (GH) in a previous pregnancy, parity, height and weight) improved prediction of gestational hypertension.

Methods
Study design and study population

This study was nested in a prospective cohort of 1010 adult pregnant women with a singleton pregnancy and without known pre-existent hypertension recruited between July 2012 and March 2014 at Ridge Regional Hospital and Maamobi General Hospital in Accra. Accra, the capital city of Ghana, is cosmopolitan with high, middle and low-income persons from different ethnic backgrounds living and working in the city [18]. Persons from all the social strata access health services, including antenatal and delivery care in these public hospitals. These hospitals were also chosen because they have a high attendance so the recruitment of pregnant women into the study could be completed in a shorter time. Eligibility criteria for this study were gestational age at enrollment of between between 8 and 13 weeks, based on ultrasound scan. This specific subset of women was selected based on evidence that prediction with these biomarkers is most appropriate at this gestational age [7–10, 19–21]. Women with gestational age at enrollment of less than 8 weeks or more than 13 weeks ($n = 411$), without PlGF MoM values ($n = 95$) or women without outcome data ($n = 131$) were excluded. We used the principle of 10 outcome events per variable for logistic and Cox regression analysis [22–25] to obtain a sample size adequate for our analysis. With an incidence of gestational hypertension of 10% in the Ghanaian population [26], and eight variables in the prediction model, a sample size of 393 women was considered adequate for the analysis.

The women were included in the study after they had given written informed consent and were interviewed by trained research assistants using a structured questionnaire for socio-demographic characteristics and obstetric history. They were followed up at each antenatal clinic visit till they delivered. None of the women who developed gestational hypertension progressed to preeclampsia. Pregnancy outcomes were obtained at delivery and from the hospital maternity register.

Variables
Independent variables

Maternal weight (measured in kilogrammes with a bathroom scale), height (measured in centimeters with a stadiometer), blood pressure (measured in millimeters of mercury) and urine protein (defined as 2+ or more on urine dipstick) were obtained at the initial and subsequent antenatal clinic visits from the maternal health record books.

Blood pressure measurements were performed by trained midwives using a mercury sphygmomanometer. The appropriate adult sized cuff was placed on the bare left upper arm with the woman comfortably seated and her back supported and legs uncrossed. The arm was at the level of the heart and neither the patient nor the observer talked during the measurement. Korotkoff phase V sounds were used [27]. Two readings were taken at interval of five minutes and the average used as the woman's blood pressure.

PAPP-A and PlGF assay

Blood specimen was obtained from women on the day of their enrollment into the study by a phlebotomist. After the blood had coagulated, it was centrifuged to obtain the serum which was stored at a temperature of -20 °C in a freezer at the Maamobi General Hospital. Serum samples from the Ridge Hospital were stored temporarily in a fridge at 4 °C and transported daily in a cold box with ice packs to the laboratory at Maamobi General Hospital for storage. The frozen serum samples were air-freighted on dried ice to the Dutch Institute for Public Health and Environment (RIVM) in Bilthoven, the Netherlands, where they were stored at a temperature of − 80 °C until they were analyzed for PlGF and PAPP-A. PAPP-A and PlGF concentrations were determined using commercially available immunoassays and the AutoDelfia automated analyzer (PerkinElmer, Turku, Finland). Details of the assay method are described elsewhere by Browne et al. [28]. PAPP-A concentrations were corrected for gestational age and maternal weight and expressed as multiple of the median (MoM) using the reference equations from the Dutch national prenatal screening programme for Down syndrome based on PAPP-A measurements between 8 to 13 weeks gestation of more than 10,000 pregnancies [29]:

PAPP-A MoM gestational age correction

$$y = 12,605.9606 - 552.53697^*$$
$$\times\ + 7.42649^* \times^2 - 0.0278^* \times^3,$$

where x = gestational age at blood sampling in days.

PAPP-A MoM weight correction; Exp (1.23234075−0.0181912*x), where x = weight in kilograms.

PlGF concentrations were also corrected for gestational age and expressed as MoM [28] by using the manufacturer's (Perkin Elmer) reference equation for gestational age in days (between 9 to 13 weeks gestation) as follows:

$$y = 75.08 - 1.7769^* \times\ + 0.01589^* \times^2$$

where x = gestational age at blood sampling in days.

PlGF was not corrected for maternal weight because serum PlGF concentration is not correlated with maternal weight [29].

Outcome

The outcome, gestational hypertension, was defined as a systolic BP of 140 mmHg or more and or a diastolic BP of 90 mmHg or more on at least two separate occasions, and present for the first time after 20 weeks of pregnancy [30].

Ethical considerations

Ethical approval for the study was granted by the Ethical Review Committee of the Ghana Health Service (GHS-ERC 07/09/11). All participating women gave written informed consent before they were enrolled in the study.

Statistical analysis

SPSS software (version 20.0, IBM SPSS Statistics Inc., Chicago, Illinois, USA) and R statistical software (R version 3.1.0 (2014−04-10). The R Foundation for Statistical Computing Platform: x86_64-w64-mingw32/×64 (64-bit)) were used for statistical analysis. The mean and standard deviation of continuous predictors were calculated for women who developed gestational hypertension and those who did not. Means were compared using the Student's t-test; percentages for categorical data were assessed by Chi-square test. The median with interquartile range was reported for non-normally distributed variables.

Logistic regression was used to derive the original prediction model using gestational hypertension as the outcome and the following maternal clinical characteristics as the predictors: maternal height, weight, parity, previous history of gestational hypertension, family history of hypertension and diastolic blood pressure. The maternal weight, height, diastolic blood pressure, parity, PAPP-A MoM and PlGF MoM were included in the logistic regression model as continuous variables. The principle of 10 events per variable for logistic and Cox regression analysis [31] was applied in model building. A history of hypertension in parents and history of gestational hypertension in a previous pregnancy were included in the logistic regression as dichotomous variables. As the variable 'previous history of gestational hypertension' was not applicable to primigravid women, a separate model was fitted for them.

PAPP-A MoM and PlGF MoM were included in the model as continuous variables so as not to lose power through categorization, and also because the appropriate cut-off value of these biomarkers for the Ghanaian population is not known [28]. The PAPP-A and PlGF as MoM values were included in turns and then together to the logistic regression. The predictive ability of each model (PAPP-A only, PlGF only, combined) was assessed. The models were internally validated using the bootstrapping technique. The resulting shrinkage factor after bootstrapping was used to adjust the regression coefficients, thus correcting for model overfitting.

The performance of the models was assessed by the area under the receiver operating characteristic curve (AUC) or c-statistic. The AUC of the original model with only maternal clinical characteristics was compared to that of the models with PAPPA and maternal clinical characteristics, PlGF with maternal characteristics and both PAPP-A, PlGF and maternal characteristics.

Results

Characteristics of the 373 study participants are presented in Table 1. Most of the women (81%) were multiparous. The mean age was 28.3 (SD 4.9) years and the mean gestational age at booking was 11.6 weeks (SD 1.4).

The flow chart for selection of study participants is shown in Fig. 1. Of 1010 women in the original cohort, 373 women met the inclusion criteria.

Table 2 compares characteristics of women who developed gestational hypertension to those who did not. Twenty-five women (6.7%) developed gestational hypertension. There was a difference in mean age between women who developed gestational hypertension and those who did not (30.3 (SD 5.3) years vs. 28.2 (SD 4.9) years, $p = 0.04$). There was no difference in mean height

Table 1 Baseline characteristics of the study population ($n = 373$)

Variable	Mean (SD) or N (%)
Age (years)	28.3 (4.9)
Height (cm)	161.2 (6.3)
Weight (kg)	66.5 (13.3)
Systolic blood pressure (mmHg)	110.5 (12.9)
Diastolic blood pressure (mmHg)	68.9 (10.3)
Gestational age at booking (weeks)	11.6 (1.4)
PlGF MoM corrected for gestational age	Median 1.28, IQR (0.96–1.88)
PAPP-A MoM corrected for gestational age	Median 2.29, IQR (1.15–3.86)
PAPP-A MoM corrected for gestational age and maternal weight	Median 2.34, IQR (1.19–3.82)
Parity:	
Primigravid women	71 (19.0%)
2–3 pregnancies	116 (31.1%)
> 4 pregnancies	186 (49.9%)

between women with and without gestational hypertension (159.1 cm (SD 7.1) vs. 161.4 cm (SD 6.3), $p = 0.08$). However, there was a difference in the mean weight of women with and without gestational hypertension (72.9 kg (SD 16.3) vs. 66.0 kg (SD 12.9), $p = 0.013$). The mean diastolic blood pressure differed between women who developed gestational hypertension and those who did not (74.3 mmHg (SD 13.6) vs. 68.5 mmHg (SD 9.9), $p = 0.006$).

Table 3 presents the median and interquartile range of MoM of PAPP-A and PlGF by gestational week. The median MoM PAPP-A (adjusted for gestational age and maternal weight) ranged between 1.68 and 4.36. The median MoM PlGF ranged between 0.90 and 1.68.

Table 4 shows the regression coefficients and the AUC of the various models for multiparous women. The AUC of the model with only maternal characteristics was 0.75 (0.64–0.86). The AUC of the model with maternal characteristics and PAPP-A was 0.78 (0.70–0.87), with maternal characteristics, and PlGF was 0.76 (0.64–0.87), and maternal characteristics with both biomarkers 0.82 (0.74–0.89). Figure 2 shows the Receiver Operating Characteristic curves for the prediction models for multiparous women. Table 5 shows the regression coefficients and the AUC of the models for primigravid women. The AUC of the model with only maternal characteristics was 0.89 (0.73- 1.00). The AUC of the model with maternal characteristics and both biomarkers was 0.95 (0.87-1.00).

Discussion

The addition of PlGF and PAPP-A together to the model markedly improved its predictive ability, with an increase in AUC from 0.75 to 0.82 for multiparous women and 0.89 to 0.95 for primigravid women, whereas adding either one of the two had only marginal effect. These findings are in line with other studies that reported improved prediction by the addition of biomarkers to maternal characteristics [5, 19, 32–34].

Several issues arise in comparing this study to other prediction studies. The first is that most prediction models predict preeclampsia rather than gestational hypertension [35]. Hence there were fewer prediction models for gestational hypertension to which we could directly compare our models. Therefore we included models for preeclampsia as well in the comparison of the model performance.

The second issue is that we derived separate models for multiparous and primigravid women. This was because the primigravid women could not respond to the question of "a previous history of gestational hypertension or preeclampsia". Being an important predictor, we maintained that variable in the model and in a sub analysis fitted a different model for primigravid women

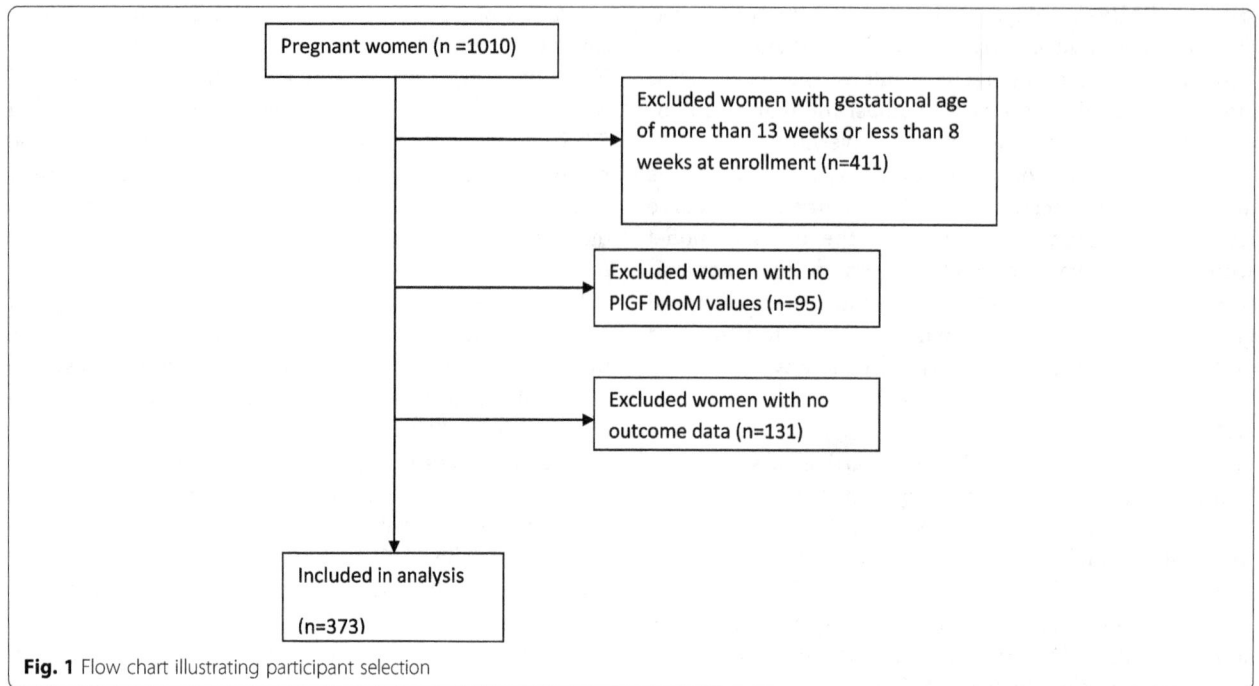

Fig. 1 Flow chart illustrating participant selection

($n = 71$). However because of the relatively small number of primigravid women and outcome events on which these estimates are based, they should be interpreted with caution The third issue is that the same types of biomarkers are not used across prediction studies. Hence finding studies with the same predictors as in this study was a challenge. A number of prediction studies also added uterine artery pulsatility index to biomarkers and maternal characteristics [19, 21, 32] because it improves prediction. For instance, Kuc et al. reported that the best detection rates for preeclampsia were obtained when maternal characteristics, biomarkers and uterine artery pulsatility index were combined [32]. Akolekar et al. also reported a three-fold increase in detection rates in screening for preeclampsia by the combination of

maternal factors, biophysical and biomarkers compared with using only maternal factors [19].

Poon et al also reported that PAPP-A and PlGF in combination with maternal characteristics and uterine artery pulsatility index improved detection rates of pre-eclampsia [21]. We did not include uterine artery pulsatility index in our study because uterine artery Doppler is not readily available in low resource settings.

Another issue is that most of the prediction studies have been conducted in Europe and North America. There are few studies in Sub Saharan African populations to which we could directly compare our results. Ukah et al in a prospective cohort study of pregnant women attending antenatal care in Maputo, Mozambique, measured the serum PlGF concentration

Table 2 Baseline characteristics of the study population by the outcome, gestational hypertension

Variable (Mean (SD))	Gestational hypertension (No) N = 348	Gestational hypertension (Yes) N = 25	p-value
Age (years)	28.2 (4.9)	30.3 (5.3)	0.04
Height(cm)	161.4 (6.3)	159.1 (7.1)	0.08
Weight (kg)	66.0 (12.9)	72.9 (16.3)	0.013
Systolic blood pressure (mmHg)	110.1 (12.7)	116.4 (14.2)	0.018
Diastolic blood pressure (mmHg)	68.5 (9.9)	74.3 (13.6)	0.006
Gestational age at booking (weeks)	11.6 (1.4)	11.3 (1.5)	0.38

Table 3 Median and interquartile range of MoM of PAPP-A and PlGF by gestational week (n = 373)

Gestational week	Number of women (%)	MoM PAPP-A, median (IQR), adjusted for gestational age and maternal weight	MoM PAPP-A, median (IQR), adjusted for maternal weight	MoM PlGF, median (IQR), adjusted for gestational age
8	17 (4.5)	4.36 (1.06–8.47)	4.46 (1.19–6.42)	1.17 (0.85–1.51)
9	40 (10.7)	1.68 (1.04–4.64)	2.04 (0.86–4.25)	0.90 (0.73–1.36)
10	86 (23.1)	2.39 (1.45–3.83)	2.33 (1.44–4.12)	1.15 (0.97–1.66)
11	71 (19.3)	1.76 (0.85–3.05)	1.96 (0.88–3.01)	1.21 (0.95–1.49)
12	66 (17.6)	2.21 (1.06–3.65)	2.26 (1.20–3.34)	1.29 (1.03–1.91)
13	93 (24.8)	2.63 (1.49–4.51)	2.55 (1.57–4.05)	1.68 (1.34–2.94)
Total	373	2.29 (1.15–3.86)	2.34 (1.19–3.82)	1.28 (0.96–1.88)

IQR Interquartile range, MoM multiple of the median
The median MoM value of the reference population by default is 1. The gestational age and weight adjusted PAPP-A median MoM was 2.29. The weight adjusted PAPP-A median MoM was 2.34 and the median PlGF MoM was 1.28

in women suspected of having preeclampsia after 20 weeks of gestation. This study had as its primary outcome, the time-to-delivery after confirmation of pre-eclampsia [36]. This study differed from ours in terms of being a diagnostic study rather than a prediction study.

The AUC is used to quantify the overall ability of a test or a logistic regression model to discriminate between two outcomes such as disease or non-disease [37–40]. It generally ranges from 0.5 to 1 and represents the prediction model's ability to correctly classify a randomly selected individual as being from one of two hypothetical populations [40–43]. An AUC value of 1.0 is considered perfect, 0.9–0.99 excellent, 0.8–0.89 good, 0.7–0.79 fair and 0.51–0.69 poor. An AUC of 0.5 is considered non-informative. Hence the AUC of 0.82 obtained in our study shows that the model with maternal characteristics and both PAPP-A and PlGF has good predictive ability.

Pencina et al. [44] and Peters et al. [33] have also indicated that increase in the AUC upon the addition of a predictor to a model shows that the predictor has improved the predictive ability of the model. In our

study, for the multiparous women, the AUC of the prediction model with only maternal clinical characteristics was 0.75 and this increased to 0.82 upon the addition of both PlGF and PAPP-A to the prediction model. For the primigravid women, the AUC of the prediction model with only maternal clinical characteristics was 0.89 and this increased to 0.95 upon the addition of both PlGF and PAPP-A to the prediction model This is an indication that the addition of both biomarkers simultaneously to the models improved the prediction performance.

The higher median MoM values of PlGF (1.28) and PAPP-A (2.29) in our study compared to the reference population of Dutch women (median MoM of 1 by default) is consistent with other studies that have shown racial and ethnic differences in the levels of these biomarkers, particularly in women of African and Asian decent [45–54]. The median MoM of PAPP-A between 8 weeks gestation to 13 weeks gestation ranged between 1.68 and 4.36. That of PlGF MoM ranged from 0.90 at gestational week 9 to 1.68 at gestational week 13. Differences in the median MoM PlGF and PAPP-A levels between some ethnic groups in Ghana have also been

Table 4 Regression coefficients and AUC of prediction models for multiparous women (n = 302)

Variable	Model with only maternal characteristics	Model with addition of PlGF MoM	Model with addition of PAPP-A MoM	Model with addition of PlGF MoM and PAPP-A MoM
Intercept	9.68	10.0	10.46	12.18
History of hypertension in parents	−1.52	−1.50	−1.60	−1.65
Previous history of hypertension in pregnancy	0.47	0.55	0.42	0.72
Weight	0.026	0.025	0.024	0.023
Height	−0.097	−0.099	−0.102	−0.112
Parity	0.29	0.29	0.33	0.34
Diastolic BP	0.036	0.036	0.037	0.042
PlGF MoM	–	−0.15	–	−0.713
PAPP-A MoM	–		0.033	0.098
AUC	0.75 (0.64–0.86)	0.76 (0.64–0.87)	0.78 (0.70–0.87)	0.82 (0.74–0.89)

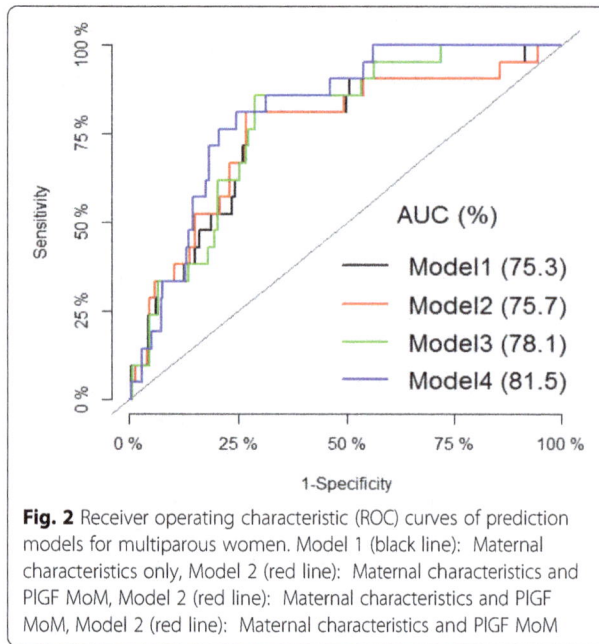

Fig. 2 Receiver operating characteristic (ROC) curves of prediction models for multiparous women. Model 1 (black line): Maternal characteristics only, Model 2 (red line): Maternal characteristics and PlGF MoM, Model 2 (red line): Maternal characteristics and PlGF MoM, Model 2 (red line): Maternal characteristics and PlGF MoM

reported in this population [28]. As a result of the higher MoM values, there is the need for a correction factor for the Ghanaian population and sub populations to prevent the under estimation of risk calculations for placental disorders and aneuploidies.

Clinical and research implications

Hypertensive disorders of pregnancy, including gestational hypertension and preeclampsia, are among the leading causes of maternal morbidity in LMICs. In Ghana they rank as the third leading cause of mortality, having overtaken hemorrhage [26]. The ability to predict this in women at increased risk (of the disorder) and thereby institute preventive measures to minimize their

impact is a useful strategy to improving maternal and perinatal outcomes.

Biomarkers have shown some promise in improving the prediction of gestational hypertension and other hypertensive disorders in pregnancy, although a lot more research is still needed. Future studies using larger sample sizes should be conducted to confirm the findings of this study. When confirmed, one factor to be considered in the use of biomarkers in prediction models in the clinical setting would be the cost of carrying out biomarker tests, especially in LMIC settings. A feasible approach in this regard would be the use of dried blood spot samples (DBS) instead of serum which requires refrigeration during storage and transport. DBS have been widely used in newborn screening for sickle cell disease [55, 56], human immunodeficiency virus screening in newborns and for other disorders [57–66]. It is cheaper than conventional serum assay and logistically simpler to implement in screening programmes because samples can be obtained and transported from remote locations where the laboratory infrastructure is limited. The technique for sample taking is also simpler and requires less training compared to venepuncture. In using DBS however, an issue to be considered is how well the concentration of the biomarkers in whole blood correlates with that of DBS. Pennings et al. [67] and Browne et al. [68] have shown that the correlation coefficient between serum and DBS concentrations for PAPP-Aand ß-hCG were both greater than 0.94. Cowans et al also reported that ß-hCG stability is improved in DBS as compared to serum storage. This makes the collection, storage, transport and assay of biomarkers using DBS feasible in low resource settings.

It is recommended that this study should be replicated locally and externally in similar settings using larger sample sizes to validate the findings of this study before possible translation to clinical practice.

Table 5 Regression coefficients and AUC of prediction models for primigravid women ($n = 71$)

Variable	Model with only maternal characteristics	Model with addition of PlGF MoM	Model with addition of PAPP-A MoM	Model with addition of PlGF MoM and PAPP-A MoM
Intercept	17.64	21.96	19.41	14.92
History of hypertension in parents	−1.47	−1.63	−1.49	−1.92
Previous history of hypertension in pregnancy	–	–	–	–
Weight	0.123	0.154	0.134	0.148
Height	−0.216	−0.264	−0.237	−0.214
Parity	–	–	–	–
Diastolic BP	0.110	0.118	0.116	0.118
PlGF MoM	–	0.323	–	0.834
PAPP-A MoM	–	–	0.098	−0.373
AUC	0.899 (0.732–1.000)	0.925 (0.808–1.000)	0.903 (0.749–1.000)	0.951 (0.870–1.000)

The feasibility and sustainability of any planned introduction and eventual scale-up in the use of biomarkers to improve prediction of hypertensive disorders has to be assessed using a cost-benefit analysis.

Conclusion

The addition of PAPP-A and PlGF to prediction models based on maternal clinical characteristics (diastolic blood pressure, family history of hypertension in parents, history of gestational hypertension in a previous pregnancy, parity, height and weight) markedly improved prediction of gestational hypertension. This study should be replicated using a larger sample size.

Abbreviations

AUC: Area under the receiver operating characteristic curve; BP: Blood Pressure; DBS: Dried Blood Spot Sample; GH: Gestational Hypertension; HDP: Hypertensive Disorder of Pregnancy; IQR: Inter Quartile Range; LMIC: Low and Middle Income Country; MoM: Multiple of the Median; PAPP-A: Pregnancy Associated Plasma Protein-A; PE: Preeclampsia; PlGF: Placental Growth Factor; RIVM: Dutch Institute for Public Health and Environment; ROC: Receiver Operating Characteristic Curve; SD: Standard Deviation

Acknowledgements

We acknowledge the midwives and the laboratory staff who played a role in the study. We also thank Dr. Justice Ahetor for assisting with aspects of the statistical analysis.

Funding

This research received funding from the UMC Utrecht Global Health Support program. The funders played no role in the study design, data collection, data analysis and interpretation as well as writing of the manuscript.

Authors' contributions

EA designed the study, collected data, carried out statistical analysis and wrote the initial draft of the manuscript. KK-G assisted with data analysis. KK-G, JLB, PCS, KAK, IAA and DEG provided scientific guidance and were also actively involved in the preparation and review of the manuscript. All the authors read and approved the final manuscript.

Competing interests

The authors declare that they have no competing interests.

Author details

[1]Julius Global Health, Julius Center for Health Sciences and Primary Care, University Medical Center Utrecht, Utrecht University, Utrecht, the Netherlands. [2]Ghana Health Service, P.M.B, Ministries, Accra, Greater Accra, Ghana. [3]Noguchi Memorial Institute for Medical Research, College of Health Sciences, University of Ghana, Legon, Accra, Ghana. [4]Division of Epidemiology & Biostatistics, School of Public Health, Faculty of Health Sciences, University of the Witwatersrand, Johannesburg, South Africa. [5]Center for Infectious Diseases Research, Diagnostics and Screening (IDS), National Institute for Public Health and the Environment (RIVM), Bilthoven, the Netherlands.

References

1. Hutcheon JA, Lisonkova S, Joseph KS. Epidemiology of pre-eclampsia and the other hypertensive disorders of pregnancy. Best Pract Res Clin Obstetr Gynaecol. 2011;25(4):391–403.
2. Peters RM, Flack JM. Hypertensive disorders of pregnancy. J Obstet Gynecol Neonatal Nurs. 2004;33(2):209–20.
3. North RA, McCowan LME, Dekker GA, Poston L, Chan EHY, Stewart AW, et al. Clinical risk prediction for pre-eclampsia in nulliparous women: development of model in international prospective cohort. BMJ. 2011;342:d1875.
4. Park H, Kim S, Jung Y, Shim S, Kim J, Cho Y, et al. Screening models using multiple markers for early detection of late-onset preeclampsia in low-risk pregnancy. BMC Pregnancy Childbirth. 2014;14(1):35.
5. Nijdam ME, Janssen KJ, Moons KG, Grobbee DE, van der Post JA, Bots ML, Franx A. Prediction model for hypertension in pregnancy in nulliparous women using information obtained at the first antenatal visit. J Hypertens. 2010;28(1):119–26.
6. Payne B, Hodgson S, Hutcheon JA, Joseph KS, Li J, Lee T, et al. Performance of the fullPIERS model in predicting adverse maternal outcomes in pre-eclampsia using patient data from the PIERS (pre-eclampsia integrated estimate of RiSk) cohort, collected on admission 3560. BJOG Int J Obstet Gynaecol. 2013;120(1):113–8.
7. Bujold E, Roberge SP, Lacasse Y, Bureau M, Audibert F, Marcoux S, et al. Prevention of preeclampsia and intrauterine growth restriction with aspirin started in early pregnancy: a meta-analysis. Obstet Gynecol. 2010;116(2, Part 1):402–14.
8. Duley L, Henderson-Smart DJ, Meher S, King JF. Antiplatelet agents for preventing pre-eclampsia and its complications. The Cochrane Library. 2007; (2):CD004659.
9. Hofmeyr GJ, Lawrie TA, Atallah AN, Duley L. Calcium supplementation during pregnancy for preventing hypertensive disorders and related problems. Cochrane Database Syst Rev. 2010;8(8):CD001059.
10. Nicolaides KH. Turning the pyramid of prenatal care. Fetal Diagn Ther. 2011; 29(3):183–96.
11. Roberge Sp VP, Nicolaides K, Giguire Y, Vainio M, Bakthi A, et al. Early administration of low-dose aspirin for the prevention of preterm and term preeclampsia: a systematic review and meta-analysis. Fetal Diagn Ther. 2012; 31(3):141–6.
12. Rolnik DL, Wright D, Poon LCY, Syngelaki A, O'Gorman N, de Paco Matallana C, Akolekar R, Cicero S, Janga D, Singh M, Molina FS, Persico N, Jani JC, Plasencia W, Papaioannou G, Tenenbaum-Gavish K, Nicolaides KH. ASPRE trial: performance of screening for preterm pre-eclampsia. Ultrasound Obstet Gynecol. 2017;50:492–95. https://doi.org/10.1002/uog.18816.
13. Bonno M, Oxvig C, Kephart GM, Wagner JM, Kristensen T, Sottrup-Jensen L, et al. Localization of pregnancy-associated plasma protein-a and colocalization of pregnancy-associated plasma protein-a messenger ribonucleic acid and eosinophil granule major basic protein messenger ribonucleic acid in placenta. Lab Investig. 1994;71(4):560–6.
14. Lawrence JB, Oxvig C, Overgaard MT, Sottrup-Jensen L, Gleich GJ, Hays LG, et al. The insulin-like growth factor (IGF)-dependent IGF binding protein-4 protease secreted by human fibroblasts is pregnancy-associated plasma protein-a. Proc Natl Acad Sci. 1999;96(6):3149–53.
15. Bersinger NA, Smárason AK, Muttukrishna S, Groome NP, Redman CW Women with preeclampsia have increased serum levels of pregnancy-associated plasma protein a (PAPP-A), inhibin a, activin a and soluble E-selectin. Hypeter Pregnan. 2003;22(1):45–55.
16. Odibo AO, Patel KR, Spitalnik A, Odibo L, Huettner P. Placental pathology, first-trimester biomarkers and adverse pregnancy outcomes. J Perinatol. 2014;34(3):186–91.
17. Antwi E, Groenwold RH, Browne JL, Franx A, Agyepong IA, Koram KA, et al. Development and validation of a prediction model for gestational hypertension in a Ghanaian cohort. BMJ Open. 2017;7(1):e012670.

18. Agyei-Mensah S, Owusu G. Segregated by neighbourhoods? A portrait of ethnic diversity in the neighbourhoods of the Accra metropolitan area, Ghana. Popul Space Place. 2010;16(6):499–516.

19. Akolekar R, Syngelaki A, Sarquis R, Zvanca M, Nicolaides KH. Prediction of early, intermediate and late pre-eclampsia from maternal factors, biophysical and biochemical markers at 11 to13 weeks. Prenat Diagn. 2011;31(1):66–74.

20. Akolekar R, Syngelaki A, Poon L, Wright D, Nicolaides KH. Competing risks model in early screening for preeclampsia by biophysical and biochemical markers. Fetal Diagn Ther. 2013;33(1):8–15.

21. Poon LC, Nicolaides KH. First-trimester maternal factors and biomarker screening for preeclampsia. Prenat Diagn. 2014;34(7):618–27.

22. Concato J, Peduzzi P, Holford TR, Feinstein AR. Importance of events per independent variable in proportional hazards analysis I. Background, goals, and general strategy. J Clin Epidemiol. 1995;48(12):1495–501.

23. Harrell FE Jr, Lee KLFAU, Mark DB. Multivariable prognostic models: issues in developing models, evaluating assumptions and adequacy, and measuring and reducing errors. Stat Med. 1996;15(0277–6715 (Print)):361–87.

24. Peduzzi P, Concato J, Feinstein AR, Holford TR. Importance of events per independent variable in proportional hazards regression analysis II. Accuracy and precision of regression estimates. J Clin Epidemiol. 1995;48(12):1503–10.

25. Peduzzi P, Concato J, Kemper E, Holford TR, Feinstein AR. A simulation study of the number of events per variable in logistic regression analysis. J Clin Epidemiol. 1996;49(12):1373–9.

26. Ghana Statistical Service (GSS), Ghana Health Service (GHS), and Macro International. Ghana Maternal Health Survey 2007. Calverton: GSS, GHS, and Macro International; 2009.

27. Pickering TG, Hall JE, Appel LJ, Falkner BE, Graves J, Hill MN, et al. Recommendations for blood pressure measurement in humans and experimental animals part 1: blood pressure measurement in humans: a statement for professionals from the Subcommittee of Professional and Public Education of the American Heart Association Council on high blood pressure research. Hypertension. 2005;45(1):142–61.

28. Browne JL, Klipstein-Grobusch K, Koster MP, Ramamoorthy D, Antwi E, Belmouden I, et al. Pregnancy associated plasma protein-a and placental growth factor in a sub-Saharan African population: a nested cross-sectional study. PLoS One. 2016;11(8):e0159592.

29. Kuc S, Koster MP, Franx A, Schielen PC, Visser GH. Maternal characteristics, mean arterial pressure and serum markers in early prediction of preeclampsia. PLoS One. 2013;8(5):e63546.

30. Report of the National High Blood Pressure Education Program Working Group on High Blood Pressure in Pregnancy. Am J Obstet Gynecol 183(1):s1-s22.

31. Harrell FE, Lee KL, Mark DB. Multivariable prognostic models: issues in developing models, evaluating assumptions and adequacy, and measuring and reducing errors. Stat Med. 1996;15(4):361–87.

32. Kuc S, Wortelboer EJ, van Rijn B, van Rijn BB, Franx A, Franx AF, Visser GH, Schielen P, Schielen PC. Evaluation of 7 serum biomarkers and uterine artery Doppler ultrasound for first-trimester prediction of preeclampsia: a systematic review. Obstet Gynecol Surv. 2011;66(4):225–39.

33. Peters SA, den Ruijter HM, Bots ML, Moons KG. Improvements in risk stratification for the occurrence of cardiovascular disease by imaging subclinical atherosclerosis: a systematic review. Heart. 2011. https://doi.org/10.1136/heartjnl-2011-300747.

34. Poon LCY, Kametas NA, Chelemen T, Leal A, Nicolaides KH. Maternal risk factors for hypertensive disorders in pregnancy: a multivariate approach. J Hum Hypertens. 2010;24(2):104–10.

35. Kleinrouweler CE, Cheong-See FM, Collins GS, Kwee A, Thangaratinam S, Khan KS, Mol BW, Pajkrt E, Moons KG, Schuit E. Prognostic models in obstetrics: available, but far from applicable. American Journal of Obstetrics & Gynecology. 2016;214(1):79-90.

36. Ukah UV, Mbofana F, Rocha BM, Loquiha O, Mudenyanga C, Usta M, Urso M, Drebit S, Magee LA, von Dadelszen P. Diagnostic Performance of Placental Growth Factor in Women With Suspected Preeclampsia Attending Antenatal Facilities in Maputo, MozambiqueNovelty and Significance. Hypertension. 2017;69(3):469-74.

37. Brown CD, Davis HT. Receiver operating characteristics curves and related decision measures: a tutorial. Chemom Intell Lab Syst. 2006;80(1):24–38.

38. Cook NR. Use and Misuse of the receiver operating characteristic curve in risk prediction. Circulation. 2007;115(7):928.

39. Hanley JA, McNeil BJ. The meaning and use of the area under a receiver operating characteristic (ROC) curve. Radiology. 1982;143(1):29–36.

40. Hosmer DW Jr, Lemeshow S, Sturdivant RX. Applied logistic regression. 3rd Edition. Wiley; 2013. p. 528. ISBN: 978-0-470-58247-3.

41. Simpson AJ, Fitter MJ. What is the best index of detectability? Psychol Bull. 1973;80(6):481.

42. Bamber D. The area above the ordinal dominance graph and the area below the receiver operating characteristic graph. J Math Psychol. 1975;12(4):387–415.

43. Zhang DD, Zhou X, Freeman DH, Freeman JL. A Nonparametric method for the comparison of partial areas under ROC curves and its application to large health care data sets. Stat Med. 2002;21(5):701–15.

44. Pencina MJ, D'agostino RB, Vasan RS. Statistical methods for assessment of added usefulness of new biomarkers. Clin Chem Lab Med. 2010;48(12):1703–11.

45. Ball S, Wright D, Sodre D, Lachmann R, Nicolaides KH. Temporal effect of afro-Caribbean race on serum pregnancy-associated plasma protein-a at 9 to 13 weeks gestation in screening for aneuploidies. Fetal Diagn Ther. 2012;31(3):162–9.

46. Cowans NJ, Spencer K. Effect of gestational age on first trimester maternal serum prenatal screening correction factors for ethnicity and IVF conception. Prenat Diagn. 2013;33(1):56–60.

47. Kagan KO, Wright D, Spencer K, Molina FS, Nicolaides KH. FirstGÇÉtrimester screening for trisomy 21 by free beta human chorionic gonadotropin and pregnancyGÇÉassociated plasma protein-A: impact of maternal and pregnancy characteristics. Ultrasound Obstet Gynecol 2008;31(5):493–502.

48. Leung TY, Spencer K, Leung TN, Fung TY, Lau TK. Higher median levels of free [beta]-hCG and PAPP-A in the first trimester of pregnancy in a Chinese ethnic group. Fetal Diagn Ther. 2006;21(1):140.

49. Manotaya S, Zitzler J, Li X, Wibowo N, Pham TM, Kang MS, et al. Effect of ethnicity on first trimester biomarkers for combined trisomy 21 screening: results from a multicenter study in six Asian countries. Prenat Diagn. 2015;35(8):735–40.

50. Nørgaard P, Wright D, Ball S, Newell P, Kirkegaard I, OBr P, et al. Autocorrelation and cross-correlation between hCGßǀ and PAPP-A in repeated sampling during first trimester of pregnancy. Clin Chem Lab Med. 2013;51(9):1781–8.

51. Pandya P, Wright D, Syngelaki A, Akolekar R, Nicolaides KH. Maternal serum placental growth factor in prospective screening for aneuploidies at 8 to13 weeks gestation. Fetal Diagn Ther. 2012;31(2):87–93.

52. Spencer K, Heath V, El Sheikhah A, Ong CYT, Nicolaides KH. Ethnicity and The need for correction of biochemical and ultrasound markers of chromosomal anomalies in the first trimester: a study of oriental, Asian and afro-Caribbean populations. Prenat Diagn. 2005;25(5):365–9.

53. Tsiakkas A, Duvdevani N, Wright A, Wright D, Nicolaides KH. Serum placental growth factor in the three trimesters of pregnancy: effects of maternal characteristics and medical history. Ultrasound Obstet Gynecol. 2015;45(5):591–8.

54. Wright D, Silva M, Papadopoulos S, Wright A, Nicolaides KH. Serum pregnancyassociated plasma protein-A in the three trimesters of pregnancy: effects of maternal characteristics and medical history. Ultrasound Obstet Gynecol. 2015;46(1):42–50.

55. Jinks DC, Minter M, Tarver DA, Vanderford M, Hejtmancik JF, McCabe ER. Molecular genetic diagnosis of sickle cell disease using dried blood specimens on blotters used for newborn screening. Hum Genet. 1989;81(4):363–6.

56. Streetly A, Latinovic R, Hall K, Henthorn J. Implementation of universal newborn bloodspot screening for sickle cell disease and other clinically significant haemoglobinopathies in England: screening results for 2005-07. J Clin Pathol. 2009;62(1):26–30.

57. Therrell BL Jr, Hannon WH, Bailey DB Jr, Goldman EB, Monaco J, Norgaard-Pedersen B, et al. Committee report: considerations and recommendations for national guidance regarding the retention and use of residual dried blood spot specimens after newborn screening. Obstet Gynecol Surv. 2011;66(11):687–9.

58. Mei JV, Alexander JR, Adam BW, Hannon WH. Use of filter paper for the collection and analysis of human whole blood specimens. J Nutr. 2001; 131(5):1631S–6S.

59. Hallack R, Doherty LE, Wethers JA, Parker MM. Evaluation of dried blood spot specimens for HIV-1 drug-resistance testing using the Trugene- HIV-1 genotyping assay. J Clin Virol. 2008;41(4):283–7.

60. Cassol SA, Lapointe N, Salas T, Hankins C, Arella M, Fauvel M, et al. Diagnosis of vertical HIV-1 transmission using the polymerase chain reaction and dried blood spot specimens. JAIDS. 1992;5(2):113–9.

61. Bellisario R, Colinas RJ, Pass KA. Simultaneous measurement of thyroxine and thyrotropin from newborn dried blood-spot specimens using a multiplexed fluorescent microsphere immunoassay. Clin Chem. 2000;46(9):1422–4.

62. Brambilla D, Jennings C, Aldrovandi G, Bremer J, Comeau AM, Cassol SA, et al. Multicenter evaluation of use of dried blood and plasma spot specimens in quantitative assays for human immunodeficiency virus RNA: measurement, precision, and RNA stability. J Clin Microbiol. 2003;41(5):1888–93.

63. Edelbroek PM, van der Heijden J, Stolk LM. Dried blood spot methods in therapeutic drug monitoring: methods, assays, and pitfalls. Ther Drug Monit. 2009;31(3):327–36.
64. Bellisario R, Colinas RJ, Pass KA. Simultaneous measurement of antibodies to three HIV-1 antigens in newborn dried blood-spot specimens using a multiplexed microsphere-based immunoassay. Early Hum Dev. 2001;64(1):21–5.
65. McCabe ER, Huang SZ, Seltzer WK, Law ML. DNA Microextraction from dried blood spots on filter paper blotters: potential applications to newborn screening. Hum Genet. 1987;75(3):213–6.
66. Parker SP, Cubitt WD. The use of the dried blood spot sample in epidemiological studies. J Clin Pathol. 1999;52(9):633.
67. Pennings JL, Siljee JE, Imholz S, Kuc S, de Vries A, Schielen PC, et al. Comparison of different blood collection, sample matrix, and immunoassay methods in a prenatal screening setting. Dis Markers. 2014;2014.509821.
68. Browne JL, Schielen PCJI, Belmouden I, Pennings JLA, Klipstein-Grobusch K. Dried blood spot measurement of pregnancyassociated plasma protein a (PAPP-A) and free ßsubunit of human chorionic gonadotropin (ßhCG) from a low resource setting. Prenat Diagn. 2015;35(6):592–7.

5

Exploring perceptions of group antenatal Care in Urban India: results of a feasibility study

R. Rima Jolivet[1][*] [iD], Bella Vasant Uttekar[2], Meaghan O'Connor[3], Kanchan Lakhwani[2], Jigyasa Sharma[4] and Mary Nell Wegner[1]

Abstract

Background: Making high-quality health care available to all women during pregnancy is a critical strategy for improving perinatal outcomes for mothers and babies everywhere. Research from high-income countries suggests that antenatal care delivered in a group may be an effective way to improve the provision, experiences, and outcomes of care for pregnant women and newborns. A number of researchers and programmers are adapting group antenatal care (ANC) models for use in low- and middle-income countries (LMIC), but the evidence base from these settings is limited and no studies to date have assessed the feasibility and acceptability of group ANC in India.

Methods: We adapted a "generic" model of group antenatal care developed through a systematic scoping review of the existing evidence on group ANC in LMICs for use in an urban setting in India, after looking at local, national and global guidelines to tailor the model content. We demonstrated one session of the model to physicians, auxiliary nurse midwives, administrators, pregnant women, and support persons from three different types of health facilities in Vadodara, India and used qualitative methods to gather and analyze feedback from participants on the perceived feasibility and acceptability of the model.

Results: Providers and recipients of care expressed support and enthusiasm for the model and offered specific feedback on its components: physical assessment, active learning, and social support. In general, after witnessing a demonstration of the model, both groups of participants—providers and beneficiaries—saw group ANC as a vehicle for delivering more comprehensive ANC services, improving experiences of care, empowering women to become more active partners and participants in their care, and potentially addressing some current health system challenges.

Conclusion: This study suggests that introducing group ANC would be feasible and acceptable to stakeholders from various care delivery settings, including an urban primary health clinic, a community-based mother and child health center, and a private hospital, in urban India.

Keywords: Antenatal care, Prenatal care, Group care, Feasibility study, Qualitative methods, India

* Correspondence: rjolivet@hsph.harvard.edu
[1]Maternal Health Task Force, Women & Health Initiative, Department of Global Health and Population, Harvard T.H. Chan School of Public Health, 651 Huntington Avenue, Boston, MA 02115, USA
Full list of author information is available at the end of the article

Plain English summary

Research from high-income countries suggests women who receive antenatal care (ANC) in a group may have better experiences and outcomes of care than those who get ANC through individual visits with a health care provider. However, there are few published studies on group ANC in low- and middle-income countries. In this study, we asked participants to share their views about whether group ANC could work and whether it would be acceptable in Vadodara, India. To conduct the study, we developed a "generic" model of group ANC, and then made sure the content matched the care guidelines from the Indian Ministry of Health and Family Welfare. We demonstrated one session of the group model to doctors, auxiliary nurse midwives, pregnant women, and support persons (mothers-in-law, mothers, husbands). These demonstrations were held in three different locations in Vadodara where ANC is typically provided: a private maternity hospital, a public health clinic, and a community-based mother and child health center. Focus group discussions, interviews, and a survey were used to learn from the participants what they thought about the group model. The feedback received through these methods showed that pregnant women and their families, as well as health care providers and administrators, thought it would be feasible and acceptable to conduct group ANC in Vadodara. Participants suggested ideas to better the chances for success in providing group ANC in this setting, including making sure that there is enough staff and space to support the model.

Background

Making high-quality health care available to all women during pregnancy is a critical strategy for improving perinatal outcomes for mothers and babies everywhere. A recent conceptual framework published by the World Health Organization (WHO) includes provision of appropriate services, assurance of positive experience of care, and effective care delivery by the health system within one comprehensive definition of quality of maternal and newborn care in facilities. The framework emphasizes the importance of three types of outcomes of high quality care: coverage of key practices, health outcomes, and people-centered outcomes. It also calls for innovations in healthcare delivery to meet achieve these outcomes [1].

Group Care in High-income Countries

Many studies from high-income countries have reported positive pregnancy experiences and improved birth outcomes among women receiving antenatal care (ANC) in a group, compared to those receiving traditional one-to-one ANC. In high-income settings, the most widespread model of group ANC with the most

extensive evidence base is CenteringPregnancy® which combines clinical care, education, and peer support in one bundled program [2]. A randomized controlled trial of group care in the United States by Ickovics et al. [3] found a 33% decrease in the odds of preterm delivery for women in group care as well as better utilization of ANC, increased prenatal knowledge, increased readiness for labor and delivery, higher satisfaction with care, and higher rates of breastfeeding initiation than women receiving individual ANC. The study also found that there were no differences in the cost of group ANC compared to usual care [3]. Similarly, Earnshaw et al. [4] analyzed data from two separate randomized controlled trials of group ANC and reported that young, urban women in group ANC demonstrated higher levels of engagement and attended more ANC visits than controls. The results of a cluster-randomized controlled trial conducted in 14 urban health centers in the United States demonstrated that women in group ANC delivered significantly fewer infants who were small for gestational age compared to women in traditional ANC [5]. Studies have also demonstrated a significant improvement in appropriate pregnancy weight gain for women in group care compared to individual ANC [6, 7]. However, a Cochrane systematic review of four randomized controlled trials (two in the United States, one in Sweden, and one in Iran) (2015) found no differences in health outcomes between women in group and individual ANC, noting that the review was limited by the small number of trials and participants [8]. The overall positive outcomes reported by group ANC studies conducted in high-income settings suggest that, with some adaptations in the number and content of sessions to meet local guidelines, the group care format might improve quality and experiences of ANC for women in low- and middle-income countries (LMICs) as well.

Group Care in low- and Middle-Income Countries

Although several researchers and programmers are currently exploring the implementation and outcomes of group ANC in LMICs, few studies have been published to date and the body of knowledge on the safety and effectiveness of group ANC in LMICs is limited [9]. Nevertheless, a few small, descriptive studies have assessed perceptions of the acceptability and feasibility of group care among various target audiences in LMICs. Patil et al. [10] assessed the feasibility and acceptability of group ANC with health care providers, decision makers, and women in Malawi and Tanzania, and reported positive responses. Ghani [11] surveyed frontline health workers in Egypt; responses indicated health workers felt the group model would have positive effects on early prevention and detection of complications, patient empowerment, and self-care behaviors, but could face barriers to implementation related to staff training requirements and cost. Arnold et al. [12] surveyed seven male partners of pregnant women who participated in group ANC in Botswana and reported positive responses such as satisfaction with care, increased access to information, and an experience of group care as respectful and sufficiently private.

The few research studies conducted to date that have evaluated the effects of group ANC in LMICs generally report positive results. In Iran, Jafari et al. [13] conducted a cluster-randomized trial of group ANC at 14 health care facilities with a total of 628 participants, 320 of whom received group ANC. The intervention resulted in reductions in the number of low birthweight babies and preterm births, intrauterine growth restriction and perinatal loss, although none of these findings was statistically significant. Women receiving group care were, however, significantly more likely to take prenatal vitamins and iron, and to be using a contraceptive method at 2 months postpartum. Women receiving group ANC also reported significantly higher satisfaction with the information they received, the relationship with their provider, and the quality of care and service delivery, and scored significantly higher on the Kotelchuck Index assessing adequacy of ANC utilization [13, 14]. The positive outcomes of group ANC reported across settings provide sufficient rationale to explore the potential for this innovation in additional LMIC settings.

This paper describes the results of a qualitative research study conducted in Vadodara, India to explore the feasibility and acceptability of a model of group ANC designed for use in LMICs. By collecting the perspectives of care providers, care managers, and care recipients (pregnant women and their accompanying family members) on the strengths and challenges related to introducing an alternative, evidence-based group model of ANC, we aimed to answer two questions:

1) What are the likely strengths and challenges of implementing an evidence-based model of group ANC in the context of three types of care-delivery settings (private, public, and community-based) in urban India?

2) Are there any context-specific modifications or adaptations that would increase the potential of this model of ANC to: a) be implemented effectively within the local health system; and b) improve patient and provider experiences by responding to specific population health needs or health system problems in Vadodara?

Methods
Study setting and design

This research was conducted in Vadodara, a city located in the western Indian state of Gujarat, with a population of 2.3 million [15]. In Vadodara, pregnant women may receive ANC at a public, district tertiary-care hospital, subdistrict hospitals, urban public health clinics (UPHCs), community-based maternal and child health centers (*anganwadis*), and private maternity hospitals. To assess stakeholder perceptions of group ANC within the unique patient populations served by these different types of facilities, we collected data in three settings: a private hospital, a UPHC, and a community-based *anganwadi*. The specific study sites were selected in collaboration with a local representative of the Indian Ministry of Health and Family Welfare (MOHFW), and permission was gained from physicians/administrators in those facilities. The study was carried out collaboratively by a team of researchers from the Centre for Operations Research and Training in Vadodara, and the Harvard T.H. Chan School of Public Health in Boston, MA.

We used a descriptive, qualitative study design to assess the feasibility and acceptability of group ANC to potential stakeholders. Given the novelty of the group ANC model in the study setting, we incorporated a demonstration of one mock session of group ANC into the study design to allow participants to visualize and directly experience the proposed innovation. The demonstration in each setting was followed immediately by data collection using qualitative methods, which are detailed below.

Model

We conducted a systematic review of the published literature and a series of key informant interviews to gather evidence on the components of group antenatal care models in current use in LMICs. Two existing group models emerged as most influential in LMIC settings: nine out of the nineteen unique models identified reportedly drew from CenteringPregnancy® [2] and four out of nineteen reported they were informed by the Home Based Lifesaving Skills (HBLSS) program [16]. We synthesized the data collected through this systematic scoping review and compiled the common elements of the group ANC models reviewed to describe a "generic" model of group ANC specifically for use in LMICs. This evidence review and synthesis is described in Sharma, et al. [9].

We then reviewed the ANC guidelines from the MOHFW and added clinical and educational content to the "generic" model to ensure compliance with the recommended standards of care in the study setting [17, 18]. Two adaptations were made:

1) The number of group sessions was set at four (not inclusive of the initial intake visit): three antenatal sessions and one post-natal care (PNC) session. This number fulfills the Indian MOHFW's minimum recommendation for four antenatal care visits (one intake visit plus three group antenatal visits) and includes the recommended PNC visit at 6 weeks postpartum.

2) The content for each of the four group sessions reflects the clinical care standards found in the most recent MOHFW maternal and newborn health register and guidelines for ANC and skilled attendance at birth.

Participants

Study participants were recruited from two groups of key stakeholders: care receivers and care providers. Care receivers included pregnant women and any support person (e.g. mother, mother-in-law, and husband) whom the women chose to accompany them. Care providers included clinicians who provide ANC (physicians and auxiliary nurse midwives) (ANMs) from each of the study sites and administrators who coordinate the provision of care at these sites. Pregnant women age 18 or older, up to 26 weeks gestation, receiving antenatal care at the study site, and who had attended at least one previous ANC visit during the current pregnancy were eligible to participate. Health care providers were eligible if they were a nurse, midwife, physician, or physician-administrator who was working at the study site and involved in the provision of antenatal care (In the Indian health system, attending physicians often also serve as facility administrators). Physicians and auxiliary nurse midwives from each site were recruited directly by the study team. Pregnant women were recruited by staff at the three study sites using convenience sampling. Each participant was given lunch and compensation for their transportation costs (200 Indian rupees, which is equivalent to approximately $3 US dollars).

Demonstration of the model

We developed an agenda for one mock session of group ANC based on our generic model components tailored to the local context, and used it to demonstrate the model for study participants. The demonstration for the care providers was conducted in English by two members of the Harvard research team (RJ and MO'C) who played the role of group facilitators, with translation into Gujarati from the CORT research team (BU and KL) as needed. A local physician and ANM were recruited to play the roles of the group facilitators during the demonstrations that were conducted for pregnant women and their support persons. These sessions were conducted in the local language (either Gujarati or Hindi) to maximize participants' understanding and participation.

A total of four demonstrations of the group ANC model were conducted: one for providers/administrators (held at a central location), and one at each of the three study sites for women and their family members. Before each demonstration, the study team provided a short introduction to the research study and its aims, requested and collected signed consent, briefly outlined the group ANC model, and clarified that the participants would not be receiving actual clinical care. In the demonstration that was staged for care providers and administrators, participants were asked to play the role of pregnant women so they could observe and experience how care is provided in the group ANC model. The content and format for all four demonstrations was the same and is described in detail in Table 1. During the first 30 min, participants took and recorded their own weight and blood pressure, completed two worksheets about their diet and discomforts during this pregnancy, and saw the clinician in rotation for a brief (mock) physical exam. The co-facilitator opened the group with a short icebreaker. The icebreaker was followed by a facilitated discussion during which participants developed and agreed on shared behavioral norms and guidelines for the group. The rest of the session focused on the interactive learning component of the model: the participants engaged in a facilitated discussion about nutrition during pregnancy and participated in a group activity and discussion of common discomforts and danger signs during pregnancy. The co-leaders guided the discussions and activities using a facilitative leadership style to encourage active participation from the women. The demonstration ended with a short activity in which each participant shared one thing they learned, designed to summarize and close the session.

Data collection

Data was collected through a mix of focus group discussions, in-depth interviews, and a written survey. The questions used to guide the focus group discussions and in-depth interviews were designed to elicit participants' perceptions regarding the feasibility and acceptability of the group ANC model in general, as well as specific elements of the model, and to capture any perceived barriers to implementation along with recommendations for how to overcome them. All physicians participated in an in-depth interview. All ANMs participated in a focus group discussion followed by an individual survey that asked the same questions as those posed in the in-depth interview. The purpose of the survey was to validate the focus group discussion findings and check for any cognitive bias, i.e., groupthink, which may have occurred during the focus group discussion. The pregnant

Table 1 Agenda for Group ANC Session Demonstration

Time	Topic	Leader	Props/Materials	Content
30	Physical self-assessment Psychosocial self-assessment	Co-leader 2 (auxiliary nurse midwife)	1. Digital scale 2. Portable blood pressure cuff 3. Mock flow chart 4. Nutrition worksheet 5. Common discomforts worksheet	• Show each participant how to take their weight and blood pressure and record the results on a mock flow chart. • Distribute two psychosocial self-assessment sheets and provide guidance on how to complete them.
	Provider physical assessment	Co-leader 1 (physician)	1. 1 charpoy and stool 2. 1 Privacy screen or curtain 3. Measuring tape 4. Fetoscope or Doppler 5. Mock chart	• Welcome women individually to the private corner where the clinical exam will take place. • Conduct a mock physical exam with each woman. • Ascertain that privacy and confidentiality are maintained.
10	Opening ice-breaker	Co-leader 2	Soft ball	• Explain the game whose aim is for everyone to introduce themselves and learn the names of others in the group. • Lead the game; help ensure everyone participates.
10	Group guidelines	Co-leader1 Co-leader 2	1. Flip chart or white board 2. Markers	• Facilitate a discussion to help the group develop its own guidelines for group conduct that is comfortable for everyone. Help the group brainstorm, offering probes. • Ask a volunteer to write the group's agreements on a flip chart, and tell the group that these guidelines will be on display during all their group sessions. • Tell the group that all members and any visitors will be asked to sign a confidentiality agreement.
30	Group discussion	Co-leader 1 Co-leader 2	Nutrition worksheet	• Use the worksheet to lead a facilitated discussion on nutrition. • Offer discussion prompts, e.g. "Does anyone know which of the foods here are high in calcium? Why is calcium important in pregnancy? What can you do if you don't like any of those foods?" • Acknowledge each participant's comment or question, refer back to the group for further reflection and discussion, then summarize or expand on the discussion. • Once the topic has been exhausted or it is time to move on, wrap up the discussion, ensuring that participants' questions have been answered satisfactorily.
10	Group learning activity	Co-leader 1 Co-leader 2	1. Common discomforts worksheet 2. Green light/red light paddles	• Use the green light/red light paddles to stimulate group discussion about common discomforts during pregnancy, share ways to address them, and discuss when a symptom should be considered a danger sign.
10	Closing ritual/activity	Co-leader 2 Co-leader 1	Yarn ball and scissors	• Explain the closing ritual designed to encourage participants to recap what they learned in the group, illustrate the connections that were made, and end the session.

women and their support persons were randomly assigned to either a focus group discussion or an in-depth interview. The only non-random assignments were to ensure that women and their support persons were not assigned to the same focus group discussion; this separation was made to avoid courtesy and other biases resulting from any potential power imbalances between women and their support persons or other factors. All focus group discussions and in-depth interviews were recorded and transcribed in Gujarati, and then translated into English. English translations were reviewed to identify themes, coded, and analyzed using Atlas.ti, version 8 software (Berlin, Germany, 2017). Themes were extracted from the participants' responses to each question in the focus group discussion, in-depth interview, and survey, and are presented below in the order they were asked. Codes were derived from the research questions and emerged from the collected data. They were color-coded and categorized into themes, and illustrative quotes were selected to represent each emergent theme. Some further quotes were selected to add in-depth understanding and capture variations in responses.

Results

Participants

There were 13 participants in the demonstration for care providers: five physicians, seven ANMs and one *anganwadi* worker. Thirty-eight individuals participated in the demonstration for care receivers: 29 pregnant women and nine support persons. The support persons included three mothers, one mother-in-law, and five husbands. Of the 29 pregnant women, nine were from a private hospital, 10 from a UPHC, and 10 from an *anganwadi*; 12 of the 29 women were primiparous and the remainder were multiparous.

Reflections on current ANC in Vadodara

Study participants were asked to share their perceptions of the strengths and challenges of the one-on-one model of ANC currently in place in Vadodara.

A typical ANC visit and goals for care

Participants were asked to describe a typical ANC visit and reflect on the goals for care during antenatal visits. Providers reported that a typical ANC visit includes confirmation of pregnancy (during the first ANC visit), lab tests, basic health measurements (weight, blood pressure, fundal height), and risk assessment to check for maternal and fetal wellbeing. In general, providers agreed that, in addition to the aforementioned physical exam and laboratory tests, ANC should include education on nutrition and self-care during pregnancy, and they emphasized the importance of attending all four recommended ANC visits. They reported that ANC services are typically provided by a physician with help from a staff nurse (in tertiary settings), an ANM or an accredited social health activist (ASHA) (in public facilities), or a second physician or medical assistant (in private hospitals). The schedule of visits is determined based on the woman's gestational age upon entry into care; she is advised to return for her next visit at least once per trimester during her pregnancy. The public facility providers reported a range of 10–40 ANC cases per day, with higher volume on days when specialty care is available or when a dedicated obstetric clinic (such as Pradhan Mantri Surakshit Matritva Yojana, or PMSMY [17]) is being held. The private hospital providers reported 20–25 cases per day on average.

Pregnant women's responses describing a typical ANC visit were congruous with those of providers, and mentioned physical exam, laboratory testing, as well as education on nutrition or recommended changes in activities of daily living. While women mentioned similar information and services that should be offered during each ANC visit as the providers did, many women also noted ($n = 14$) that assurance from the doctor was critical for wellbeing. Most pregnant women ($n = 16$) reported that ANC was provided either by a physician alone or a physician in combination with a staff nurse ($n = 13$). Pregnant women reported wait times ranging from 15 min to 4 hours. Women who had attended the ANC clinic at the tertiary hospital reported that the entire process (wait time plus visit) could take up to 6 hours. The majority of the pregnant women ($n = 24$) reported visiting more than one facility for ANC during their pregnancy: UPHCs were generally used to confirm the pregnancy and higher-level public facilities (hospitals) were used to address any complications. Women also noted that they would change facilities if they moved from their in-laws' home to their natal home. In Vadodara, and India more broadly, many women adhere to the custom of *sava-mahina*: a woman experiencing her first pregnancy (although occasionally during subsequent pregnancies as well) will live primarily at her parents' home and only return to her in-laws' home 6 weeks after delivery. This custom can affect facility choice.

Strengths and challenges of the current model

Participants were asked about their views on the strengths of the current model of ANC in Vadodara. Providers cited outreach efforts that allowed them to provide access to care for more women, expanded service capacity (more facilities are able to do more advanced laboratory tests), the convenience that electronic health records in the urban primary health centers provide particularly for the management of high-risk pregnancies, and the provision of free services (e.g. delivery services, iron and calcium tablets) in public facilities. One physician remarked, "The current model is good in all ways, like we give tablets free of cost, all services are free of cost. Besides, we give all guidance based on the [MOHFW] guideline which is fully authorized and prepared by experts."

When asked explicitly about any challenges perceived with the current model of ANC, the majority of providers ($n = 8$) and women ($n = 26$) did not report any challenges or frustrations. However, some providers noted frustration with a shortage of personnel at their facilities ($n = 2$) as well as problems with time management given the high volume of their caseloads ($n = 3$); this was noted as a problem particularly at the UPHCs where ANC is provided at the same time as the general outpatient clinic day (OPD). A provider from a UPHC stated, "I have to see 40 to 50 [OPD] patients and around 15 ANC [patients] in three and a half hours. [It is] ...not only pregnant women—I have other patients also to whom I am not able to give sufficient time." For their part, women expressed their dislike for the long wait times but also noted they were used to it.

Reflections on the group ANC model

Following questions about the current model of ANC in Vadodara, participants were asked to share their reflections about what they had just seen and experienced during the group ANC demonstration.

Physical assessment

Participants were asked what they thought about the physical assessment component of the group ANC demonstration. Both providers and pregnant women were generally comfortable with all aspects of the physical assessment, including the time and attention given to each woman's "belly check," and having that exam done in a private area within the group space. Providers reported that they thought doing the clinical checkup in the group space worked well and would be feasible in their respective facilities. They also felt it was possible to maintain privacy and confidentiality despite being in a shared space. One physician and two ANMs noted they liked the low mat for women's exams on the floor (versus an exam table) as it was easier for the pregnant women to get onto it. Regarding the checkup in the group space, one physician stated, "Yes, it is good, it is in the corner, so women don't feel shy. All the patients are checked so they know that everybody is going to be checked, all enjoyed the process."

The majority of women ($n = 17$) also agreed that the checkup in the group space worked well and was done in a way that maintained their privacy and confidentiality. One woman explained, "It was good, [the doctor] was talking all the time and I did not feel that... there was lots of noise in the room or that she was not able to listen to what I said. I did not feel anything like that. She talked softly yet I did not feel that I was in the same room [with everyone else]." However, three women, two of whom were from the private clinic and one from a public site, expressed discomfort with having their checkup done in the group space and stated that they would have preferred a private room.

Self-assessment

Participants were asked their opinions on the self-assessment components of the group ANC model. Overall, the self-assessment activities were well received by all participants. In general, providers felt that having the women take their own blood pressure (BP) and weight measurements was a novel idea, and helped women pay more attention and develop a feeling of ownership of their health information. One physician explained, "When [the women] measured their own weight they felt that they also can do something. There is empowerment of women. Because they had first time taken BP machine in hand. As we just taught them, they themselves used it so they felt happy from inside." Another physician noted, "That was a great idea I think, because when we tell them that your BP is this much, we don't know whether it registers with them or not. Here when they did [it] on their own, they notice their BP more. And peers are doing the same thing so they compare with them."

The pregnant women also enjoyed taking their own BP and weight, noting that it made them pay closer attention to what the numbers meant and how those numbers can affect their health. According to one woman, "It was good we weighed ourselves and wrote in the report [worksheet] ourselves. We got to know how to check BP. I liked that I measured my BP on my own; in the hospital, we would not come to know [that information] as provider would just write it on their own. They do not tell us, so we do not realize." The majority of the providers ($n = 10$) also felt that the self-assessment worksheets worked well. While they did express concerns that some women—particularly in less literate communities—may need assistance with completing the worksheets, they were confident that overall, women would get used to it and, when necessary, they could receive help. None of the women reported any difficulty or discomfort with the self-assessment worksheets used during the demonstration, even though a few had required assistance from their peers or the co-facilitator to complete the written worksheets.

Peer support and education

Participants were asked for their opinions about the learning component of the group ANC demonstration. Providers and pregnant women responded positively to the group discussion and group activities. The providers were highly enthusiastic about the peer support and education aspects of the model. They felt that group ANC could accomplish all of the goals of high-quality ANC while also providing more time for counseling and learning. Providers appreciated the interactive learning style that the discussion promoted. The physician who acted as a group leader for the demonstrations noted her surprise at how willing the women were to engage in the discussion: "Initially I was little skeptical whether I would be able to get answers [from the women]. But when we finally tried it, lot of information came from them, especially in the private [hospital] the level of knowledge was too good [meaning "very good"]. Even in the public [settings], in slums, though knowledge was not so much, we could encourage women to talk and many of the answers came from them."

The women also reportedly enjoyed the discussion and stated that it gave them the opportunity to learn from the provider as well as each other. One pregnant woman explained, "Everyone gets chance to speak [and] due to that, a good atmosphere is also created. If only the service provider speaks, after sometime it feels like a lecture. As everyone speaks and shares their experience, we get to learn from that also. If I'm not suffering at present but some other lady is suffering and I hear her experiences, and after some time if I have a similar problem then I will remember about the discussion at that time." Another pregnant woman noted that the group discussion was helpful for participants who were shy; although they did not speak up themselves, they had the chance to learn from others who might be going through similar situations.

Both providers and pregnant women also felt that the group activity was an effective, entertaining way to learn about information related to pregnancy (in the demonstration the topic was common discomforts and danger signs). Providers liked that the activity was fun and interactive while still being informative. One demonstrator remarked, "[This activity was a] good one. You learn when you are having fun. I didn't find that women were getting bored or were in hurry, everyone was pretty attentive. I could see that they were happy playing games and learning. It is a better way of teaching." The same demonstrator noted that she had been worried that women might copy one another's answers or could be unwilling to share personal information about discomforts but that the women proved otherwise, offering their original thoughts and experiences.

The pregnant women also reported positive feedback on the group activity. One woman said that she preferred it to a one-on-one meeting with the physician: "If we all are together we do enjoy having fun (*masti ho jaati hai*) and we also learn. We like to learn more in the form of games rather than sitting alone, waiting for the doctor; that I don't like."

Other aspects of the model
Participants were asked for feedback on other aspects of the model, including a set schedule of visits and the duration of each session. Five providers expressed concerns about introducing a set schedule of visits for group ANC. Three providers were worried about what would happen if they were called away to attend an emergency during a scheduled group sessions. They also expressed concern about women forgetting pre-scheduled sessions. Pregnant women, on the other hand, expressed a preference for the idea of a set schedule of appointments, and thought it would allow them to better manage their time. One woman explained: "That would be good that

in advance we know the schedule, so we can finish other work and come."

When asked for their opinions on the length of the group sessions (90–120 min), providers stated that it would be feasible and acceptable in each of their settings, although some thought it might present a challenge to manage OPD patients at the same time. Still, they reported that they would appreciate the increased efficiency of seeing 10–12 ANC patients in that period of time. However, providers from public facilities believed that 120 min would likely be necessary in settings serving less educated women in order to allow more time for discussion. A provider commented, "Initially again, I was doubtful that women will be ready to spend two hours, but we didn't feel any time that any one of them was bored or was not attentive or was in a hurry to go home. In fact, I had an experience that they wanted to keep on talking. I didn't feel that anyone felt like leaving even when session was over. I think if they have a good experience they would take out time." And, "In a way we see, group ANC is good. Together for all 10 women, physical checkups are done and their BP, weight, etc. is completed in one and half hour to two hours. Otherwise in individual visit women come one by one so our lot of time goes in that. If we call women together, it will save our time, and they will get to know each other."

Overall, pregnant women expressed satisfaction with the proposed session duration of 90–120 min because it was spent actively participating, rather than simply waiting to see the doctor. One woman remarked, "It is better to come over here rather than watching TV at home, at least by coming here we felt good and learnt something new." In their focus group discussion, all of the husbands ($n = 5$) also agreed with that sentiment.

Solutions to potential barriers
Participants were asked to identify any potential barriers to implementation in their setting, and to share their ideas about solutions that could help overcome those barriers. Providers made several concrete suggestions:

a) Conduct sessions in the afternoons as most women are occupied with chores and household responsibilities in the mornings
b) In addition to grouping women by similar gestational age, be sure to organize groups based on a common language (demonstration sessions showed that not all women attending a facility in Vadodara speak the same language)
c) To ensure consistency of leadership, if one group leader is unable to join a session due to an unforeseen event, ensure that the co-facilitator, who

is familiar with the group and its concerns, is available to lead the session

d) To ensure continuity of care, if a pregnant woman is unable to join a session due to an unforeseen event, ensure that she can schedule an individual ANC visit so that her care is not interrupted

e) Consider engaging an additional support person (not clinical staff) at the facility to manage the logistical aspects of the group (i.e. scheduling, pre-session reminders to the women)

f) Engage leadership at a higher level in the (public) system to help support the implementing facilities and their staff

The providers from the public facilities felt that support from leadership at the health system level would be essential to the successful implementation of the group model. One ANM explained: "Yes, we can do [group ANC] but we need support for that. Meeting space for all the people, making groups [with a] minimum [of] 8–12 women."

Three pregnant women felt that pre-session reminders (phone call or text) would help group ANC participants remember to attend each group visit, and one woman suggested that it might be helpful to have a physiotherapist join the sessions.

The potential barriers to implementing group ANC in Vadodara as well as the concrete solutions offered to overcome them, while hypothetical, provide useful insights and suggestions grounded in knowledge of an urban health system in the Indian context that should be tested through implementation research.

Discussion

To our knowledge, this is the first study to evaluate the feasibility and acceptability of group ANC in India and the first study in Asia to evaluate a group model for pregnant women that includes a clinical care component. The findings provide evidence to support the rationale for future studies designed to evaluate the effects of group ANC on health outcomes, experiences of care, and system performance in India. The results of this qualitative assessment of stakeholders' perceptions about the potential feasibility and acceptability of introducing group ANC in India were positive following participation in a demonstration of one mock session of the model.

While some participants expressed initial skepticism about the group model in concept, after participating in the demonstration the reaction of both providers and recipients of care was generally enthusiastic. Overall, pregnant women who participated were more open to the novel experience. Ultimately, both groups of participants saw group ANC as a vehicle for delivering more comprehensive ANC services, improving experiences of

care, empowering women to become more active partners and participants in their care, and potentially addressing some current health system challenges. For example, both women and providers felt that group ANC might help to reduce wait times for women while care providers and administrators also expressed optimism that group ANC could improve patient retention in facilities. Care administrators identified patient retention as a priority goal as well as a challenge in Vadodara. The feedback gathered through the various qualitative methods also suggests some concrete system requirements that, if met, could help to ensure effective implementation of this model.

This study has some limitations. Due to resource and time constraints, we were only able to demonstrate one session of the full four-session model and participants' responses and perceptions may have been different following a longer exposure to the model. Our study had a relatively small number of participants although the number was likely adequate given the qualitative methods used; however, we cannot fully ascertain the adequacy of the sample size as our study was not designed to test saturation. Our study instruments (focus group discussion guides, in-depth interview guides, and written survey) were not validated prior to use in this study. In addition, because the researchers were involved in the model demonstration as well as the data collection, there is a possibility of social desirability bias in the responses. Finally, because our study was conducted only in three urban facilities, the outcomes may not be transferable to other settings. Future research on group ANC in India could assess its feasibility and acceptability in a broader variety of settings, and evaluate outcomes of the model in both rural and urban facilities.

Our research complements and builds on the small but growing evidence base of studies assessing the feasibility of group ANC in LMICs. Similar to the findings of the three studies published to date that have collected stakeholder responses to group ANC [10–12], our research also recorded positive responses from study participants. The results of our study provide support for testing the group ANC model in urban India, as they indicate that the model would be both possible and welcome in this setting. We also gathered some specific suggestions to improve the feasibility of implementing group ANC in urban India. These include ensuring adequate staffing ratios to handle the volume and range of patients presenting to the clinics who are not enrolled in group ANC; hiring dedicated personnel to help with group ANC logistics and scheduling; giving attention to the space requirements for effective group ANC; and initiation of a system of appointment reminders for women. These insights could be useful to others planning to implement the model in similar LMIC settings.

This study is particularly timely given the recently updated WHO ANC recommendations (2016), which identify group ANC as a health systems intervention with the potential to improve the utilization and quality of ANC. The WHO report offers the following context-specific research recommendation:

"Group antenatal care provided by qualified healthcare professionals may be offered as an alternative to individual antenatal care for pregnant women in the context of rigorous research, depending on a woman's preferences and provided that the infrastructure and resources for delivery of group antenatal care are available" [1].

Conclusions

This qualitative research study collected the perceptions of care providers, care administrators, pregnant women and their family support persons to assess the feasibility and acceptability of a model of group ANC that was developed through a systematic scoping review of group care in LMICs. It demonstrates positive responses from stakeholders of all types in a variety of care delivery settings following active participation in a demonstration of the model. It provides specific feedback from participants on each of the major components of the group care model: physical assessment, active learning, and peer support. It suggests concrete ways to facilitate the introduction of the group ANC model in urban India and to overcome potential system barriers to implementation.

Abbreviations
ANC: Antenatal care; ANM: Auxiliary nurse midwife; ASHA: Accredited social health activist; BP: Blood pressure; CORT: Centre for operations research and training; LMICs: Low- and middle-income countries; MOHFW: Ministry of Health and Family Welfare; OPD: Out-patient clinic day; PMSMY: Pradhan mantri surakshit matritva yojana; PNC: Postnatal care; UPHC: Urban primary care clinic; WHO: World Health Organization

Acknowledgements
The authors would like to thank the following people for their contributions to the development of the research study described in this paper and for their support during its implementation: Ana Langer, Maternal Health Task Force, Women & Health Initiative, Harvard T.H. Chan School of Public Health; M.E. Khan, CORT; Sandhya Barge, CORT; Jashoda Sharma, CORT; Shoba Ramanadhan, Harvard Catalyst consultant; and the two individuals who acted as co-facilitators in the demonstrations of the group ANC model that were conducted with the study participants.

Funding
Funding for this study was provided by the John D. and Catherine T. MacArthur Foundation. The funding body had no role in the design of the study or the collection, analysis, and interpretation of data or in writing the manuscript.

Authors' contributions
RRJ, MO'C, and MNW developed the concept and study design. RRJ, BVU, MO'C, JS, and KL participated in the conception, design, analysis and/or interpretation of data. RRJ and BVU served as primary investigators and project directors in the US and India, respectively. MO'C and KL served as research coordinators and project managers in the US and India, respectively. BVU and MO'C managed the IRB applications, with inputs from other members of the team, in the US and India, respectively. RRJ, MO'C, JS, BVU and KL contributed to the development of the demonstration model, and the study instruments. RRJ, BVU, MO'C and KL participated in the model demonstration. BVU and KL led participant and demonstrator recruitment, selection of study sites, carried out the data collection, transcribed and translated the data into English, and analyzed the results. All authors participated in writing the manuscript by reviewing drafts and approving the final version.

Competing interests
The authors declare that they have no competing interests.

Author details
[1]Maternal Health Task Force, Women & Health Initiative, Department of Global Health and Population, Harvard T.H. Chan School of Public Health, 651 Huntington Avenue, Boston, MA 02115, USA. [2]Centre for Operations Research and Training, 402 Woodland Apartment, Race Course Circle, Vadodara, Gujarat 390 007, India. [3]Maternal Health Task Force, Women & Health Initiative, Harvard T.H. Chan School of Public Health, 651 Huntington Avenue, Boston, MA 02115, USA. [4]Department of Global Health and Population, Harvard T. H. Chan School of Public Health, 677 Huntington Ave, Boston, MA 02115, USA.

References
1. WHO Recommendations on Antenatal Care for a Positive Pregnancy Experience. Geneva: World Health Organization; 2016.
2. Rising SS. Centering pregnancy: an interdisciplinary model of empowerment. J Nurse Midwifery. 1998;43(1):9.
3. Ickovics JR, Kershaw TS, Westdahl C, Magriples U, Massey Z, Reynolds H. Rising SS: group prenatal care and perinatal outcomes: a randomized controlled trial. Obstet Gynecol. 2007;110(2 Pt 1):330–9.
4. Earnshaw VA, Rosenthal L, Cunningham SD, Kershaw T, Lewis J, Rising SS, Stasko E, Tobin J, Ickovics JR. Exploring group composition among young, urban women of color in prenatal care: implications for satisfaction, engagement, and group attendance. Womens Health Issues. 2016;26(1):110–5.
5. Ickovics JR, Earnshaw V, Lewis JB, Kershaw TS, Magriples U, Stasko E, Rising SS, Cassells A, Cunningham S, Bernstein P, et al. Cluster randomized controlled trial of group prenatal care: perinatal outcomes among adolescents in new York City health centers. Am J Public Health. 2016; 106(2):359–65.
6. Magriples U, Boynton MH, Kershaw TS, Lewis J, Rising SS, Tobin JN, Epel E, Ickovics JR. The impact of group prenatal care on pregnancy and postpartum weight trajectories. Am J Obstet Gynecol. 2015;213(5): 688 e681–9.
7. Tanner-Smith EE, Steinka-Fry KT, Gesell SB. Comparative effectiveness of group and individual prenatal care on gestational weight gain. Matern Child Health J. 2014;18(7):1711–20.

8. Catling CJ, Medley N, Foureur M, Ryan C, Leap N, Teate A, Homer CS. Group versus conventional antenatal care for women. Cochrane Database Syst Rev. 2015;2:CD007622.

9. Sharma J, O'Connor M, Jolivet RR. Group antenatal care in low- and middle-income countries: a systematic evidence synthesis. Reprod Health. 2018; 15(1):38. https://doi.org/10.1186/s12978-018-0476-9.

10. Patil CL, Abrams ET, Klima C, Kaponda CP, Leshabari SC, Vonderheid SC, Kamanga M, Norr KF. CenteringPregnancy-Africa: a pilot of group antenatal care to address millennium development goals. Midwifery. 2013;29(10):1190–8.

11. Ghani RMA. Perception toward conducting the centering pregnancy model in the Egyptian teaching hospitals: a step to improve the quality of antenatal care. Eur J Biol Med Sci Res. 2014;2(2):45–54.

12. Arnold J, Morgan A, Morrison B. Paternal perceptions of and satisfaction with group prenatal Care in Botswana. Online J Cult Competence Nurs Healthc. 2014;4(2):17–26.

13. Jafari F. Maternal and neonatal outcomes of group prenatal care: a new experience in Iran. Early Hum Dev. 2010;86:S140.

14. Jafari F, Eftekhar H, Mohammad K, Fotouhi A. Does group prenatal care affect satisfaction and prenatal care utilization in Iranian pregnant women? Iran J Public Health. 2010;39(2):52–62.

15. Population of Vadodara. 2017. http://indiapopulation2017.in/population-of-vadodara-2017.html. Accessed 28 Mar 2018.

16. Buffington ST, Sibley LM, Beck DR, Armbruster DA. Home based life saving skills - second edition. Silver Spring: American College of Nurse-Midwives; 2010.

17. Maternal Health Division. Pradhan Mantri Surakshit Matritva Abhiyan. New Delhi: Ministry of Health and Family Welfare, Government of India; 2016.

18. Maternal Health Division. Guidelines for antenatal care and skilled attendance at birth by ANMs/LHVs/SNs. New Delhi: Ministry of Health and Family Welfare, Government of India; 2010.

6

Urinary phthalate metabolites in relation to serum anti-Müllerian hormone and inhibin B levels among women from a fertility center

Yao-Yao Du[1], Na Guo[1], Yi-Xin Wang[2,3], Xiang Hua[1], Tao-Ran Deng[1], Xue-Mei Teng[1], Yang-Cheng Yao[1] and Yu-Feng Li[1*]

Abstract

Background: Phthalates, a class of endocrine disruptors, have been demonstrated to accelerate loss of ovarian follicle pool via disrupting folliculogenesis, and lead to diminished ovarian reserve. However, human data are limited. Here, we aimed to examine whether urinary phthalate metabolites are correlated with markers of ovarian reserve among women attending a fertility clinic.

Methods: We measured eight phthalate metabolites in urine samples collected from 415 women seeking infertility treatment at the Reproductive Medicine Center of Tongji Hospital, Wuhan, China. Data on measures of ovarian reserve, as indicated by serum anti-Müllerian hormone (AMH) and inhibin B (INHB) levels, were retrieved retrospectively through electronic medical charts. Multivariate linear models were performed to estimate the associations of urinary phthalate metabolites and serum AMH and INHB. We further explored the potential nonlinearity of the relationships with restricted cubic spline analysis.

Results: Overall, we found largely null associations between urinary phthalate metabolites and serum AMH. The multivariable adjusted differences in serum INHB levels comparing the highest quartile of urinary MEHP to the lowest were − 18.29% (95% CI: − 31.89%, − 1.98%; *P*-trend = 0.04). Women in the second to fourth quartiles of MEOHP had a significant decrease of − 23.74% (95% CI: −35.85%, − 9.24%), − 19.91% (95% CI: −33.30%, − 3.82%) and − 20.23% (95% CI: −34.43%, − 2.96%), respectively, in INHB levels compared to the first quartile. In the spline analysis, we identified a nonlinear relationship between MEOHP exposure and serum INHB.

Conclusions: We provided evidence for a negative association between urinary concentrations of certain phthalate metabolites and serum INHB levels, suggesting an adverse effect of phthalates exposure on growing antral follicles. Whether phthalates exposure at environmentally level will pose a risk for ovarian reserve needs further investigation.

Keywords: Phthalates, Anti-Müllerian hormone, Inhibin B, Ovarian reserve, Endocrine disruptors

* Correspondence: yufengli64@tjh.tjmu.edu.cn
[1]Reproductive Medicine Center, Tongji Hospital, Tongji Medical College, Huazhong University of Science and Technology, 1095 JieFang Avenue, Wuhan, Hubei, People's Republic of China
Full list of author information is available at the end of the article

Plain English summary

Ovarian reserve is reflected by the resting follicle pool. Accelerated depletion of ovarian follicles, manifested as increased rate of ovarian aging, has serious consequences. It will not only lead to reduced fertility but also to non-reproductive health problems through early menopause. Phthalates are a group of synthetic industrial chemicals. Environmental exposure to phthalates in the general population is ubiquitous, and has aroused growing public health concern based on their endocrine disrupting potency. Evidence from toxicological studies has suggested a role for phthalates in accelerating loss of ovarian follicle pool via disrupting follicular development, and consequently leading to diminished ovarian reserve. However, human data are limited, and whether they can execute comparable effects in humans needs to be elucidated. Therefore, in this retrospective study, we measured eight phthalate metabolites in urine samples collected from 415 women attending a fertility clinic in China, and examined whether phthalate exposure is correlated with serum anti-Müllerian hormone (AMH) and inhibin B (INHB) levels—two well-established markers of ovarian reserve. Our study provided evidence for a negative association between urinary concentrations of certain phthalate metabolites and serum INHB levels, suggesting an adverse effect of phthalate exposure on growing antral follicles. Moreover, we identified a similar decrease in INHB after a threshold level of select phthalates was met, and younger women had larger decrease in INHB levels compared to those of advanced age. However, we found largely null associations between urinary phthalate metabolites and serum AMH. Whether phthalate exposure at environmentally level will pose a risk for ovarian reserve needs further investigation.

Background

Ovarian reserve is established early in life with a finite number of oocytes. It gradually declines across the reproductive lifespan of a woman until the menopause, paralleled with a reduction in oocyte quality [1]. Apart from age, there are other factors contributing to the depletion of ovarian reserve, including genetic factors, iatrogenic causes, and autoimmune diseases. Recent research has raised concerns that environmental exposure may pose a risk for ovarian function, leading to reduced fertility, premature ovarian failure, and even long-term health problems through early onset of menopause [2]. Among the toxicants of concern is one class of the endocrine disrupting chemicals (EDCs)—phthalates, which have been linked to a broad range of adverse reproductive outcomes in epidemiological and toxicological studies [3].

Phthalates are produced in high volume worldwide and used in the synthesis of polyvinyl chloride products,

for example, building supplies, food packaging, and medical devices, to impart flexibility and durability. They are also applied in the formation of cosmetics, personal care products and the coatings of medications, as solvents or excipients [4]. Importantly, they have the potential to leach out from these materials during transportation and storage, and enter the body through ingestion, dermal absorption and inhalation. 'Every day' exposure to phthalates, at home or in workplace, is ubiquitous corroborated by the fact that many phthalates or their metabolites are found at measurable concentrations in the biological fluids within most of the general population [5–7].

In recent years, accumulated data from experimental studies has demonstrated that certain phthalates have the potential to accelerate loss of ovarian follicle pool via disrupting folliculogenesis at different stages [8]. Di(2-ethylhexyl) phthalate (DEHP) has been shown to deplete the pool of primordial follicles either by disrupting primordial follicle assembly via dysregulated gene expression or by accelerating initial follicular recruitment through altered PI3K signaling [9, 10]. In vivo or in vitro exposed to DEHP, di-n-butyl phthalate (DBP) or their monoesters increased atresia of antral follicles through mechanisms of decreased estradiol (E_2) production, elevated apoptosis gene expression or oxidative stress damage [11–13]. In animal models, gestational exposure to mono(2-ethylhexyl) phthalate (MEHP), a metabolite of DEHP, resulted in premature ovarian aging in female offspring manifested as shortened reproductive lifespan, which may be a result of increased rate of follicle recruitment and maturation [14]. As the ovarian reserve reflects primarily the resting pool of primordial follicles, together with follicles recruited into the later preantral and antral stages, reduction in the number of follicles at any stage may lead to reduced ovarian reserve [1]. Notably, in our previous study, phthalates have been detected in the follicular fluid of women seeking infertility treatment [15], a population at higher reproductive risk due to the possibility that they may have the highest exposures or more vulnerable to phthalate-induced toxicity. Thus, it is reasonable to hypothesize that phthalates may be capable of interfering the folliculogenesis process, and result in diminished ovarian reserve.

Nevertheless, although the results from basic research are consistent enough to imply a relationship between phthalate exposure and impaired folliculogenesis, the data from clinical studies are scarce. An earlier study has reported a significant decrease in antral follicle count (AFC) toward higher levels of DEHP metabolites in women seeking infertility treatment [16]. While AFC is a routine biomarker of ovarian reserve in clinical practice, its inherent limitations derived from difficulties in standardized measurement and incapability of reflecting the health status of follicles, for example, inclusion of atretic follicles, suggest that a more accurate and robust indicator would be needed [17, 18]. Produced predominantly by preantral and small antral follicles, anti-Müllerian hormone (AMH) acts as a regulator of follicular recruitment [18]. Interest in AMH's role in reproduction has heightened of late. Emerging data have shown that, with the development of fully automated assays, AMH becomes a substantially better indicator of ovarian reserve than AFC, not only because of its objectivity and potential standardization of analysis but also its advantage of reflecting both the quantity and quality aspects of the follicle pool [19]. Inhibin B (INHB), secreted by granulosa cells of small growing follicles, is also a biomarker of ovarian aging. With its ability to suppress the rise in follicle-stimulating hormone (FSH), INHB is thought to represent the early event in reproductive senescense [20]. Therefore, in the present study, we aimed to examine whether urinary phthalate metabolites are correlated with diminished ovarian reserve (DOR), as indicated by serum AMH and INHB levels among women attending a fertility clinic.

Methods

Study participants

This retrospective cohort study was conducted at the Reproductive Medicine Center of Tongji Hospital, Wuhan, China between November 2016 and December 2016. We recruited participants based on the following criteria: 1) women aged between 20 and 45 years, with indications for in vitro fertilization (IVF) or intracytoplasmic sperm injection (ICSI); 2) women who provided one urine sample and signed an informed consent on the day of ovum pick-up; 3) women who had a serum hormone measurement at the first consultation and the tests were within the 4-month period before urine collection. Women who had an oophorectomy ($n = 2$) or gonadotoxic therapy, or with chromosomal abnormality (n = 2), or had oral contraceptive use in the last three months before hormone measurement were excluded from the study, leaving 415 women eligible for participation. At enrollment, the participants completed detailed questionnaires on their demographics, medical history, diets, smoking habits, and other lifestyle factors under the guidance of an investigator. Approval of the study was obtained from the Institutional Review Board of Tongji Hospital.

Hormone measurement and clinical data

All women had serum AMH, INHB, and AFC measured as a routine fertility assessment at the clinic. Serum AMH was determined at the initial visit of the clinic. Serum INHB and AFC were assessed between day 2 and 4 of a menstrual cycle prior to stimulation. The AMH and INHB assays were conducted using the enzyme-linked immunuosorbent assay (ELISA) kit (Ansh Labs, Webster, TX, USA) based on the automated DS2 (Dynex Technologies, Chantilly, USA) ELISA processing system. For both AMH and INHB assays, six standards and two quality controls of high and low concentrations were run with serum samples in each assay to monitor accuracy and precision. The standard calibration curves were linear ($r^2 > 0.99$) with a measuring range of 0.06–18 ng/mL for AMH, and a range of 10–1500 pg/mL for INHB. The relative standard deviations (RSD) of both assays were less than 10%. The inter-assay and intra-assay coefficient of variations determined by quality control samples were ≤15% and ≤10%, respectively. AFC was determined through trans-vaginal ultrasound and defined as the total amount of 2–9 mm follicles in both ovaries. Women with polycystic ovary (PCO) morphology or polycystic ovary syndrome (PCOS) were diagnosed according to the Rotterdam criteria [21]. Other clinical data on age, BMI, and causes of infertility were retrieved from electronic medical records.

Urine collection and exposure assessment

On the day of ovum pick-up, 10 mL spot urine specimen was collected with a sterile polypropylene container from each participant. The median interval between the day of blood collection for AMH and INHB assays and the day of the urine collection for the phthalate assays were 72 d [interquartile range (IQR): 46–93.5 d]. Urine samples were aliquoted into 2 mL specimens and stored at – 80 °C prior to phthalate metabolites measurement. All urine samples were assayed for eight phthalate metabolites using solid-phase extraction coupled with high-performance liquid chromatography and tandem mass spectrometry, as previously described [22]. The eight metabolites included monomethyl phthalate (MMP), monoethyl phthalate (MEP), mono-n-butyl phthalate (MBP), monobenzyl phthalate (MBzP), MEHP, mono(2-ethyl-5-hydroxyhexyl) phthalate (MEHHP), mono(2-ethyl-5-oxohexyl) phthalate (MEOHP) and mono-n-octyl phthalate (MOP). For each batch of 60–110 samples, one blank, two quality control samples and six standards were processed along with the urine samples. The blank control contained 1-mL water was used to assess the contaminations during sample processing and analysis. Two quality control samples spiked with 5 and 50 ng/mL of the target phthalates, respectively, were used to determine the validation of intraday method accuracy by calculating the recovery. The average recovery for target compounds ranged from 88.06% to 110.93%, and RSD was less than 10.00%. The calibration curve generated from six analytical standards had a linearity of > 0.99, with a range of 0.5–200 ng/mL. If any metabolites in urine samples had much higher concentrations than the linear range of the calibration curves, the samples were re-analyzed after dilution of remaining samples to ensure the accuracy of measurements. The limits of detection (LOD) ranged from 0.01 to 0.04 ng/mL for targeted analytes. Additionally, we calculated the molar sum of the DEHP metabolites (ΣDEHP)—MEHP, MEHHP, and MEOHP, by converting the individual metabolite into molar concentration (μmol/L). To standardize the measures, we determined urinary creatinine concentrations using an automated clinical chemistry analyzer.

Statistical analysis

In descriptive analyses, we used median (IQR) or number (%) to describe the demographic and clinical characteristics of the study population. Urinary phthalate metabolites were standardized by creatinine. The creatinine-adjusted concentrations were expressed as microgram per gram creatinine. We calculated geometric means, medians and selected percentiles to summarize the distributions of phthalate metabolites. Urinary concentrations below the LOD were assigned a value of LOD/$\sqrt{2}$. Because more than 70% MOP were below the LOD, we dichotomized the concentrations of MOP as either being below or above the LOD and considered it as a dichotomous variable in subsequent analysis.

Multivariable linear regression was performed to estimate the associations of phthalate metabolites with serum AMH and INHB. AMH and INHB levels were natural logarithm transformed to achieve normality. Based on the distribution of the subjects, phthalate metabolites (unadjusted) were categorized into quartiles and estimates for each outcome measure were obtained by comparing each higher quartile to the lowest one (reference category). Tests for trend were performed to explore the potential dose-response relationships between phthalate metabolites and the hormones using the exposure quartiles as ordinal categorized variables with integer values (1–4). The associations between MOP and the hormone measures were also evaluated with concentrations of MOP < LOD as the reference value. We have constructed two types of regression models by adjusting different sets of covariates, and selected covariates based on their biological relevance. Although ethnicity and current smoking were suggested to be potential confounders, they were not considered for inclusion due to their low presentation (< 5%) in the total population. Considering that age and BMI were related to both phthalate exposure and hormone levels as previously outlined [23–25], they were selected to enter the regression models. We considered for urine dilution adjustment by adding creatinine as a separate covariate in the multivariable regression models instead of creatinine-corrected concentrations (i.e. μg/g Cr) because creatinine levels have been suggested to associate with age, gender, race/ethnicity, BMI, muscle mass, diet, activity,

etc., thus modeling creatinine-corrected metabolite levels may introduce bias [26, 27]. Therefore, age, BMI and creatinine were entered into model 1 as covariates. Since women diagnosed with PCOS or PCO morphology tend to have altered AMH and INHB levels [28, 29], infertility diagnosis of PCO/PCOS (yes or no) were adjusted in model 2 as a binary variable, together with covariates from model 1. Given that in the regression analysis serum AMH and INHB were ln-transformed, we calculated the percent change with the regression coefficients (β) to allow for easier interpretation of the results. The percent change and corresponding 95% confidence intervals (CI) were calculated as follows: [exp (β)-1]*100, which indicates a percent difference in the outcome comparing each of the higher category of exposure to the lowest one (reference category).

To further explore the potential nonlinearity of the relationship between urinary phthalates and the hormones, we used restricted cubic splines (RCS) with 3 knots at the 5th, 50th, and 95th percentiles of natural logarithm transformed phthalate distributions and set the median level as reference. The optimal number of knots was selected based on model fit and biologic plausibility. We chose the 3-knot RCS function because it had lower Akaike Information Criteria (AIC), which suggests that the model could better explain the observation, while easier for interpretation in the biological context. The location of knots was selected as usually recommended, because it has been suggested to have a little impact on the shape of the dose-response association compared to the number of knots [30]. The Wald chi-square test was used to assess the overall and nonlinear associations between phthalate exposure and the hormones [31]. Taking into account the underlying effect modification by age, we reran the multiple regression models by dividing the participants into young and advanced age groups (< 35 years versus ≥35 years). We examined whether age modifies the effect of urinary phthalate metabolites on serum AMH and INHB levels by adding a product term between metabolite quartiles modeled as ordinal variables and strata of age in the regression models.

Since serum AMH levels could be dichotomized at a cut-off value of 1.1 ng/mL to indicate women with diminished or normal ovarian reserve [32], we additionally explored the effect of urinary phthalate concentrations on this clinically relevant endpoint using multivariable logistic regressions. In addition to hormone biomarkers of ovarian reserve, in the secondary analysis, we fitted multivariable generalized linear models with a Poisson distribution and log-link function to evaluate the associations of urinary phthalate concentrations with AFC. All data analyses were performed using either the Predictive Analytics Suite Workstation (PASW) version 22.0 (IBM Corporation, Armonk, NY) or SAS 9.4 software (SAS

Institute, Inc., Cary, NC, USA). Statistical significance was assumed for $P < 0.05$.

Results

The present study comprised 415 women with an average age of 30 years and BMI of 21.5 kg/m^2. Most of them were Han (96.9%) and non-smokers (94.9%). A total of 229 women (55.2%) were nulliparous. Nearly half of the subjects underwent IVF or ICSI due to tubal or pelvic infertility (40.0%), followed by male factor (23.9%) and diminished ovarian reserve (13.5%). The median (IQR) concentrations of serum AMH and INHB were 3.90 (1.96–6.99) ng/mL and 82 (59–104) pg/mL, respectively, and AFC was 12 on average. Since eleven women had missing values on serum INHB levels, they were excluded from relevant analysis. Other basic characteristics of the participants were summarized in Table 1.

Table 1 Demographics and clinical characteristics of the subjects ($n = 415$)

Characteristics	Data
Age (years)	30 (27–35)
BMI (kg/m^2)	21.5 (19.8–23.7)
Ethnicity	
Han	402 (96.9)
Other	13 (3.1)
Smoking	
Non-smoker	394 (94.9)
Former smoker	19 (4.6)
Current smoker	2 (0.5)
Gravidity	
Yes	186 (44.8)
No	229 (55.2)
Duration of infertility (years)	3 (1.5–5.0)
IVF/ICSI treatment indication	
Tubal or pelvic factor infertility	166 (40.0)
Ovulation disorders	40 (9.6)
Diminished ovarian reserve	56 (13.5)
Endometriosis	23 (5.5)
Uterine disorders	13 (3.1)
Male factor	99 (23.9)
Unexplained	18 (4.3)
AFC	12 (8–18)
AMH (ng/mL)	3.90 (1.96–6.99)
INHB[a] (pg/mL)	82 (59–104)

BMI: body mass index; IVF: in vitro fertilization; ICSI: intracytoplasmic sperm injection; AFC: antral follicle count; AMH: anti-Müllerian hormone; INHB: inhibin B
Data are median [IQR (interquartile range)] or number (%)
[a]Serum INHB levels were measured in 404 women

Table 2 presents the creatinine-adjusted concentrations of urinary phthalate metabolites. The detection frequencies of most phthalate metabolites were considerably high, ranging from 95.4% to 100%, except for MOP with 28.7% samples had concentration below the LOD. Metabolite concentrations in the urine varied widely. Among them, MBP had the highest median level (112.74 µg/g Cr), followed by metabolites of DEHP—-MEHHP (median 12.30 µg/g Cr), MEHP (median 10.75 µg/g Cr) and MEOHP (median 10.27 µg/g Cr).

Overall, no significant dose-response associations were observed between urinary phthalate metabolites and serum AMH in linear models, after adjusting for age, BMI and creatinine (Table 3). Similar results were obtained when additionally adjusted for PCO/PCOS diagnosis (yes or no) in model 2, except for an increase in AMH levels comparing MOP > LOD to those below the LOD. Moreover, we examined the validity of the linearity assumption between phthalates and serum AMH with restricted cubic spline analysis. In spline regression models, the overall and nonlinear spline terms were both non-significant, thus further corroborating our null findings between urinary phthalates and serum AMH (Additional file 1: Figure S1). In the age-stratified analysis, the associations between phthalates and AMH were not modified by age (P for interaction > 0.05). Urinary concentrations of metabolites were consistently not related to serum AMH neither among women < 35 years nor among those ≥35 years (Additional file 2: Table S1).

In the linear regression models adjusted for age, BMI and creatinine, we found a suggestive trend for lower serum INHB among women with higher urinary MEHP concentrations (P-trend = 0.06) (Table 4). Compared to the lowest quartile, women in the highest quartile of MEHP had a significant decrease of – 17.55% (95% CI: – 31.34%, – 0.90%) in INHB levels. When controlling for the covariates in model 2, the dose-response trend between MEHP and serum INHB reached significance (P-trend = 0.04), with a larger decrease of percent difference in quartile 4 from quartile 1 (– 18.29%; 95% CI: – 31.89%, – 1.98%). For MEOHP, significant decrease in serum INHB was observed across the second to fourth quartiles compared with quartile one in adjusted model 2. The adjusted differences in INHB levels for quartile 2, 3 and 4 compared with quartile 1 of MEOHP were – 23.74% (95% CI: –35.85%, – 9.24%), – 19.91% (95% CI: –33.30%, – 3.82%) and – 20.23% (95% CI: –34.43%, – 2.96%), respectively. The largest decrease found in quartile two suggested that there might exist a threshold value. Decrease in INHB seemed to reach a plateau when concentrations exceeded the threshold, reflecting a potential nonlinear relationship. Among the remaining six phthalate metabolites and ΣDEHP, no consistent change in serum INHB levels was observed. In the age-

Table 2 Distribution of urinary phthalate metabolites[a] ($n = 415$)

Metabolites	% > LOD	GM	Median	Selected percentiles	
				25%	75%
MMP	96.6	7.23	6.86	3.65	15.86
MEP	100	10.73	8.81	4.16	22.28
MBP	100	106.40	112.74	66.61	180.82
MBzP	95.4	0.08	0.07	0.03	0.17
MEHP	98.8	9.99	10.75	5.44	20.68
MEHHP	100	13.40	12.30	8.16	20.46
MEOHP	100	10.42	10.27	6.36	16.91
MOP	28.7	0.04	<LOD	<LOD	0.12
ΣDEHP	–	0.13	0.12	0.08	0.20

LOD: the limits of detection; GM: geometric mean; MMP: monomethyl phthalate; MEP: monoethyl phthalate; MBP: monobutyl phthalate; MBzP: monobenzyl phthalate; MEHP: mono(2-ethylhexyl) phthalate; MEHHP: mono(2-ethyl-5-hydroxyhexyl) phthalate; MEOHP: mono(2-ethyl-5-oxohexyl) phthalate; MOP: mono-n-octyl phthalate; DEHP: di(2-ethylhexyl) phthalate
ΣDEHP: Molar sum of DEHP metabolites (MEHP, MEHHP and MEOHP) expressed in μmol/g creatinine (Cr)
% > LOD: Phthalate metabolites above the limits of detection
[a]Urinary phthalate metabolites concentrations were creatinine adjusted (μg/g Cr)

stratified analyses, women in the younger subgroup had apparent decrease in INHB levels for MEHP, MEOHP and ΣDEHP quartiles, whereas women ≥35 years had no significant change in INHB levels (Additional file 3: Table S2). Although the product terms were not statistically significant (P for interaction > 0.05), this finding may imply a potential effect modification by age.

When the metabolites were modeled as continuous variables in the spline analysis, we identified a nonlinear relationship between MEOHP exposure and serum INHB among women < 35 years of age (Fig. 1). The test for the overall association between MEOHP and INHB in the younger subgroup was significant (P for overall association < 0.05), which means whatever the shape of the association is, MEOHP was significantly correlated with INHB. The null hypothesis of the test for nonlinearity that assumed a linear relationship between MEOHP and INHB was rejected (P for nonlinear association = 0.01), suggesting there exists a nonlinear association. Collectively, we observed that within a range of relatively low levels of exposure, serum INHB was negatively associated with urinary MEOHP in a dose dependent pattern. However, when a threshold level was met, the decline in INHB was attenuated.

In logistic regression models comparing women with low (defined as an AMH value of < 1.1 ng/mL) versus normal ovarian reserve, urinary phthalate concentrations were not associated with an increased odds of DOR after adjusting for potential confounders (Additional file 4: Table S3). In the secondary analysis using AFC as a biomarker of ovarian reserve, a positive dose-response

Table 3 Associations between urinary phthalate metabolite concentrations and serum AMH[1] in multivariable linear models ($n = 415$)

Metabolite	Model 1[4]	Model 2[5]
	β (95% CI)	β (95% CI)
MMP[2]		
1[6] (< 5.18)	Ref	Ref
2 (5.18–12.21)	− 0.06 (− 0.29, 0.17)	0.03 (− 0.19, 0.24)
3 (12.21–25.78)	− 0.10 (− 0.34, 0.14)	0.05 (− 0.17, 0.27)
4 (> 25.78)	0.02 (− 0.22, 0.25)	0.04 (− 0.18, 0.26)
MEP[2]		
1[6] (< 6.02)	Ref	Ref
2 (6.02–12.80)	− 0.10 (− 0.35, 0.14)	− 0.08 (− 0.30, 0.15)
3 (12.80–33.98)	− 0.05 (− 0.30, 0.20)	− 0.10 (− 0.32, 0.13)
4 (> 33.98)	− 0.08 (− 0.33, 0.17)	− 0.12 (− 0.34, 0.11)
MBP[2]		
1[6] (< 73.85)	Ref	Ref
2 (73.85–184.55)	**0.28 (0.04, 0.52)**	0.18 (−0.03, 0.40)
3 (184.55–342.12)	0.01 (− 0.24, 0.27)	− 0.08 (− 0.31, 0.16)
4 (> 342.12)	0.18 (− 0.10, 0.47)	0.11 (− 0.15, 0.37)
MBzP[2]		
1[6] (< 0.035)	Ref	Ref
2 (0.035–0.102)	0.04 (−0.20, 0.27)	0.04 (−0.17, 0.26)
3 (0.102–0.27)	−0.06 (− 0.31, 0.20)	0.02 (−0.21, 0.25)
4 (> 0.27)	0.12 (−0.14, 0.38)	0.15 (−0.08, 0.38)
MEHP[2]		
1[6] (< 6.95)	Ref	Ref
2 (6.95–17.21)	0.12 (−0.11, 0.35)	0.10 (−0.11, 0.31)
3 (17.21–36.01)	0.06 (− 0.18, 0.31)	0.01 (−0.21, 0.24)
4 (> 36.01)	0.20 (−0.05, 0.45)	0.16 (−0.07, 0.39)
MEHHP[2]		
1[6] (< 10.94)	Ref	Ref
2 (10.94–19.09)	0.08 (−0.16, 0.33)	0.09 (−0.14, 0.31)
3 (19.09–34.68)	0.12 (−0.15, 0.39)	0.12 (−0.13, 0.36)
4 (> 34.68)	0.24 (−0.04, 0.52)	0.17 (−0.08, 0.43)
MEOHP[2]		
1[6] (< 7.41)	Ref	Ref
2 (7.41–15.34)	0.02 (−0.22, 0.26)	−0.03 (− 0.26, 0.19)
3 (15.34–27.72)	−0.03 (− 0.29, 0.22)	− 0.05 (− 0.29, 0.18)
4 (> 27.72)	0.16 (− 0.11, 0.44)	0.05 (− 0.21, 0.30)
ΣDEHP[2]		
1[6] (< 0.10)	Ref	Ref
2 (0.10–0.19)	0.14 (−0.10, 0.39)	0.07 (−0.15, 0.29)
3 (0.19–0.35)	0.01 (−0.25, 0.26)	−0.02 (− 0.25, 0.21)
4 (> 0.35)	0.19 (−0.08, 0.46)	0.12 (− 0.13, 0.36)
MOP[3]	0.16 (−0.02, 0.34)	**0.20 (0.04, 0.37)**

Statistically significant results comparing a specific category to the reference are bolded
[1]Serum AMH levels were natural logarithm transformed
[2]Phthalate metabolite concentrations were categorized into quartiles
[3]Dichotomous variable based on above/below limits of detection
[4]Model 1 was adjusted for age, BMI and creatinine
[5]Model 2 was adjusted for age, BMI, creatinine and PCO/PCOS diagnosis (yes or no)
[6]Reference category

Table 4 Associations between urinary phthalate metabolite concentrations and serum INHB[1] in multivariable linear models ($n = 404$)

Metabolite	Model 1[4] Percent change[6] (95% CI)	Model 2[5] Percent change[6] (95% CI)
MMP[2]		
1[7] (< 5.18)	Ref	Ref
2 (5.18–12.21)	−2.47 (− 17.72, 15.49)	− 0.30 (− 15.80, 17.94)
3 (12.21–25.78)	−1.00 (− 16.72, 17.70)	3.15 (− 13.24, 22.75)
4 (> 25.78)	4.71 (− 11.75, 24.23)	5.23 (− 11.13, 24.73)
MEP[2]		
1[7] (< 6.02)	Ref	Ref
2 (6.02–12.80)	−4.40 (− 19.83, 14.00)	− 3.92 (− 19.27, 14.34)
3 (12.80–33.98)	3.36 (− 13.50, 23.49)	1.82 (− 14.62, 21.41)
4 (> 33.98)	0.50 (− 16.31, 20.56)	− 0.80 (− 17.22, 18.89)
MBP[2]		
1[7] (< 73.85)	Ref	Ref
2 (73.85–184.55)	− 9.79 (− 24.19, 7.47)	−11.84 (− 25.84, 4.81)
3 (184.55–342.12)	− 16.56 (− 30.65, 0.50)	**−18.62 (− 32.23, − 2.18)**
4 (> 342.12)	− 14.02 (− 30.16, 5.87)	−15.46 (− 31.20, 3.87)
MBzP[2]		
1[7] (< 0.035)	Ref	Ref
2 (0.035–0.102)	−9.43 (− 23.59, 7.36)	− 9.34 (− 23.43, 7.25)
3 (0.102–0.27)	− 7.78 (− 23.28, 10.96)	−5.45 (− 21.34, 13.54)
4 (> 0.27)	3.46 (− 13.84, 24.23)	4.39 (− 12.89, 25.23)
MEHP[2]		
1[7] (< 6.95)	Ref	Ref
2 (6.95–17.21)	− 13.32 (− 26.80, 2.53)	− 13.58 (− 26.88, 2.12)
3 (17.21–36.01)	− 12.89 (− 26.95, 3.87)	−14.02 (− 27.75, 2.33)
4 (> 36.01)	**− 17.55 (− 31.34, − 0.90)**	**− 18.29 (− 31.89, − 1.98)***
MEHHP[2]		
1[7] (< 10.94)	Ref	Ref
2 (10.94–19.09)	−7.78 (− 23.05, 10.52)	− 7.41 (− 22.59, 10.74)
3 (19.09–34.68)	1.61 (−16.56, 23.61)	1.71 (− 16.31, 23.61)
4 (> 34.68)	− 3.63 (− 21.42, 18.18)	−5.07 (− 22.43, 16.18)
MEOHP[2]		
1[7] (< 7.41)	Ref	Ref
2 (7.41–15.34)	**− 22.74 (− 35.14, − 7.87)**	**−23.74 (− 35.85, − 9.24)**
3 (15.34–27.72)	**− 19.59 (− 33.17, − 3.25)**	**−19.91 (− 33.30, − 3.82)**
4 (> 27.72)	−17.80 (− 32.56, 0.20)	**− 20.23 (− 34.43, − 2.96)**
∑DEHP[2]		
1[7] (< 0.10)	Ref	Ref
2 (0.10–0.19)	−9.43 (− 23.97, 7.90)	−11.04 (− 25.25, 5.87)
3 (0.19–0.35)	−13.58 (− 28.18, 3.87)	− 14.10 (− 28.39, 3.15)
4 (> 0.35)	−12.10 (− 27.75, 6.82)	− 13.76 (− 28.97, 4.71)
MQP[3]	2.76 (14.62, 10.74)	−1.78 (− 13.67, 11.74)

*Tests for linear trend with P-value < 0.05. Statistically significant results comparing a specific category to the reference are bolded
[1]Serum INHB levels were natural logarithm transformed
[2]Phthalate metabolite concentrations were categorized into quartiles
[3]Dichotomous variable based on above/below limits of detection
[4]Model 1 was adjusted for age, BMI and creatinine
[5]Model 2 was adjusted for age, BMI, creatinine and PCO/PCOS diagnosis (yes or no)
[6]Percent change and 95% CI were calculated as follows: [exp (β)-1]*100
[7]Reference category

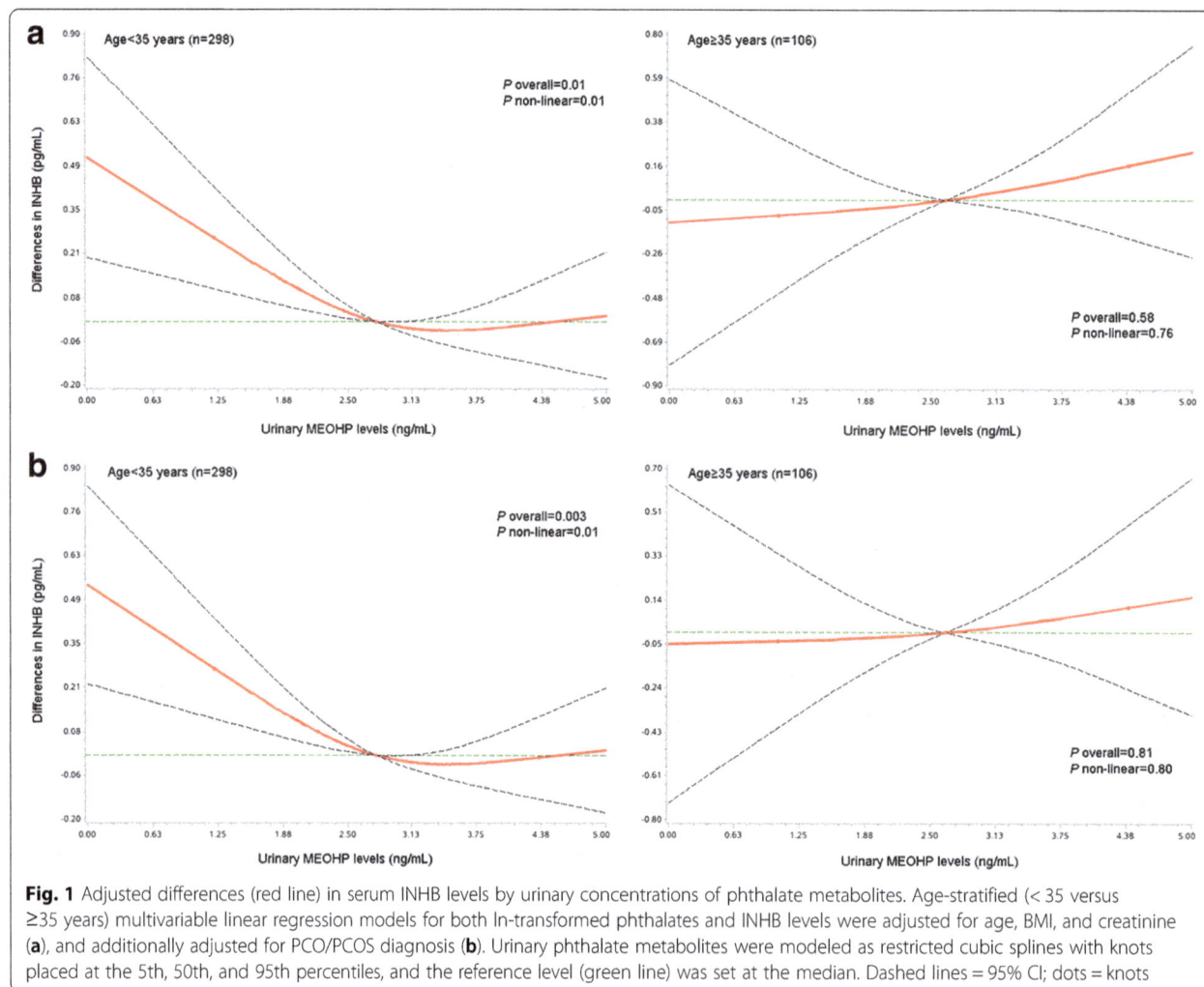

Fig. 1 Adjusted differences (red line) in serum INHB levels by urinary concentrations of phthalate metabolites. Age-stratified (< 35 versus ≥35 years) multivariable linear regression models for both ln-transformed phthalates and INHB levels were adjusted for age, BMI, and creatinine (**a**), and additionally adjusted for PCO/PCOS diagnosis (**b**). Urinary phthalate metabolites were modeled as restricted cubic splines with knots placed at the 5th, 50th, and 95th percentiles, and the reference level (green line) was set at the median. Dashed lines = 95% CI; dots = knots

relationship between quartiles of urinary MEHHP and MEOHP levels in relation to AFC was observed with the adjustment for age, BMI and creatinine (P-trend for MEHHP = 0.001; P-trend for MEOHP = 0.004). However, when further adjusting for diagnosis of PCO/PCOS in model 2, these positive associations appeared non-significant (Additional file 5: Table S4).

Discussion

Although a growing number of in vitro and animal studies are emerging linking phthalates with altered ovarian reserve, we found largely null associations between urinary phthalate metabolites and serum AMH levels, considered one of the best markers of ovarian reserve, in this large retrospective study comprised of 415 women undergoing IVF. Another major finding in this study was that urinary MEHP was associated with lower serum INHB levels. We also found evidence of a nonlinear relationship between MEOHP concentrations and INHB.

As the number of activated follicles is dependent upon primordial follicle pool, serum AMH is considered to reflect the ovarian reserve, despite the fact that AMH is produced by small growing follicles rather than by non-growing primordial follicles [33]. Therefore, though AMH is a relatively acute marker of ovarian reserve currently available in clinical practice, its indirect reflection of primordial follicles in nature may contribute to the lack of association between serum AMH and phthalate exposure observed in our study. In one study comprising menopausal women, urinary concentrations of MEHHP and MEOHP were related to earlier age at natural menopause [34]. The ovarian reserve declines with increasing age, culminating in menopause with a virtual exhaustion of follicle numbers. Therefore, to reveal the actual effect of phthalate exposure on ovarian aging, a more direct marker or the endpoint of ovarian pool exhaustion, for example menopause, might be needed. Another explanation for our null findings is that the accelerated follicle loss caused by phthalates may date back to early life exposure [1]. Given that fetal organ development during pregnancy is susceptible to the intrauterine environment, it is possible that prenatal exposure to phthalates may heighten the risk of reduced ovarian reserve in adulthood. In support of our speculation, one animal study demonstrated that maternal exposure to DEHP has sped up the recruitment of primordial follicles in F1 and F2 offspring, leading to premature ovarian failure [35]. Hart et al. reported that girls who experienced in utero exposure to MEP exhibited lower serum AMH levels in their adolescence, suggesting that early life exposure has the potential to modify the trajectory of ovarian reserve in adult life [36]. Thus, it is possible that with a prospective longitudinal study design and exposure assessment at early life stages, the effect of phthalates on ovarian aging would be elucidated. Finally, we observed a positive association between urinary MOP and higher levels of AMH, which was the sole finding that reached statistical significance. Nevertheless, it should be noted that because of the low levels and detection rates of urinary MOP, as well as the multiple comparisons made in the analysis, the result might be spurious or a chance finding.

As a functional unit of the ovary, the abnormal growth and atresia of antral follicles may cause defects in hormone production. Evidence from toxicological studies has established antral follicles as a target of phthalates. With an in vitro culture system, Gupta et al. demonstrated that DEHP and its bioactive metabolite MEHP had the potential to inhibit antral follicle growth and disrupt steroidogenesis manifested as a decline in estradiol production [37]. Moreover, DEHP were also shown to induce follicle atresia in cultured mouse antral follicles via mechanisms involving imbalanced pro- and anti-apoptotic pathways and dysregulated expression of genes involved in cell cycle [11]. Consequently, our observations of decreased serum INHB in relation to MEHP might be a result of increased astresia and growth arrest of antral follicles. A paucity of human data has been gathered regarding the effect of phthalate exposure on ovarian reserve. One prospective cohort study involving women seeking infertility treatment has demonstrated that a significant decrease in AFC was associated with higher urinary concentrations of DEHP metabolites [16]. Our findings of reduced INHB levels and higher MEHP is corroborated by their findings to some extent, because AFC determined by trans-vaginal ultrasound are comprised of follicles with a size of 2 to 10 mm, which is equivalent to the follicles secreting INHB [38]. It has been established that women with PCOS has higher concentrations of serum INHB which reflects the increased number of antral follicles [29]. Thus, it is plausible that the associations between MEHP and INHB became more evident when we additionally controlled for PCO/

PCOS diagnosis. In addition, we identified a nonlinear association between MEOHP and serum INHB, which appeared more apparent among younger women. Within a low level of exposure, urinary MEOHP was inversely correlated with INHB until it reached a potential threshold value at the second quartile. This finding is also supported by a research showing a similar decrease in AFC after a threshold level of DEHP metabolites was met [16]. Nonlinear effect is not uncommon in studies of natural hormones and EDCs. Grande et al. revealed a threshold effect of DEHP exposure during gestation and lactation on the delay of pubertal onset in female offspring [39]. Similarly, in adult mice, DEHP exposure induced prolonged estrous cycles in a non-monotonic dose response [40]. Although the specific mechanisms by which phthalates affect ovarian function remains unclear, there is evidence that phthalates could exert their effects through binding steroid receptors [41]. Thus, one possible explanation for the attenuated decrease in INHB at higher MEOHP level might be that the receptors at the target tissue or cells are gradually saturated, leading to the observed nonlinear biological effect. In addition, our findings do show some cause for concern over the low-dose effect of phthalate exposure and need further verification in both animal and human studies. In line with the study reported by Messerlian and Souter et al. [16], younger women were at higher risk of phthalate-induced ovarian toxicity, as indicated by the stratified analysis. Among women of advanced age, the null associations between phthalate exposure and INHB may be explained by the fact that the effect magnitude of phthalate is relatively small when compared with age which is of greater value in influencing ovarian function. In contrast, younger women may be more sensitive to other factors, and the influence of age has not preponderated over others. Thus, the effect of phthalates appeared evident.

The discrepancy between serum AMH and INHB in relation to phthalate metabolites was in agreement with an animal study exploring the effect of acute DEHP exposure on fecundability and ovarian aging [40]. In this study, adult mice treated with DEHP orally for 10 days exhibited dysregulated folliculogenesis and decreased serum levels of INHB at 9-months postdosing, while serum AMH levels were not affected. The differences in hormone results were explained by the observation that acute exposure to DEHP did not alter the number of preantral follicles, but increased the percentage of atretic antral follicles. Still, the divergent finding was somewhat puzzling. Nevertheless, several potential explanations were considered. Although both serum AMH and INHB are secreted by small growing follicles, follicles that contribute the most to AMH and INHB levels are differed by diameter. Follicles of 1–2 mm in diameter are probably the main contributors to serum AMH levels with the evidence that the intrafollicular concentrations of AMH decreased gradually with increasing follicle diameters [18], concomitant with the observation that granulosa cells of secondary, preantral and small antral follicles < 4 mm in diameter expressed the highest level of AMH [42]. In contrast, concentrations of INHB increased with the growth of follicles until they reached a diameter of 9 mm [43]. Hence, larger antral follicles at later developmental stage constitute the primary source of serum INHB. Based on these facts, if a patient whose AFC is mostly represented by small follicles (i.e. 1–2 mm), while phthalates target larger antral follicles, the discrepant findings between serum AMH and INHB relative to urinary phthalate concentrations might occur. Another explanation is probably that women included in the present study had different status of ovarian reserve manifested as altered concentrations of gonadotropin hormones [i.e. FSH and luteal hormone (LH)] in the early follicular phase. While AMH function as a paracrine factor independent of endogenous hormones, the biosynthesis of INHB is regulated by FSH and LH, and involved in the pituitary gland feedback loop [44]. Therefore, the different characteristics of ovarian reserve in the study population may be a potential reason for inconsistency between the AMH and INHB results.

In the secondary analysis, the findings of AFC and phthalates were inconsistent with that of INHB which is contrary to our expectation. The divergent observations between AFC and INHB might be partially ascribed to their different characteristics in reflecting ovarian reserve. Because AFC could not distinguish healthy from atretic follicles [18], when phthalate exposure increases follicle atresia and consequently affects hormone production, the occurrence of the discrepant results seems plausible.

Our relatively large sample size of 415 women gave us more than 85% power to detect a correlation between phthalate concentrations and hormone levels when the correlation coefficient was assumed 0.15 and the two-sided significance level was set at 0.05. With regard to the serum AMH and INHB measurement in the present study, the well-established automated assay platform in routine clinical practice minimized the inter- and intra-operator variability. Meanwhile, it is worth noting that our retrospective study design precluded us from drawing a causality of exposure and altered ovarian function. Additionally, since urine collection for exposure measurement was conducted up to 4 months after AMH and INHB assays, there is a possibility of reverse causation. Phthalates could be found in a wide range of personal care products, foodstuffs, certain types of oral medications and medical devices [4], thus we could not exclude the possibility that urinary phthalate concentrations

might be influenced by changes in daily care routines and dietary habits, as well as medical interventions during the 4-month period. Additionally, misclassification of exposure was likely to occur not only from timing of exposure and outcome but also from our single measurement of spot urine because of short half-life of phthalates and variability in individual behaviors. However, it has been suggested that one spot urine measurement has moderate capacity to reflect average exposure within 4 months (sensitivity ranging from 0.58 to 0.77), when a surrogate category analysis was performed [45]. Given that the median time intervals between blood collection for AMH and INHB assays and urine collection for phthalate measurement were 72 d (IQR: 46–93.5 d) in the study, the single measurement might allow for a moderately reliable ranking of a few months exposure preceding the urine collection. Finally, our findings drawn from women undergoing IVF may not extrapolate to the general population, and the possibility of bias from uncontrolled confounding may also exist.

Conclusions

In this large retrospective study, we provided evidence for a negative association between higher urinary concentrations of certain phthalate metabolites and serum INHB levels, suggesting an adverse effect of phthalates exposure on growing antral follicles. However, little evidence of an association was observed between urinary phthalates and serum AMH. Whether phthalates exposure at environmentally level will pose a risk for ovarian reserve could not be determined from the present data, and further studies with a prospective design and more direct indicators of primordial follicle pool might reveal the potential effect.

Additional files

Additional file 1: Figure S1. Adjusted differences (red line) in serum AMH levels by urinary concentrations of phthalate metabolites. Multivariable linear regression models for both ln-transformed phthalates and AMH levels were adjusted for age, BMI, and creatinine. Urinary phthalate metabolites were modeled as restricted cubic splines with knots placed at the 5th, 50th, and 95th percentiles, and the reference level (green line) was set at the median. Dashed lines = 95% CI; dots = knots.

Additional file 2: Table S1. Associations between urinary phthalate metabolites and serum AMH[1] in multivariable linear models stratified by age.

Additional file 3: Table S2. Associations between urinary phthalate metabolites and serum INHB[1] in multivariable linear models stratified by age.

Additional file 4: Table S3. Adjusted odds ratios (95% CI) for polycystic ovarian morphology (PCOM) and diminished ovarian reserve (DOR) by urinary phthalate metabolites ($n = 415$).

Additional file 5: Table S4. Associations between urinary phthalate metabolites and AFC in multivariable generalized linear models ($n = 415$).

Abbreviations

ΣDEHP: Molar sum of DEHP metabolites (MEHP, MEHHP and MEOHP) expressed in μmol/L; AFC: Antral follicle count; AIC: Akaike information criteria; AMH: Anti-Müllerian hormone; BMI: Body mass index; DBP: Di-n-butyl phthalate; DEHP: Di(2-ethylhexyl) phthalate; E_2: Estradiol; EDCs: Endocrine-disrupting chemicals; ELISA: Enzyme-linked immunuosorbent assay; FSH: Follicle-stimulating hormone; ICSI: Intracytoplasmic sperm injection; INHB: Inhibin B; IQR: Interquartile range; IVF: in vitro fertilization; LH: Luteal hormone; LOD: The limits of detection; MBP: Monobutyl phthalate; MBzP: Monobenzyl phthalate; MEP: Monoethyl phthalate; MEHP: Mono(2-ethylhexyl) phthalate; MEHHP: Mono(2-ethyl-5-hydroxyhexyl) phthalate; MEOHP: Mono(2-ethyl-5-oxohexyl) phthalate; MMP: Monomethyl phthalate; MOP: Mono-n-octyl phthalate; PCO: Polycystic ovary; PCOS: Polycystic ovary syndrome; RCS: Restricted cubic spline

Acknowledgements

We sincerely thank the nurses and technicians in the Reproductive Medicine Center of Tongji Hospital in Wuhan for clinical data collection and hormone measurement.

Funding

This study was supported by the National Natural Science Foundation of China (grant number: 81571508 and 81771654).

Authors' contributions

YD performed the statistical analyses and drafted the manuscript. NG participated in the design of the study, assisted in the statistical analyses, and critically revised the manuscript. XH, TD and XT were involved in recruitment of study participants, sample collection, and retrieve of data. YW and YY carried out the measurement of urinary phthalate metabolites. YL designed the study, and revised critically for the manuscript. All authors made significant contributions to the manuscript and approved the final version for submission.

Competing interests

The authors declare that they have no competing interests.

Author details

[1]Reproductive Medicine Center, Tongji Hospital, Tongji Medical College, Huazhong University of Science and Technology, 1095 JieFang Avenue, Wuhan, Hubei, People's Republic of China. [2]Department of Occupational and Environmental Health, School of Public Health, Tongji Medical College, Huazhong University of Science and Technology, Wuhan, Hubei, People's Republic of China. [3]Key Laboratory of Environment and Health, Ministry of Education & Ministry of Environmental Protection, and State Key Laboratory of Environmental health (incubating), School of Public Health, Tongji Medical College, Huazhong University of Science and Technology, Wuhan, Hubei, People's Republic of China.

References

1. Richardson MC, Guo M, Fauser BC, Macklon NS. Environmental and developmental origins of ovarian reserve. Hum Reprod Update. 2014;20: 353–69.
2. Vabre P, Gatimel N, Moreau J, Gayrard V, Picard-Hagen N, Parinaud J, Leandri RD. Environmental pollutants, a possible etiology for premature ovarian insufficiency: a narrative review of animal and human data. Environ Health. 2017;16:37.
3. Kay VR, Chambers C, Foster WG. Reproductive and developmental effects of phthalate diesters in females. Crit Rev Toxicol. 2013;43:200–19.
4. Katsikantami I, Sifakis S, Tzatzarakis MN, Vakonaki E, Kalantzi OI, Tsatsakis AM, Rizos AK. A global assessment of phthalates burden and related links to health effects. Environ Int. 2016;97:212–36.
5. Hines EP, Calafat AM, Silva MJ, Mendola P, Fenton SE. Concentrations of phthalate metabolites in milk, urine, saliva, and serum of lactating North Carolina women. Environ Health Perspect. 2009;117:86–92.
6. Silva MJ, Barr DB, Reidy JA, Malek NA, Hodge CC, Caudill SP, Brock JW, Needham LL, Calafat AM. Urinary levels of seven phthalate metabolites in the U.S. population from the National Health and nutrition examination survey (NHANES) 1999-2000. Environ Health Perspect. 2004;112:331–8.
7. Guo Y, Wu Q, Kannan K. Phthalate metabolites in urine from China, and implications for human exposures. Environ Int. 2011;37:893–8.
8. Hannon PR, Flaws JA. The effects of phthalates on the ovary. Front Endocrinol (Lausanne). 2015;6:8.
9. Zhang T, Li L, Qin XS, Zhou Y, Zhang XF, Wang LQ, De Felici M, Chen H, Qin GQ, Shen W. Di-(2-ethylhexyl) phthalate and bisphenol a exposure impairs mouse primordial follicle assembly in vitro. Environ Mol Mutagen. 2014;55: 343–53.
10. Hannon PR, Peretz J, Flaws JA. Daily exposure to di(2-ethylhexyl) phthalate alters estrous cyclicity and accelerates primordial follicle recruitment potentially via dysregulation of the phosphatidylinositol 3-kinase signaling pathway in adult mice. Biol Reprod. 2014;90:136.
11. Hannon PR, Brannick KE, Wang W, Gupta RK, Flaws JA. Di(2-ethylhexyl) phthalate inhibits antral follicle growth, induces atresia, and inhibits steroid hormone production in cultured mouse antral follicles. Toxicol Appl Pharmacol. 2015;284:42–53.
12. Craig ZR, Hannon PR, Wang W, Ziv-Gal A, Flaws JA. Di-n-butyl phthalate disrupts the expression of genes involved in cell cycle and apoptotic pathways in mouse ovarian antral follicles. Biol Reprod. 2013;88:23.
13. Wang W, Craig ZR, Basavarajappa MS, Hafner KS, Flaws JA. Mono-(2-ethylhexyl) phthalate induces oxidative stress and inhibits growth of mouse ovarian antral follicles. Biol Reprod. 2012;87:152.
14. Moyer B, Hixon ML. Reproductive effects in F1 adult females exposed in utero to moderate to high doses of mono-2-ethylhexylphthalate (MEHP). Reprod Toxicol. 2012;34:43–50.
15. Du YY, Fang YL, Wang YX, Zeng Q, Guo N, Zhao H, Li YF. Follicular fluid and urinary concentrations of phthalate metabolites among infertile women and associations with in vitro fertilization parameters. Reprod Toxicol. 2016; 61:142–50.
16. Messerlian C, Souter I, Gaskins AJ, Williams PL, Ford JB, Chiu YH, Calafat AM, Hauser R. Urinary phthalate metabolites and ovarian reserve among women seeking infertility care. Hum Reprod. 2016;31:75–83.
17. Iliodromiti S, Anderson RA, Nelson SM. Technical and performance characteristics of anti-Mullerian hormone and antral follicle count as biomarkers of ovarian response. Hum Reprod Update. 2015;21:698–710.
18. Dewailly D, Andersen CY, Balen A, Broekmans F, Dilaver N, Fanchin R, Griesinger G, Kelsey TW, La Marca A, Lambalk C, et al. The physiology and clinical utility of anti-Mullerian hormone in women. Hum Reprod Update. 2014;20:370–85.
19. Fleming R, Seifer DB, Frattarelli JL, Ruman J. Assessing ovarian response: antral follicle count versus anti-Mullerian hormone. Reprod BioMed Online. 2015;31:486–96.
20. Sowers M, McConnell D, Gast K, Zheng H, Nan B, McCarthy JD, Randolph JF. Anti-Mullerian hormone and inhibin B variability during normal menstrual cycles. Fertil Steril. 2010;94:1482–6.
21. Revised 2003 consensus on diagnostic criteria and long-term health risks related to polycystic ovary syndrome (PCOS). Hum Reprod. 2004;19:41–7.

22. Wang YX, You L, Zeng Q, Sun Y, Huang YH, Wang C, Wang P, Cao WC, Yang P, Li YF, Lu WQ. **Phthalate exposure and human semen quality: results from an infertility clinic in China.** Environ Res. 2015;142:1–9.

23. Blount BC, Silva MJ, Caudill SP, Needham LL, Pirkle JL, Sampson EJ, Lucier GW, Jackson RJ, Brock JW. Levels of seven urinary phthalate metabolites in a human reference population. Environ Health Perspect. 2000;108:979–82.

24. Hatch EE, Nelson JW, Qureshi MM, Weinberg J, Moore LL, Singer M, Webster TF. Association of urinary phthalate metabolite concentrations with body mass index and waist circumference: a cross-sectional study of NHANES data, 1999-2002. Environ Health. 2008;7:27.

25. Freeman EW, Gracia CR, Sammel MD, Lin H, Lim LC, Strauss JF 3rd. Association of anti-mullerian hormone levels with obesity in late reproductive-age women. Fertil Steril. 2007;87:101–6.

26. Barr DB, Wilder LC, Caudill SP, Gonzalez AJ, Needham LL, Pirkle JL. Urinary creatinine concentrations in the U.S. population: implications for urinary biologic monitoring measurements. Environ Health Perspect. 2005;113:192–200.

27. Johns LE, Cooper GS, Galizia A, Meeker JD. Exposure assessment issues in epidemiology studies of phthalates. Environ Int. 2015;85:27–39.

28. Homburg R, Ray A, Bhide P, Gudi A, Shah A, Timms P, Grayson K. The relationship of serum anti-Mullerian hormone with polycystic ovarian morphology and polycystic ovary syndrome: a prospective cohort study. Hum Reprod. 2013;28:1077–83.

29. Anderson RA, Groome NP, Baird DT. Inhibin a and inhibin B in women with polycystic ovarian syndrome during treatment with FSH to induce mono-ovulation. Clin Endocrinol. 1998;48:577–84.

30. Durrleman S, Simon R. Flexible regression models with cubic splines. Stat Med. 1989;8:551–61.

31. Desquilbet L, Mariotti F. Dose-response analyses using restricted cubic spline functions in public health research. Stat Med. 2010;29:1037–57.

32. Ferraretti AP, La Marca A, Fauser BC, Tarlatzis B, Nargund G, Gianaroli L. ESHRE consensus on the definition of 'poor response' to ovarian stimulation for in vitro fertilization: the bologna criteria. Hum Reprod. 2011;26:1616–24.

33. Anderson RA, Nelson SM, Wallace WH. Measuring anti-Mullerian hormone for the assessment of ovarian reserve: when and for whom is it indicated? Maturitas. 2012;71:28–33.

34. Grindler NM, Allsworth JE, Macones GA, Kannan K, Roehl KA, Cooper AR. Persistent organic pollutants and early menopause in U.S. women. PLoS One. 2015;10:e0116057.

35. Zhang XF, Zhang T, Han Z, Liu JC, Liu YP, Ma JY, Li L, Shen W. Transgenerational inheritance of ovarian development deficiency induced by maternal diethylhexyl phthalate exposure. Reprod Fertil Dev. 2015;27:1213–21.

36. Hart R, Doherty DA, Frederiksen H, Keelan JA, Hickey M, Sloboda D, Pennell CE, Newnham JP, Skakkebaek NE, Main KM. The influence of antenatal exposure to phthalates on subsequent female reproductive development in adolescence: a pilot study. Reproduction. 2014;147:379–90.

37. Gupta RK, Singh JM, Leslie TC, Meachum S, Flaws JA, Yao HH. Di-(2-ethylhexyl) phthalate and mono-(2-ethylhexyl) phthalate inhibit growth and reduce estradiol levels of antral follicles in vitro. Toxicol Appl Pharmacol. 2010;242:224–30.

38. Broekmans FJ, de Ziegler D, Howles CM, Gougeon A, Trew G, Olivennes F. The antral follicle count: practical recommendations for better standardization. Fertil Steril. 2010;94:1044–51.

39. Grande SW, Andrade AJ, Talsness CE, Grote K, Chahoud I. A dose-response study following in utero and lactational exposure to di(2-ethylhexyl)phthalate: effects on female rat reproductive development. Toxicol Sci. 2006;91:247–54.

40. Hannon PR, Niermann S, Flaws JA. Acute exposure to di(2-Ethylhexyl) phthalate in adulthood causes adverse reproductive outcomes later in life and accelerates reproductive aging in female mice. Toxicol Sci. 2016;150:97–108.

41. Craig ZR, Wang W, Flaws JA. Endocrine-disrupting chemicals in ovarian function: effects on steroidogenesis, metabolism and nuclear receptor signaling. Reproduction. 2011;142:633–46.

42. Weenen C, Laven JS, Von Bergh AR, Cranfield M, Groome NP, Visser JA, Kramer P, Fauser BC, Themmen AP. Anti-Mullerian hormone expression pattern in the human ovary: potential implications for initial and cyclic follicle recruitment. Mol Hum Reprod. 2004;10:77–83.

43. Andersen CY, Schmidt KT, Kristensen SG, Rosendahl M, Byskov AG, Ernst E. Concentrations of AMH and inhibin-B in relation to follicular diameter in normal human small antral follicles. Hum Reprod. 2010;25:1282–7.

44. Wunder DM, Bersinger NA, Yared M, Kretschmer R, Birkhauser MH. Statistically significant changes of antimullerian hormone and inhibin levels during the physiologic menstrual cycle in reproductive age women. Fertil Steril. 2008;89:927–33.

45. Dewalque L, Pirard C, Vandepaer S, Charlier C. Temporal variability of urinary concentrations of phthalate metabolites, parabens and benzophenone-3 in a Belgian adult population. Environ Res. 2015;142:414–23.

7

Women's attitudes and beliefs towards specific contraceptive methods in Bangladesh and Kenya

Kazuyo Machiyama[1]*[ID], Fauzia Akhter Huda[2], Faisal Ahmmed[2], George Odwe[3], Francis Obare[3], Joyce N. Mumah[4], Marylene Wamukoya[4], John B. Casterline[5] and John Cleland[1]

Abstract

Background: Missing from the huge literature on women's attitudes and beliefs concerning specific contraceptive methods is any detailed quantitative documentation for all major methods in low- and middle-income countries. The objectives are to provide such a documentation for women living in Matlab (rural Bangladesh), Nairobi slums and Homa Bay (rural Kenya) and to compare the opinions and beliefs of current, past and never users towards the three most commonly used methods (oral contraceptives, injectables and implants).

Methods: In each site, 2424 to 2812 married women aged 15–39 years were interviewed on reproduction, fertility preferences, contraceptive knowledge and use, attitudes and beliefs towards family planning in general and specific methods. We analysed the data from round one of the prospective cohort study.

Results: While current users typically expressed satisfaction and held more positive beliefs about their method than past or never users, nevertheless appreciable minorities of current users thought the method might pose serious damage to health, might impair fertility and was unsafe for prolonged use without taking a break. Larger proportions, typically between 25% and 50%, associated their method with unpleasant side effects. Past users of pills and injectables outnumbered current users and their beliefs were similar to those of never users. In all three sites, about half of past injectable users reported satisfaction with the method and the satisfaction of past implant users was lower.

Conclusions: High levels of contraceptive use can clearly co-exist with widespread misgivings about methods, even those that are widely used. Serious concerns about damage to health, long term fertility impairment, and dangers of prolonged use without taking a break were particularly common in the Kenyan sites and these beliefs may explain the high levels of discontinuation observed in Kenya and elsewhere in Africa. This documentation of beliefs provides useful guidance for counselling and informational campaigns. The generally negative views of past users imply that programmes may need not only to improve individual counselling but also strengthen community information campaign to change the overall climate of opinion which may have been influenced by dissatisfaction among past users.

Keywords: Contraception, Contraceptive methods, Attitude, Belief, Satisfaction, Kenya, Bangladesh

* Correspondence: Kazuyo.Machiyama@lshtm.ac.uk
[1]Faculty of Epidemiology and Population Health, London School of Hygiene and Tropical Medicine, Keppel Street, London WC1E 7HT, UK
Full list of author information is available at the end of the article

Plain english summary

In low- and middle-income countries, women's beliefs about specific contraceptive methods are not well understood. This study documents the beliefs about eight contraceptive methods among women living in Matlab (rural Bangladesh), Nairobi slums and Homa-Bay (rural Kenya) and compares the opinions of current, past and never users of the most commonly used methods (oral contraceptives, injectables and implants). In each site, we interviewed 2424 to 2812 married women aged 15–39 years. As expected, we found that current contraceptive users were typically satisfied and had more positive beliefs about their method than past or never users. Nevertheless, large minorities of current users thought that their method might cause serious health problems, impair future childbearing and was unsafe to use for a long time; higher proportions (25–50%) reported that their method use caused unpleasant side effects. Past users of pills and injectables outnumbered current users and their beliefs were similar to never users. In all three sites, about half of past injectable users reported satisfaction with the method but the satisfaction of past implant users was lower. Despite high contraceptive use in these populations, adverse and inaccurate beliefs about the major methods persist, particularly in Kenya. This study provides useful guidance for counselling and informational campaigns. The generally negative views of past users imply that programmes may need not only to improve individual counselling but also strengthen community information campaign to change the overall climate of opinion which may have been influenced by dissatisfaction among past users.

Background

Over the past half century, an extensive literature has been accumulated on women's attitudes and beliefs concerning contraception in general and specific methods. The extensive evidence for low- and middle-income countries (LMICs) falls into four main categories. The most common category comprises studies that examine attitudes towards and beliefs about contraception in general, with little or no distinction between specific methods [1–6]. The emphasis in many papers is on negative perceptions, often labelled as myths and misinformation. Commonly reported themes include the belief that use of modern methods will cause long term infertility, serious health damage, such as cancer and foetal abnormalities. In some studies, respondents associated contraception with promiscuity [2].

The second category concerns specific methods. Owing to the HIV pandemic, a huge literature on beliefs about condoms has been generated, much of which has been summarised by Maticka-Tyndale [7]. A review of perspectives on intra-uterine devices

(IUDs) identified 14 studies from Africa, Asia and Latin America [8]. Positive features of this method included its high effectiveness and long-acting nature while commonly expressed concerns were health risks including cancer, ectopic pregnancy, infertility and harm to the husband during intercourse. A study in Kenya found that postpartum women preferred implants over IUDs because of less pain, less infringement of modesty and preference for a superficial insertion in the upper arm than in the uterus [9]. The literature on hormonal methods shows the dominant concerns to be side effects such as nausea, dizziness and weight change, menstrual disruption and infertility [10–12]. In both Mali and Kenya, many women believed that oral contraceptives accumulate inside the body, causing infertility or a variety of diseases [13, 14].

The most influential, though indirect, body of evidence on views about contraceptive methods is based on self-reported reasons for non-use or discontinued use of contraception. The dominant source of data is the Demographic and Health Surveys (DHSs). The most recent analysis of reasons for non-use among married women not wishing to get pregnant found that, in most of the 52 countries studied, 20–33% cited side effects or health concerns. In 21 countries, this category of reason was the most common [15]. Moreover, in many countries, the majority of women giving this reason for contraceptive avoidance had previously used a modern method. Thus fear of side effects (and perhaps concerns about health) is partly based on personal experience and partly on hearsay evidence from friends or from media [16].

Table 1 Selected Background of Respondents

Characteristics	Matlab	Nairobi	Homa Bay
Educational attainment (%)			
Primary or less	30.4	60.4	77.5
Secondary or higher	69.6	39.6	22.5
Current FP method use (%) (1)			
No use	40.7	24.6	35.5
Pills	25.4	8.4	2.7
Injectables	17.7	32.4	26.8
Implants	2.2	19.8	17.9
Condoms	5.5	1.7	8.1
Other	8.5	13.2	8.9
Women want no more children (%)	44.8	27.0	29.2
Mean age of women	29.3	29.1	27.9
Mean number of living children	1.9	2.3	3.4
Total Number of Respondents	2605	2812	2424

(1) If more than one method is used, only the most effective method is included in this table

Table 2 Percentage of women with specific opinions, amongst those who have heard of methods (Matlab)

Attributes	Pills	Injectables	Implants	IUD	Condoms	Female sterilisation
Access						
Easy	97.2	90.4	66.1	69.5	87.1	71.5
Hard	2.2	8.0	24.9	24.1	9.6	23.9
Don't know/unsure	0.6	1.6	9.0	6.4	3.3	4.6
Effectiveness						
Yes	99.3	98.6	97.0	97.3	88.0	97.6
No	0.5	1.0	0.5	0.5	8.3	0.8
Don't know	0.2	0.4	2.5	2.2	3.7	1.6
Cause health problems						
Yes, serious	3.0	7.3	8.3	10.3	3.5	6.7
Yes, not serious	20.5	33.0	15.3	15.1	3.0	8.6
No	69.1	40.2	11.1	8.0	58.6	27.3
Don't know	7.4	19.5	65.3	66.6	34.9	57.4
Interfere with menstruation						
Yes	7.6	56.8	15.7	16.5	–	4.3
No	84.4	21.6	12.9	12.0	–	33.5
Don't know	8.0	21.6	71.4	71.5	–	62.3
Cause unpleasant side effect						
Yes	26.2	37.8	18.7	21.5	7.9	7.7
No	66.1	41.7	12.2	9.0	54.1	30.8
Don't know	7.7	20.5	69.1	69.5	38.0	61.5
Unsafe to use for a long time						
Yes, should take a break	21.2	23.4	20.4	21.2	23.4	–
No, safe for long time	74.3	67.1	52.7	53.7	53.7	–
Don't know	4.5	9.5	26.9	25.1	22.9	–
Cause infertility						
Yes, perhaps	8.8	6.5	4.1	4.1	–	–
No	85.2	84.8	74.8	76.2	–	–
Don't know	6.0	8.7	21.1	19.7	–	–
FP use among friend, relatives						
Most	25.0	17.0	0.7	0.9	1.2	0.8
About half	11.8	14.9	1.3	1.3	0.3	0.7
Few	54.2	52.2	41.2	36.1	31.1	52.3
None	4.2	8.2	28.1	31.8	14.5	21.1
Don't know	4.8	7.7	28.6	29.9	52.9	25.1
Experiences of friend, relatives (1)						
Satisfactory	95.6	89.5	77.2	75.5	82.4	87.5
Unsatisfactory	2.2	5.6	8.6	10.2	3.2	2.0
Mixed/Don't know	2.2	4.8	14.2	14.3	14.4	10.5
Husband's approval						
Approve	89.4	71.2	19.9	22.0	37.5	14.2
Disapprove	7.5	22.6	64.2	64.4	52.7	70.8
Don't know	3.1	6.2	15.9	13.6	9.8	15.0

Table 2 Percentage of women with specific opinions, amongst those who have heard of methods (Matlab) *(Continued)*

Attributes	Pills	Injectables	Implants	IUD	Condoms	Female sterilisation
Mean net positive score (2)	61.9	36.2	24.5	23.6	45.8	31.8
Mean % of don't know (3)	4.9	11.2	36.7	36.4	26.0	35.4
TOTAL(N)	2600	2583	2253	1917	2572	2544

(1) Amongst those knowing some friends were using the methods
(2) Mean percent difference between percentages of women who gave positive and negative responses among the above attributes except husband's approval
(3) Mean percent of women who said "don't know" to the above attributes except experiences of a method in social network and husband's approval

Reasons for discontinued use is more useful than reasons for non-use in distinguishing method-specific concerns. For oral contraceptives, injectables and IUDs, side effects or health concerns are the most common reason for stopping use. For condoms, objections from the husband or desire for a more effective method are the key reasons while for withdrawal and periodic abstinence accidental pregnancy dominates [17]. One limitation of this type of evidence is lack of comparable data for continuing users who perhaps are equally concerned about side effects or health risks as discontinued users but persist with use because of stronger motivation to avoid pregnancy or for some other reason.

The final main type of studies addresses the characteristics of contraceptive technology that women judge to be important. The single largest study of this type involved focus group discussions with 576 women in seven countries, six of which were LMICs [18]. Widespread agreement was found on the key importance of effectiveness and reversibility. Opinions varied by site on the desirability of a quick return to fertility after stopping the method and of the possibility of clandestine use. Most women found amenorrhea as a result of hormonal method use to be disturbing and similar results were found in Ghana and Nigeria [19, 20]. In a systematic review of contraceptive attributes that women take into account when choosing a method drawing on studies in USA and Europe as well as LMICs, ease of use, frequency of use, return to fertility, and side effects and health concerns were the most commonly mentioned [21].

Conspicuously and surprisingly lacking from the evidence-base for LMICs is detailed, quantitative documentation of the beliefs of women concerning all major methods of contraception. Our study addresses the omission by presenting descriptive survey data on method-specific beliefs in three populations. The data presented here form part of a wider prospective cohort study whose aims are to advance the understanding of reasons for unmet need for contraception and measurement of fertility preferences. The detailed rationale and study protocol may be found elsewhere [22]. In brief, its conceptual underpinnings posit that adverse method-specific beliefs constitute one cause of unmet need and

unintended pregnancy, alongside four other factors (generic hostility to contraception, partner-related factors, weak or inconsistent fertility preferences and low perceived risk of pregnancy). The prospective design of the study will permit assessment of the relative power of these factors to predict method-specific adoption, continuation and pregnancy-incidence. Here, however, we present data from round one with the aim of documenting method-specific beliefs and of comparing the beliefs concerning oral contraceptives, injectables and implants of current, past and never users.

Methods

The survey was conducted in the icddr,b service area and the government service area of the Matlab Health and Demographic Surveillance System (HDSS), Bangladesh, the Nairobi Urban Health and Demographic Surveillance System (NUHDSS) in two slums in Nairobi, Kenya, and Homa Bay County in rural Western Kenya. Details of the three study population have been published [22], but, in summary, contraception has been well established in Matlab for decades and the total fertility rate (TFR) is 2.7 [23]. The population is predominantly Muslim. In Nairobi slums, the TFR is 3.5 and HIV prevalence is 8% in the adult population [24, 25]. In the two slums covered by the NUHDSS, the population is ethnically diverse, the majority belong to a Christian faith and mobility is high. Homa Bay's population is predominantly rural, Christian and of Luo ethnicity. It has a high TFR of 5.2, high unmet need for contraception and a severe HIV epidemic with an infection level in the adult population of 26% [26]. All married or cohabiting women aged between 15 and 39 years residing in the three sites were eligible for the study. We set a target sample size for each site of 2600. The sample size was determined to detect a 30% difference in reproductive outcomes (pregnancy, use and non-use of contraceptives) at 95% confidence level and 80% power with an assumption of 10% non-response rate [27].

Data collection was carried out between August and December 2016. Respondents were randomly sampled from eligible female residents from the HDSS

Table 3 Percentage of women with specific opinions by use status (Matlab)

Attributes	Pills			Injectables			Implants		
	Current users	Past users	Never users	Current users	Past users	Never users	Current users	Past users	Never users
Access									
Easy	98.6	98.3	92.4	98.5	95.5	84.0	96.5	87.5	64.7
Hard	1.4	1.5	5.0	1.5	4.2	13.0	1.8	12.5	25.8
Don't know/unsure	0.0	0.2	2.6	0.0	0.3	3.0	1.7	0.0	9.5
Effectiveness									
Yes	99.8	99.4	98.5	98.9	99.1	98.1	100.0	96.4	96.9
No	0.2	0.6	0.6	1.1	0.8	1.1	0.0	3.6	0.5
Don't know	0.0	0.0	0.9	0.0	0.1	0.8	0.0	0.0	2.6
Cause health problems									
Yes, serious	0.9	3.8	3.3	2.2	11.0	6.7	1.8	28.6	8.0
Yes, not serious	10.6	23.6	24.7	22.6	43.3	29.5	24.6	35.7	14.5
No	88.5	72.4	36.6	75.3	45.5	23.6	71.9	28.6	9.0
Don't know	0.0	0.2	35.4	0.0	0.2	40.2	1.7	7.1	68.5
Interfere with menstruation									
Yes	6.0	9.0	5.8	67.9	72.2	41.8	43.9	53.6	14.0
No	93.8	90.6	56.6	31.0	27.5	14.0	52.6	39.3	11.1
Don't know	0.2	0.4	37.6	1.1	0.3	44.2	3.5	7.1	74.9
Cause unpleasant side effect									
Yes	14.1	31.9	26.5	26.3	52.3	31.8	29.8	57.1	17.4
No	85.8	67.7	37.9	73.3	47.3	26.0	66.7	37.5	10.1
Don't know	0.2	0.4	36.6	0.4	0.4	42.2	3.5	5.4	72.5
Unsafe to use for a long time									
Yes, should take a break	18.9	24.7	14.8	24.5	27.0	20.5	36.8	37.5	19.4
No, safe for long time	79.8	73.4	69.9	74.4	72.1	60.9	61.4	53.6	52.5
Don't know	1.3	1.9	15.2	1.1	0.9	18.6	1.8	8.9	28.1
Cause infertility									
Yes, perhaps	6.5	10.3	7.6	6.1	7.1	6.2	3.5	0.0	4.3
No	90.9	85.9	76.6	91.8	89.9	78.6	87.7	91.1	74.0
Don't know	2.6	3.8	15.8	2.1	3.0	15.2	8.8	8.9	21.7
FP use among friends, relatives									
Most	32.5	24.2	18.0	27.8	20.3	10.7	1.8	1.8	0.7
About half	15.0	10.5	11.3	18.0	14.7	13.8	7.0	5.3	1.1
Few	48.8	56.1	55.8	47.9	54.3	52.3	71.9	67.9	39.7
None	1.8	5.0	5.2	3.0	6.2	11.6	8.8	21.4	28.8
Don't know	1.9	4.2	9.7	3.3	4.5	11.6	10.5	3.6	29.7
Experiences of friends, relatives (1)									
Satisfactory	98.4	95.3	92.4	95.8	88.8	87.3	93.5	71.4	76.6
Unsatisfactory	0.5	3.5	1.3	2.6	9.7	3.7	4.3	21.4	8.2
Mixed/Don't know	1.1	1.3	6.3	1.6	1.5	9.0	2.2	7.1	15.1
Husband's approval									
Approve	98.8	94.9	63.8	97.6	88.9	48.9	96.5	67.9	16.6
Disapprove	1.2	4.6	22.7	2.4	10.6	38.6	3.5	25.0	66.8
Don't know	0.0	0.5	13.5	0.0	0.5	12.5	0.0	7.1	16.6

Table 3 Percentage of women with specific opinions by use status (Matlab) *(Continued)*

Attributes	Pills			Injectables			Implants		
	Current users	Past users	Never users	Current users	Past users	Never users	Current users	Past users	Never users
Satisfied with use									
Satisfied	92.2	69.7	–	91.3	51.1	–	87.7	39.3	–
Unsatisfied	4.8	27.7	–	8.0	47.2	–	10.5	51.8	–
Mixed/Neither	3.0	2.6	–	0.7	1.7	–	1.8	8.9	–
Mean net positive score (2)	74.8	60.9	48.8	53.3	34.7	31.0	45.8	19.2	24.0
Mean % of don't know (3)	0.8	1.4	19.2	1.0	1.2	22.0	3.9	5.1	38.4
TOTAL(N)	662	1399	539	461	877	1245	57	56	2140

(1) Amongst those knowing some friends were using the methods
(2) Mean percent difference between percentages of women who gave positive and negative responses among the above attributes except husband's approval
(3) Mean percent of women who said "don't know" to the above attributes except experiences of a method in social network and husband's approval
Note: Chi-square test was conducted to assess associations between each of the above attributes and use status. The *p*-values were all 0.01 or smaller except the perceptions on effectiveness of injectables (*p* = 0.067)

databases in the Matlab and Nairobi sites. In Homa Bay two-stage cluster sampling was used. A total of 34,308 women were identified as being married and aged between 15 and 39 years in the Matlab HDSS database. Out of these, 3109 were randomly selected and 2605 women completed the interviews. The Nairobi HDSS database identified a total of 5905 married or cohabiting women who were eligible for inclusion. Out of these, 3093 women were randomly sampled and interviews were completed with 2812 of the eligible women.

In Homa-Bay, we randomly selected 12 sub-locations (the smallest administrative unit in Kenya) in each three purposely identified sub-counties in Homa Bay County. All households with currently married or co-habiting women aged 15–49 years in the selected sub-locations were identified with the help of the local administration. Subsequently, the sampling frame was generated by listing all individuals in these households. In the second stage, 3118 were randomly sampled out of 5424 eligible women. A total of 2424 women completed the interviews.

All respondents provided written consents after having been informed about the objectives, procedures, benefits and risks of the study using an information sheet and informed consent form. All married and co-habiting adolescents aged 15–17 years were considered emancipated minors for whom parental permission is not required.

The questionnaire was developed through literature review and consultation with experts. We reviewed existing literature and more than 30 questionnaires on fertility preferences and reasons for non-use of family planning fielded in high-, middle- and low-income countries including instruments from the DHS, the Determinants of Unintended Pregnancy Risk study in New Orleans; the US- based National Survey of Family

Growth (NSFG); and the Fog Zone study by the Guttmacher Institute. A questionnaire was developed and reviewed through consultation with dozens of experts in the field. The questionnaire was further refined after pre-testing.

Structured interviews, lasting on average for 45–60 min, were conducted using the local languages following a 7 to 10-day training. Very similar questionnaires were used in all three sites covering the following topics: background, reproduction, contraceptive knowledge and use, beliefs and attitudes towards contraception in general and specific methods and fertility preferences of the women. Two summary measures of method-specific beliefs were generated. A net positive score is the mean percent difference between positive and negative responses across nine women's attributes, ignoring "don't know" and perceived husband's approval. Positive responses refer to perceptions that a method is easy to obtain and to use, very effective in preventing pregnancy and safe to use for a long time without a break, does not cause health problems, unpleasant side effects, menstrual disruption or infertility, and that half or more of friends, relatives, neighbours (i.e. social network) had used the method and their experiences were satisfactory. A familiarity measure which is simply the mean percent responding "don't know" across eight attributes excluding experiences of method use among women's social network and perceived husband's approval. In addition, past and current users of a method were asked whether they were satisfied or dissatisfied with use.

Descriptive analysis and chi-square tests were carried out to assess differences in beliefs and attitudes among current, past and never users of pills, injectables and implants. Clustering was taken into account for the statistical analyses when analysing the data from Homa-Bay. We used STATA SE version 15.0 for the data analysis.

Table 4 Percentage of women with specific opinions, amongst those who have heard of methods (Nairobi)

Attributes	Pills	Injectables	Implants	IUD	Condoms	Female sterilisation
Access						
Easy	92.3	96.7	89.7	70.0	88.3	41.8
Hard	7.4	3.1	10.0	28.7	11.0	56.7
Don't know/unsure	0.4	0.2	0.3	1.3	0.7	1.4
Effectiveness						
Yes	69.8	89.1	89.2	70.0	61.1	68.4
No	29.9	10.8	10.5	28.1	38.1	31.1
Don't know	0.3	0.1	0.3	1.8	0.8	0.5
Cause health problems						
Yes, serious	12.5	18.5	23.2	35.4	4.0	30.0
Yes, not serious	28.8	37.1	36.2	24.6	11.6	13.5
No	58.2	44.2	40.1	38.1	83.4	54.2
Don't know	0.6	0.2	0.5	1.9	1.1	2.3
Interfere with menstruation						
Yes	40.5	78.0	66.5	48.9	–	30.3
No	58.5	21.5	32.6	47.3	–	63.8
Don't know	1.0	0.5	0.9	3.8	–	5.9
Cause unpleasant side effect						
Yes	47.2	59.9	58.7	58.7	18.0	40.6
No	52.4	40.0	41.0	39.7	81.2	56.5
Don't know	0.5	0.1	0.3	1.5	0.8	2.9
Unsafe to use for a long time						
Yes, should take a break	70.1	62.9	56.9	65.2	48.8	–
No, safe for long time	29.5	36.7	42.7	33.3	49.6	–
Don't know	0.4	0.4	0.4	1.5	1.6	–
Cause infertility						
Yes, perhaps	13.8	28.0	21.8	18.9	–	–
No	85.6	71.6	77.4	79.2	–	–
Don't know	0.5	0.4	0.8	1.9	–	–
FP use among friends, relatives						
Most	20.2	63.5	38.2	5.7	11.4	1.7
About half	7.1	9.9	13.7	2.9	2.4	0.6
Few	52.2	21.1	39.3	49.4	28.2	32.5
None	19.7	4.8	8.3	40.9	54.8	64.5
Don't know	0.7	0.7	0.5	1.0	3.1	0.7
Experiences of friends, relatives (1)						
Satisfactory	55.1	60.2	59	50.7	70.6	71.1
Unsatisfactory	24.3	14.8	19.2	30.1	15.2	20.5
Mixed/Don't know	20.6	25	21.9	19.2	14.3	8.3
Husband's approval						
Approve	63.6	77.4	62.6	30.6	29.4	14.0
Disapprove	35.9	22.1	36.5	68.0	70.0	84.9
Don't know	0.5	0.5	0.8	1.4	0.6	1.1

Table 4 Percentage of women with specific opinions, amongst those who have heard of methods (Nairobi) *(Continued)*

Attributes	Pills	Injectables	Implants	IUD	Condoms	Female sterilisation
Mean net positive score (2)	20.3	21.6	19.2	0.9	31.2	5.5
Mean % of don't know (3)	0.5	0.3	0.5	1.9	1.4	2.3
TOTAL (N)	2787	2808	2789	2664	2792	2423

(1) Amongst those knowing some friends were using the methods
(2) Mean percent difference between percentages of women who gave positive and negative responses among the above attributes except husband's approval
(3) Mean percent of women who said 'don't know' to the above attributes except experiences of a method in social network and husband's approval

Ethical approvals for this study were obtained from the Institutional Review Boards of the countries and three participating institutions.

Results

The number of women successfully interviewed was 2424 in Homa Bay, 2605 in Matlab, and 2812 in Nairobi (Additional file 1: Table S1). The average ages of women in the three sites were closely similar, 28 or 29 years (Table 1). About 70% in Matlab had secondary or higher schooling, compared with 40% in Nairobi and 23% in Homa Bay. The mean number of surviving children was lowest in Matlab, highest in Homa Bay and intermediate in Nairobi. Women in Matlab were much more likely to express a desire to stop childbearing than those in the Kenyan sites. In Nairobi, 75% were currently using a method of contraception, with injectables followed by implants, as the dominant methods. In Homa Bay, the level of current use was 65%, with a method-mix similar to that in Nairobi. Current use was lowest in Matlab (59%), where oral contraception pills and injectables were the favoured methods. But this unexpected result, in view of the far lower fertility rate in Matlab, may largely reflect the fact that 34% of husbands had been away for three months or longer preceding the date of interview, mainly as migrant workers, thus reducing the need for pregnancy-protection.

Generic attitudes

Though the focus of this paper is on method-specific beliefs, we start by presenting information on attitudes towards contraceptive use in general. In all three sites, over 90% of women reported that they supported family planning, but 25% in Homa Bay and 12% in Nairobi perceived their husbands to be opposed (Additional file 1: Table S2). Use of contraception by women's social network of friends, neighbours, and relatives was thought to be common and their attitudes were favourable in all three sites. Conversely, only around half in Matlab (51%) and Homa Bay (47%) and three-fourths (76%) in Nairobi perceived that their religion supports family planning.

Large majorities considered the following features of methods to be very important: effectiveness, no health risk, lack of unpleasant side effects, no effect on menstruation, and ease of access and use (Additional file 1: Table S3). The amenability of a method for clandestine use and use for a long time without the need for re-supply were endorsed as very important by smaller majorities.

Method-specific beliefs and opinions: Matlab

A total of ten opinions and beliefs was ascertained for all women who have ever heard of each of six modern methods (Tables 2, 3, 4, 5, 6 and 7) and two traditional methods (Additional file 1: Table S4). Because of the wide array of information, the discussion here will be highly selective.

In Matlab, implants, IUDs and female sterilisation were rarely used and unfamiliarity was reflected in the high proportions of respondents who said "don't know" on attributes of these methods. Thus over half of women did not know whether these methods might cause health problems, unpleasant side effects or menstrual disruption. However, nearly all women acknowledged these three methods to be effective and two-thirds or more thought access would be easy. Among those knowing social network members who had used these methods, over three-quarters deemed their experience to be satisfactory. Yet a majority considered that their husband would disapprove of using these methods.

Oral contraceptives followed by injectables dominate the method-mix. Pills attracted more favourable opinions than injectables. For instance, 40% and 38% thought injectables might cause health problems and unpleasant side effects, respectively, compared with 24% and 26% for pills. Nearly one-quarter thought that their husbands would disapprove of their use of injectables compared with 8% for pills. The two methods were rated similarly on other dimensions. Both were regarded as easy to obtain and effective. The experience of their social network with use of either method was judged to be satisfactory by over 90%. Very few thought that either method might cause infertility and almost equal proportions considered long term use to be safe.

We compared the views of current, past and never users of pills, injectables and implants (Table 3). The largest consistent difference between current and past users across all three methods was the view that the method

Table 5 Percentage of women with specific opinions by use status (Nairobi)

Attributes	Pills			Injectables			Implants		
	Current users	Past users	Never users	Current users	Past users	Never users	Current users	Past users	Never users
Access									
Easy	98.3	94.0	90.6	99.1	96.9	93.0	96.7	92.4	87.1
Hard	1.7	6.0	8.8	0.9	3.0	6.3	3.3	7.6	12.5
Don't know/unsure	0.0	0.0	0.6	0.0	0.1	0.7	0.0	0.0	0.4
Effectiveness									
Yes	93.6	70.9	65.9	97.7	86.0	83.4	98.2	89.0	86.6
No	6.4	29.0	33.7	2.3	14.0	16.2	1.8	11.0	12.9
Don't know	0.0	0.1	0.4	0.0	0.0	0.4	0.0	0.0	0.4
Cause health problems									
Yes, serious	5.1	14.2	12.6	10.6	23.0	21.1	9.7	35.5	24.5
Yes, not serious	18.4	32.7	28.2	33.4	38.5	39.4	31.9	35.9	37.6
No	76.5	52.9	58.4	55.9	38.5	38.9	58.5	28.4	37.2
Don't know	0.0	0.2	0.8	0.1	0.0	0.6	0.0	0.2	0.7
Interfere with menstruation									
Yes	25.2	40.7	42.5	73.0	82.3	77.1	59.6	75.1	66.7
No	74.8	59.0	55.9	27.0	17.7	21.0	40.4	24.9	31.9
Don't know	0.0	0.2	1.6	0.0	0.0	1.9	0.0	0.0	1.4
Cause unpleasant side effect									
Yes	30.3	51.4	47.3	50.6	65.8	61.7	44.8	70.9	60.1
No	69.7	48.6	51.9	49.4	34.2	37.9	55.2	28.9	39.5
Don't know	0.0	0.0	0.8	0.0	0.0	0.4	0.0	0.2	0.4
Unsafe to use for a long time									
Yes, should take a break	46.2	69.2	74.0	49.0	70.0	69.0	37.9	61.6	61.6
No, safe for long use	53.8	30.8	25.4	50.9	29.9	29.8	61.9	38.4	37.9
Don't know	0.0	0.0	0.7	0.1	0.2	1.2	0.2	0.0	0.5
Cause infertility									
Yes, perhaps	9.8	13.1	14.7	26.1	30.0	26.9	16.0	22.7	23.4
No	89.3	86.8	84.6	73.6	69.8	72.1	83.4	77.0	75.7
Don't know	0.9	0.1	0.7	0.3	0.2	1.0	0.5	0.2	0.9
FP use among friends, relatives									
Most	34.2	26.1	15.3	72.6	63.0	52.1	56.3	46.9	30.8
About half	10.7	7.5	6.5	9.2	10.0	10.7	14.9	14.7	13.1
Few	45.3	50.6	54.0	15.2	22.3	26.9	25.9	33.0	44.7
None	9.8	15.2	23.5	2.5	4.2	9.0	2.7	4.6	10.8
Don't know	0.0	0.6	0.8	0.4	0.5	1.3	0.2	0.7	0.6
Experiences of friends, relatives (1)									
Satisfactory	83.4	52	52.2	74.9	52.9	52.7	75.2	48.8	56
Unsatisfactory	5.2	27.9	25.3	4.6	19.3	20.9	6.6	25.1	21.9
Mixed/Don't know	11.4	20.1	22.4	20.4	27.8	26.4	18.2	26.1	22.1
Husband's approval									
Approve	92.3	71.8	55.3	91.5	77.5	58.4	90.0	68.5	53.1
Disapprove	7.69	28.19	43.82	8.4	22.4	39.8	9.8	31.5	45.7
Don't know	0.0	0.0	0.8	0.1	0.1	1.8	0.2	0.0	1.2

Table 5 Percentage of women with specific opinions by use status (Nairobi) *(Continued)*

Attributes	Pills			Injectables			Implants		
	Current users	Past users	Never users	Current users	Past users	Never users	Current users	Past users	Never users
Satisfied with use									
Satisfied	90.2	41.3	–	87.7	44.9	–	86.5	32.3	–
Unsatisfied	8.5	55.8	–	10.5	53.2	–	10.7	64.8	–
Mixed/Neither	1.3	2.3	–	1.3	1.3	–	2.0	2.0	–
Missing	0.0	0.6	–	0.6	0.6	–	0.7	1.0	–
Mean net positive score (2)	53.4	19.8	15.8	38.0	14.1	13.0	44.5	11.8	13.2
Mean % of don't know (3)	0.1	0.2	0.8	0.1	0.1	1.0	0.1	0.2	0.7
TOTAL(N)	234	869	1684	909	1218	681	549	409	1831

(1) Amongst those knowing some friends were using the methods
(2) Mean percent difference between percentages of women who gave positive and negative responses among the above attributes except husband's approval
(3) Mean percent of women who said "don't know" to the above attributes except experiences of a method in social network and husband's approval
Note: Chi-square test was conducted to assess associations between each of the above attributes and use status. The p-values were all 0.01 or smaller except the perceptions on risk of infertility of pills ($p = 0.061$) and injectables ($p = 0.015$).

caused unpleasant side effects, though appreciable minorities (from 14% for the pill to 30% for the implant) of current users acknowledged side effects. Notably, 29% of past implant users thought that the method caused serious health problems. Furthermore, past implant users were more likely to rate their experience as unsatisfactory than past injectable or pill users.

Method-specific beliefs and opinions: Nairobi

As indicated by the mean net positive scores, beliefs about methods were less favourable in Nairobi than in Matlab and the proportions giving "don't know" responses were much lower. With the exception of sterilisation, large majorities considered methods easy to obtain (Table 4). Injectables and implants were judged to be effective by 90%. However, in a clear departure from objective evidence, this level falls to about 70% for IUDs and sterilisation. The view that a method might cause serious health problems was widespread (with the exception of condoms), rising from 13% for pills to 30% for sterilisation and 35% for IUDs. Similarly, about 60% associated injectables, implants, and IUDs with unpleasant side effects, as did over 40% for pills and sterilisation. Only minorities were of the view that the hormonal methods and IUDs could be safely used for a long time without taking a break. Between 14% (pills) and 28% (injectables) of women thought that a method might cause infertility. Despite these views, between 51% and 71% rated the experience of social network members with use of methods as satisfactory. While most women thought that their partners would approve of their use of pills, injectables and implants, perceived approval dropped to 30% for IUDs and condoms and further to 14% for sterilisation.

Analysis of opinions by use status showed sharp divides between current users and past or never users (Table 5). For instance, 11% of current injectable users (the dominant method in this site) believed that the method caused serious health problems compared with over 20% of past or never users. This difference was more pronounced for implants: 10% for current users versus 36% for past users and 25% for never users. Similarly, about three quarters of current users of injectables, pills and implants reported satisfactory experience of their social network compared with about 50% of past and never users. A clear gradient in perceived partner's approval is apparent for all three methods, with 90% approval for current users, around 70% for past users and 50–60% for never users. Nevertheless, appreciable proportions of current users held negative views about their method: 30%, 51% and 45% of pill, injectable and implant users, respectively, thought that the method caused unpleasant side effects. Around 40% of current users considered their method to be unsafe for prolonged use. Despite these reservations, close to 90% of current users rated their method as satisfactory compared with 32–44% of past users.

Method-specific beliefs and opinions: Homa Bay

Condoms received a much higher mean net positive score than other methods and perceived partner's approval of this method was higher in this site with high adult HIV prevalence than in Matlab or Nairobi. The experience of social network members with use of condoms was more likely to be rated as satisfactory than other methods: 73% for condoms compared with 54–58% for the two dominant methods, injectables and implants (Table 6). Condoms were more likely to be considered as effective than pills, though less likely than injectables and implants.

With the exception of condoms, about 30% thought that other methods caused serious health problems; between 38% (sterilisation) and 63% (injectables)

Table 6 Percentage of women with specific opinions, amongst those who have heard of methods (Homa Bay)

Attributes	Pills	Injectables	Implants	IUD	Condoms (4)	Female sterilisation (5)
Access						
Easy	79.4	90.4	84.5	52.8	93.9	41.7
Hard	12.5	7.9	10.5	25.8	3.6	40.3
Don't know/unsure	8.1	1.6	5.0	21.4	2.5	18.0
Effectiveness						
Yes	62.6	91.6	90.3	66.1	77.5	82.5
No	23.8	5.6	3.7	8.6	17.4	5.4
Don't know	13.5	2.8	6.0	25.3	5.1	12.1
Cause health problems						
Yes, serious	37.8	31.2	28.3	36.0	11.4	32.7
Yes, not serious	21.5	31.0	25.9	16.0	11.3	12.2
No	23.0	30.1	30.5	18.7	70.0	31.5
Don't know	17.7	7.7	15.4	29.3	7.3	23.6
Interfere with menstruation						
Yes	56.5	80.2	60.1	35.6	–	–
No	22.1	14.7	22.5	25.1	–	–
Don't know	21.4	5.2	17.4	39.2	–	–
Cause unpleasant side effect						
Yes	57.5	63.2	51.7	44.7	14.0	38.3
No	21.6	28.7	30.1	20.9	77.6	36.0
Don't know	20.9	8.2	18.2	34.4	8.4	25.7
Unsafe to use for a long time						
Yes, should take a break	66.9	68.5	60.8	62.5	37.3	–
No, safe for long time	20.3	26.3	31.7	17.4	56.4	–
Don't know	12.8	5.2	7.6	20.0	6.3	–
Cause infertility						
Yes, perhaps	15.6	17.1	12.7	16.2	–	–
No	72.9	77.3	78.1	63.4	–	–
Don't know	11.6	5.7	9.2	20.5	–	–
FP use among friends, relatives						
Most	13.9	64.6	49.1	3.9	30.3	3.3
About half	7.4	8.3	8.7	3.5	7.7	2.7
Few	49.3	19.0	31.8	42.4	26.0	51.3
None	13.8	2.1	3.7	26.9	6.1	26.0
Don't know	15.7	6.0	6.8	23.4	30.0	16.7
Experiences of friends, relatives (1)						
Satisfactory	38.0	54.1	57.7	39.4	72.9	59.1
Unsatisfactory	28.5	11.2	13.1	27.2	10.6	17.3
Mixed/Don't know	33.5	34.7	29.2	33.4	16.5	17.1
Husband disapprove						
Approve	45.5	64.4	52.2	25.2	53.3	18.1
Disapprove	43.7	30.2	38.7	58.8	41.2	70.5
Don't know	10.8	5.5	9.1	15.9	5.5	11.4

Table 6 Percentage of women with specific opinions, amongst those who have heard of methods (Homa Bay) *(Continued)*

Attributes	Pills	Injectables	Implants	IUD	Condoms (4)	Female sterilisation (5)
Mean net positive score (2)	−2.5	16.6	20.1	−3.4	49.8	5.6
Mean % of don't know (3)	15.2	5.3	10.7	26.7	9.9	19.2
TOTAL(N)	2358	2405	2391	1973	1338	2080

(1) Amongst those knowing some friends were using the methods
(2) Mean percent difference between percentages of women who gave positive and negative responses among the above attributes except husband's approval
(3) Mean percent of women who said "don't know" to the above attributes except experiences of a method in social network and husband's approval
(4) 1008 responses missing owing to error in electronic data capture program
(5) The question on interference with menstruation was not asked for female sterilisation in Homa-Bay

considered that methods caused unpleasant side effects and about two-thirds judged methods to be unsafe for prolonged use without taking a break.

As in Nairobi, current users of pills, injectables and implants were much more likely to express positive views about their method than past or never users, except with regard to fears among a minority of women about infertility. However, the prevalence of adverse views even among current users was striking. Thus, 14%, 24% and 16% of current pill, injectable and implant users, respectively, considered that their method caused serious health problems and between 34% and 55% associated the method with unpleasant side effects. These adverse beliefs did not translate into dissatisfaction with the current method: on the contrary, between 77% and 88% judged their method to be satisfactory while only 31–45% of past users were satisfied with the use.

Discussion

In view of the principle of cognitive dissonance—the tendency to align beliefs and attitudes to behaviour—it is no surprise that most current users of a method consider it to be satisfactory and express more positive views than past or never users. In apparent contradiction to high overall satisfaction is the finding that appreciable proportions of these current users appear to be concerned about serious health effects and acknowledge that the method causes unpleasant side effects. The view that it is unsafe to use a method for a long time without taking a break is widespread among current users, particularly in the Kenyan sites. Follow-up surveys will establish the impact of these perceptions on discontinuation.

Dissatisfaction among past users, who tend to outnumber current users, may be a powerful influence on the overall climate of opinion; indeed the views of past and never users tend to be similar. The low level of overall satisfaction among past users of injectables, pills and implants in Kenyan sites, associated with health worries and side effects, is a concern, particularly with implant users of whom only about 30% in Nairobi reported satisfaction. A continuation of the steep rise in the use of implants in Kenya, therefore, could be in jeopardy. Similarly in Matlab, the results imply considerable potential resistance to long-acting reversible methods (IUDs and implants), the promotion of which is a national priority.

The study is not without limitations. Information on perceived partner's approval of specific methods is difficult to interpret. While close to 90% reported partner's support of family planning in general, perceived approval is low in Matlab for use of implants, IUDs and female sterilisation, and also low in the Kenyan sites for use of IUDs and sterilisation. Whether or not, these results reflect women's own misgivings about these methods remains unclear.

The value of this detailed information in explaining reproductive and contraceptive behaviour is uncertain and a verdict must await the results of follow-up surveys. Nevertheless, the results are of considerable interest because this study, to our knowledge, is the first to have obtained comparable quantitative information in LMICs on attitudes and beliefs on each of eight major family planning methods. Many of the findings from this study are consistent with earlier studies that have documented fears about side effects and damage to health to be widespread. The result regarding the belief that it is unsafe to use a method for a long term without taking a break is simiar to the common behaviours observed in the Philippines [28]. Other findings are new and have considerable possible implications for behaviour.

Moreover, the ability of this study to contrast the beliefs of current, past and never users of the three more prevalent methods represents a major contribution. In 2015 an expert meeting on misperceptions about contraceptives called for a revitalization of discussion on this issue. Participants identified the need for quantitative data that distinguish concerns stemming from documented side effects from those resulting from rumours or myths and the need for evidence about links between misperceptions and method choice [29]. This paper starts to address these gaps in evidence and further progress is expected when follow-up survey data become available.

Table 7 Percentage of women with specific opinions by use status (Homa Bay)

Attributes	Pills			Injectables			Implants		
	Current users	Past users	Never users	Current users	Past users	Never users	Current users	Past users	Never users
Access									
Easy	92.3	84.7	77.1	93.7	90.6	87.0	93.9	88.7	81.1
Hard	7.7	12.5	12.7	6.2	8.7	8.4	6.2	8.3	12.1
Don't know/unsure	0.0	2.8	10.3	0.2	0.7	4.6	0.0	3.0	6.9
Effectiveness									
Yes	86.2	66.8	60.3	97.1	92.1	85.2	98.6	89.9	88.1
No	10.8	28.5	22.8	2.1	7.0	6.8	1.1	5.7	4.0
Don't know	3.1	4.7	16.9	0.8	0.8	8.0	0.2	4.5	7.9
Cause health problems									
Yes, serious	13.9	42.7	37.0	24.2	36.8	29.4	16.4	36.3	29.9
Yes, not serious	33.9	22.9	20.6	30.1	32.3	30.0	24.6	26.2	26.1
No	46.2	26.2	21.0	40.9	27.7	23.3	51.5	31.9	24.4
Don't know	6.2	8.2	21.4	4.8	3.3	17.3	7.5	5.7	19.6
Interfere with menstruation									
Yes	40.0	59.6	56.1	80.2	84.1	74.0	62.9	67.9	57.6
No	53.9	32.5	17.4	19.0	14.2	11.2	35.3	24.4	18.7
Don't know	6.2	8.0	26.5	0.8	1.8	14.8	1.8	7.7	23.7
Cause unpleasant side effect									
Yes	33.9	63.0	56.5	55.3	68.7	62.2	41.0	59.8	53.0
No	60.0	29.0	17.7	39.9	27.8	19.2	51.7	31.9	23.9
Don't know	6.2	8.0	25.8	4.8	3.6	18.6	7.3	8.3	23.1
Unsafe to use for a long time									
Yes, should take a break	47.7	70.5	66.4	58.0	73.7	70.6	50.8	65.2	62.6
No, safe for long time	40.0	22.4	18.9	37.3	23.6	19.9	47.2	29.8	27.9
Don't Know	12.3	7.1	14.7	4.7	2.7	9.5	2.1	5.1	9.6
Cause infertility									
Yes, perhaps	15.4	15.6	15.6	15.4	16.8	19.3	10.7	13.4	13.1
No	80.0	77.4	71.1	80.5	80.0	69.8	83.4	81.0	76.1
Don't know	4.6	6.9	13.4	4.1	3.2	11.0	5.9	5.7	10.8
FP use among friends, relatives									
Most	18.5	19.1	11.9	73.6	66.7	52.6	70.8	53.9	42.1
About half	10.8	8.0	7.1	6.8	7.7	10.6	6.6	6.6	9.7
Few	50.8	45.1	50.6	14.7	17.6	25.3	18.2	30.4	35.7
None	7.7	13.4	14.2	0.9	2.4	2.8	1.8	2.7	4.5
Don't know	12.3	14.4	16.2	4.1	5.5	8.7	2.5	6.6	8.0
Experiences of friends, relatives (1)									
Satisfactory	65.4	39.7	36.2	69.0	48.2	47.9	77.6	49.2	53.6
Unsatisfactory	11.5	34.9	27.0	4.0	15.4	11.7	3.8	21.6	14.1
Mixed/Don't know	23.1	25.5	36.7	27.0	36.4	40.4	18.6	29.2	32.3
Husband's approval									
Approve	76.9	55.6	40.9	77.2	67.5	47.0	77.7	59.8	43.7
Disapprove	20.0	38.4	46.4	20.7	29.1	41.1	20.7	36.0	44.2
Don't know	3.1	6.1	12.6	2.1	3.4	12.0	1.6	4.2	12.1

Table 7 Percentage of women with specific opinions by use status (Homa Bay) *(Continued)*

Attributes	Pills			Injectables			Implants		
	Current users	Past users	Never users	Current users	Past users	Never users	Current users	Past users	Never users
Satisfied with use									
Satisfied	76.9	38.4	–	86.1	44.9	–	87.7	31.0	–
Unsatisfied	16.9	43.6	–	6.3	38.7	–	7.1	30.1	–
Mixed/Neither	3.1	6.3	–	5.1	9.0	–	5.2	3.3	–
Missing (4)	3.1	11.8	–	2.4	7.3	–	0.0	35.7	–
Mean net positive score (2)	31.1	−0.3	−4.5	29.7	12.8	9.6	42.1	16.6	14.8
Mean % of don't know (3)	6.3	7.5	18.1	3.0	2.7	11.5	3.4	5.8	13.7
TOTAL(N)	65	576	1717	662	1066	677	439	336	1616

(1) Amongst those knowing some friends were using the methods
(2) Mean percent difference between percentages of women who gave positive and negative responses among the above attributes except husband's approval
(3) Mean percent of women who said "don't know" to the above attributes except experiences of a method in social network and husband's approval
(4) The missing occurred due to initial technical errors in the electronic data capture
Note: Chi-square test was conducted to assess associations between each of the above attributes and use status. The p-values were all 0.002 or smaller

Conclusions

In conclusion, high levels of contraceptive use can clearly co-exist with widespread misgivings about methods, even those that are widely used. Serious concerns about damage to health, long term fertility impairment, and dangers of prolonged use without taking a break were particularly common in the Kenyan sites and these beliefs may explain the high levels of discontinuation observed in Kenya and elsewhere in Africa. This documentation of beliefs provides useful guidance for counselling and informational campaigns. The generally negative views of past users imply that programmes may need not only to improve individual counselling but also strengthen community information campaign to change the overall climate of opinion which may have been influenced by dissatisfaction among past users.

Acknowledgements
The authors thank the women who participated in this study and the teams worked at the three study sites, Matlab, Nairobi and Homa-Bay, and at icddr, b, APHRC, Population Council, Kenya. We would like to thank the members of the STEP UP Consortium Advisory Group and Senior Management Team for their invaluable feedback in the design and implementation of the study.

Funding
The *Improving Measurement of Unintended Pregnancy and Unmet Need for Family Planning study* was funded by the UK Department for International Development (DFID) through the Strengthening Evidence for Programming on Unintended Pregnancy (STEP UP).

Authors' contributions
KM was the principal investigator (PI) and responsible for the overall study coordination and implementation of the study. JC, KM and JBC conceptualized the study and led development of study design, questionnaire and analysis plans. JNM, FAH and FO are the site PIs and were responsible for the implementation of the study in the respective sites. FA, GO and MW conducted the analysis and the results were reviewed by KM, FAH, JNM and JC. JC and KM prepared the first draft and tables for the manuscript, FAH, GO, JNM, JBC, FA reviewed and provided inputs for revisions. All authors read and approved the final manuscript.

Ethics approvals and consent to participate
Ethical approvals for this study were granted from the Institutional Review Boards of the London School of Hygiene and Tropical Medicine and Population Council as well as by the AMREF Ethics and Scientific Review Committee for the Nairobi site, Kenyatta National Hospital-University of Nairobi Ethics and Research Committee for the Homa-Bay site and icddr,b Institutional Review Board (Research Review Committee and Ethical Review Committee) for the Matlab site, respectively. All adolescents aged 15–17 years who were married or co-habiting with a partner were considered emancipated minors for which parental permission is not required. All study participants gave written informed consent to participate in the study.

Competing interests
The authors declare that they have no competing interests.

Author details
[1]Faculty of Epidemiology and Population Health, London School of Hygiene and Tropical Medicine, Keppel Street, London WC1E 7HT, UK. [2]icddr,b, Dhaka, Bangladesh. [3]Population Council, Nairobi, Kenya. [4]African Population and Health Research Center, Nairobi, Kenya. [5]Institute for Population Research, Ohio State University, Columbus, USA.

References
1. Kabagenyi A, Reid A, Ntozi J, Atuyambe L. Socio-cultural inhibitors to use of modern contraceptive techniques in rural Uganda: a qualitative study. Pan Afr Med J. 2016. https://doi.org/10.11604/pamj.2016.25.78.6613.
2. Ochako R, Mbondo M, Aloo S, Kaimenyi S, Thompson R, Temmerman M, Kays M. Barriers to modern contraceptive methods uptake among young women in Kenya: a qualitative study. BMC Public Health. 2015. https://doi.org/10.1186/s12889-015-1483-1.
3. Gueye A, Speizer IS, Corroon M, Okigbo CC. Belief in family planning myths at the individual and community levels and modern contraceptive use in urban Africa. Int Perspect Sex Reprod Health. 2015. https://doi.org/10.1363/4119115.
4. Morse JE, Rowen TS, Steinauer J, Byamugisha J, Kakaire O. A qualitative assessment of Ugandan women's perceptions and knowledge of contraception. Int J Gynaecol Obstet. 2014. https://doi.org/10.1016/j.ijgo.2013.07.014.
5. Chipeta EK, Chimwaza W, Kalilani-Phiri L. Contraceptive knowledge, beliefs and attitudes in rural Malawi: misinformation, misbeliefs and misperceptions. Malawi Med J. 2010.

6. Mosha I, Ruben R, Kakoko D. Family planning decisions, perceptions and gender dynamics among couples in Mwanza, Tanzania: a qualitative study. BMC Public Health. 2013. https://doi.org/10.1186/1471-2458-13-523.

7. Maticka-Tyndale E. Condoms in sub-Saharan Africa. Sex Health. 2012. https://doi.org/10.1071/SH11033.

8. Daniele MAS, Cleland J, Benova L, Ali M. Provider and lay perspectives on intra-uterine contraception: a global review. Reprod Health. 2017. https://doi.org/10.1186/s12978-017-0380-8.

9. Hubacher D, Masaba R, Manduku CK, Veena V. Uptake of the levonorgestrel intrauterine system among recent postpartum women in Kenya: factors associated with decision-making. Contraception. 2013. https://doi.org/10.1016/j.contraception.2013.03.001.

10. Grubb GS. Women's perceptions of the safety of the pill: a survey in eight developing countries. Report of the perceptions of the pill survey group. J Biosoc Sci. 1987;19(3):313–21.

11. Williamson LM, Parkes A, Wight D, Petticrew M, Hart GJ. Limits to modern contraceptive use among young women in developing countries: a systematic review of qualitative research. Reprod Health. 2009. https://doi.org/10.1186/1742-4755-6-3.

12. Hardon A. Women's views and experiences of hormonal contraceptives: what we know and what we need to find out. Beyond acceptability: users' perspectives on contraception. London: Reproductive Health Matters; 1997. Accessed.

13. Castle S. Factors influencing young Malians' reluctance to use hormonal contraceptives. Stud Fam Plan. 2003. https://doi.org/10.1111/j.1728-4465.2003.00186.x.

14. Rutenberg N, Watkins SC. The buzz outside the clinics: conversations and contraception in Nyanza Province, Kenya. Stud Fam Plan. 1997;28(4):290–307.

15. Sedgh G, Ashford LS, Hussain R. Unmet need for contraception in developing countries: examining women's reasons for not using a method. New York: Guttmacher Institute; 2016. https://www.guttmacher.org/sites/default/files/report_pdf/unmet-need-for-contraception-in-developing-countries-report.pdf. Accessed 4 Apr 2018.

16. Diamond-Smith N, Campbell M, Madan S. Misinformation and fear of side-effects of family planning. Cult Health Sex. 2012; https://doi.org/10.1080/13691058.2012.664659.

17. Ali MM, Cleland JG, Shah IH. Causes and consequences of contraceptive discontinuation: evidence from 60 demographic and health surveys. Geneva: WHO; 2012. http://apps.who.int/iris/bitstream/handle/10665/75429/9789241504058_eng.pdf;jsessionid=85F4F8A8BE3BBE2AF2CAB109A0D5AE78?sequence=1. Accessed 4 Apr 2018.

18. Snow R, Garcia S, Kureshy N, Sadana R, Singh S, Becerra-Valdivia M, Lancaster S, Mofokeng M, Hoffman M, Aitken I. Attributes of contraceptive technology: women's preferences in seven countries. Beyond acceptability: users' perspectives on contraception. London: Reproductive Health Matters; 1997. Accessed.

19. Hindin MJ, McGough L, Misperceptions AR. Misinformation and myths about modern contraceptive use in Ghana. J Fam Plann Reprod Health Care. 2014. https://doi.org/10.1136/jfprhc-2012-100464.

20. Glasier AF, Smith KB, van der Spuyb Z, Ho PC, Cheng L, Dada K, Wellings K, Bairda DT. Amenorrhea associated with contraception-an international study on acceptability. Contraception. 2003. https://doi.org/10.1016/S0010-7824(02)00474-2.

21. Wyatt KD, Anderson RT, Creedon D, Montori VM, Bachman J, Erwin P, LeBlanc A. Women's values in contraceptive choice: a systematic review of relevant attributes included in decision aids. BMC Womens Health. 2014. https://doi.org/10.1186/1472-6874-14-28.

22. Machiyama K, Casterline JB, Mumah JN, Huda FA, Obare F, Odwe G, Kabiru CW, Yeasmin S, Cleland J. Reasons for unmet need for family planning, with attention to the measurement of fertility preferences: protocol for a multi-site cohort study. Reprod Health. 2017. https://doi.org/10.1186/s12978-016-0268-z.

23. icddr, b. Health and demographic surveillance system-Matlab: registration of health and demographic events 2015. Scientific report no 135. Dhaka. Icddr, b. 2015.

24. National Aids Control Council. Kenya HIV Country Profiles. Nairobi. National Aids Control Council. 2014. Accessed.

25. African Population and Health Research Center. Population and Health Dynamics in Nairobi's Informal Settlements: Report of the Nairobi Cross-sectional Slums Survey (NCSS) 2012. Nairobi. APRHC; 2014. http://aphrc.org/wp-content/uploads/2014/08/NCSS2-FINAL-Report.pdf. Accessed 4 Apr 2018.

26. Kenya Bureau of Statistics, Ministry of Health, national AIDS control council, Kenya medical research institute, National Council for population and development, ICF international. Kenya demographic and health survey 2014. Rockville: ICF International; 2015.

27. Fleiss JL, Levin B, Paik MC. Statistical methods for rates and proportions. Third ed. Hoboken: Wiley; 2003.

28. Henry R. Contraceptive practice in Quirino Province. Philippines: Experiences of Side Effects. Calverton: University of the Philippines Population Institute, University of La Salette, Macro International; 2001. https://pdf.usaid.gov/pdf_docs/PNACM416.pdf. Accessed 4 Apr 2018.

29. Wells E. Countering myths and misperceptions about contraceptives. PATH: Outlook on Reproductive Health. Seattle; 2015. https://www.path.org/publications/files/RH_outlook_myths_mis_june_2015.pdf. Accessed 4 Apr 2018.

8

Sexual and reproductive health behavior and unmet needs among a sample of adolescents living with HIV in Zambia

Sumiyo Okawa[1*], Sylvia Mwanza-Kabaghe[2,3], Mwiya Mwiya[3], Kimiyo Kikuchi[4], Masamine Jimba[1], Chipepo Kankasa[3] and Naoko Ishikawa[5]

Abstract

Background: Adolescents living with HIV face challenges, such as disclosure of HIV status, adherence to antiretroviral therapy, mental health, and sexual and reproductive health (SRH). These challenges affect their future quality of life. However, little evidence is available on their sexual behaviors and SRH needs in Zambia. This study aimed at assessing their sexual behaviors and SRH needs and identifying factors associated with marriage concerns and a desire to have children.

Methods: This cross-sectional study was conducted at the University Teaching Hospital from April to July 2014. We recruited 200 adolescents aged 15–19 years who were aware of their HIV-positive status. We collected data on their first and recent sexual behavior, concerns about marriage, and desire to have children. We used the Generalized Linear Model to identify factors associated with having concerns about marriage and desire to have children. We performed thematic analysis with open-ended data to determine their perceptions about marriage and having children in the future.

Results: Out of 175 studied adolescents, 20.6% had experienced sexual intercourse, and only 44.4% used condoms during the first intercourse. Forty-eight percent had concerns about marriage, and 87.4% desired to have children. Marriage-related concerns were high among those who desired to have children (adjusted relative risk [ARR] = 2.51, 95% CI = 1.02 to 6.14). Adolescents who had completed secondary school were more likely to desire to have children (ARR = 1.35, 95% CI = 1.07 to 1.71). Adolescents who had lost both parents were less likely to want children (ARR = 0.80, 95% CI = 0.68 to 0.95). Thematic analysis identified that major concerns about future marriage were fear of disclosing HIV status to partners and risk of infecting partners and/or children. The reasons for their willingness to have children were the desire to be a parent, having children as family assets, a human right, and a source of love and happiness.

Conclusions: Zambian adolescents living with HIV are at risk of engaging in risky sexual relationships and have difficulties in meeting needs of SRH. HIV care service must respond to a wide range of needs.

Keywords: HIV, Adolescents, Sexual behavior, Sexual and reproductive health, Zambia

* Correspondence: sumiyo@m.u-tokyo.ac.jp
[1]Department of Community and Global Health, Graduate School of Medicine, The University of Tokyo, Tokyo, Japan
Full list of author information is available at the end of the article

Plain English summary

Adolescents living with HIV face difficulties including sexual and reproductive health (SRH). Physical growth and psychosocial development during adolescence could complicate the challenges. This study examined these adolescents' sexual behaviors, needs, and concerns regarding SRH in Zambia.

This cross-sectional study was conducted at the University Teaching Hospital from April to July 2014. We collected data from 200 adolescents aged 15–19 years who were aware of their HIV-positive status and analyzed their sexual behavior and SRH needs with focus on whether they have concerns about marriage and desires for having children and the details of concerns and the reasons for desires.

Out of 175 adolescents, 20.6% had experienced sexual intercourse, 48.8% had concerns about their marriage, and 87.4% desired to have children. Adolescents who desired to have children were more likely to have concerns about marriage (ARR = 2.51). Adolescents who had completed secondary school were more likely to desire to have children (ARR = 1.35). Adolescents who had lost both parents were less likely to want children (ARR = 0.80). Major concerns about future marriage identified by the adolescents were fear of disclosing HIV status to partners and risk of infecting partners and/or children. The main reasons for their willingness to have children were the desire to be a parent, having children as family assets, a human right, and a source of love and happiness.

In conclusion, Zambian adolescents living with HIV have unmet needs regarding SRH. HIV care for adolescents should respond to a wide range of needs.

Background

Human immunodeficiency virus (HIV) care and antiretroviral therapy (ART) services have significantly reduced AIDS-related deaths [1]. Adolescents are defined as those aged 10–19 years by the World Health Organization (WHO) [2]. They are one of the vulnerable populations affected by HIV. In 2015, 1.8 million adolescents were living with HIV, and this number is still growing globally [3]. About half of them contracted HIV infections from their mothers [4], and HIV is the second most common cause of death among them [5]. Even though they are living with HIV, they are healthier and live longer than those in previous decades. However, staying healthy remains a great challenge due to delayed diagnosis, limited access to treatment, adherence to lifelong treatment, and chronic complications caused by treatment [6, 7].

Adolescents living with HIV face challenges such as recognition of HIV status, adherence to ART, mental health, and sexual and reproductive health (SRH) [8–11]. Rapid physical and psychosocial development throughout adolescence [5] could complicate such challenges. In addition, delayed puberty onset is commonly observed among perinatally-infected adolescents, which can result in low self-image, depression, and reproductive consequences [12]. For example, they make themselves targets for sexual abuse or they may easily engage in sexual intercourse to prove their worth. However, little evidence is available on sexual behaviors of adolescents living with HIV. In high-income counties, 27–46% of adolescents and young adults (ages 13–24) living with HIV have experienced sexual intercourse [13–16]. In low- and middle-income countries, it is less prevalent; for example, 25% of Ugandan adolescents and young adults (ages 11–21) and 5% of Thai adolescents (ages 11–18) living with HIV have experienced sexual intercourse [17, 18].

HIV infection affects primary needs of SRH during adolescence and adulthood. The WHO's definitions of sexual health and reproductive health emphasize "having pleasurable and safe sexual experiences, free of coercion, discrimination and violence" [19] and "having the capability to reproduce and the freedom to decide if, when and how often to do so" [20]. Although they are basic human needs, it would be difficult for people living with HIV to meet these needs. Adolescents may experience various threats such as the risk of HIV transmission to partners, difficulties in disclosing HIV status to an intimate partner, managing subsequent rejection by partners, and optimal and consistent use of condoms [21, 22]. They may be particularly vulnerable to the risk of unsafe sexual activity due to peer pressure, poverty, stigma about HIV, ignorance by sexual partners, and alcohol consumption [17].

Despite multiple barriers to meeting their SRH needs, most adolescents living with HIV, at least in the United States, intended to have children [14]. Although few studies have assessed adolescents' fertility intention in African countries, the rates of fertility intention among male and female adults were ranged between 37 and 51%, and the fertility intention was higher among those who were younger, had fewer children, were taking ART, and perceived themselves to have good health status [23–25]. However, the majority have not discussed their fertility intentions with health care workers [23, 25]. This implies that information and counselling on safe and timely pregnancy and childbirth are not widely provided to adolescents and adults living with HIV in African countries. The WHO has published two guidelines to promote client-friendly SRH services and respond to the complex needs of SRH and rights for adolescents living with HIV [2, 26]. However, little evidence is available to understand adolescents' needs regarding intimate relationships, sexual behavior, marriage, and fertility intention in African countries.

The republic of Zambia has been affected by a high burden of HIV. In 2016, an estimated 12.4% of the adult population was living with HIV while 11,000 adolescents were newly infected [3]. The majority of young adolescents contracted HIV through mother-to-child transmission [27] whereas older adolescents are more likely to get HIV infection through sexual transmission or other routes [4]. Major adolescent health issues in the country are lack of knowledge about HIV, early initiation of sexual intercourse, sexually transmitted diseases, and teenage pregnancy [28, 29]. Qualitative studies have identified the difficulties of disclosing HIV status to a partner [30] and the unmet needs for information on HIV and SRH among adolescents living with HIV [31]. More than 870 health care facilities provided HIV care and treatment services across the country [32], and 67% of adults and 52% of children were receiving ART in 2016 [3]. The University Teaching Hospital is the central hospital in the capital city of Lusaka, which houses the Paediatric and Adult Centers of Excellence in HIV care and treatment. Although HIV care and treatment services have become widely available in the country, the existing services do not address challenges and needs of adolescents adequately. Particularly, limited evidence is available on sexual behaviors and SRH needs, and the quality of care in this area remains underdeveloped. We conducted this study to assess sexual behavior and SRH needs among adolescents living with HIV in Zambia and to identify factors associated with having concerns about marriage and desire to have children.

Methods

Study design and setting

We conducted this cross-sectional study at the Paediatric HIV Centre of Excellence and the Adult HIV Centre of Excellence at the University Teaching Hospital from April to July 2014. The two centres are the national referral centres and the model hospitals for adolescent HIV care and treatment services. The two centres equip various specialists and infrastructure to provide care, laboratory test, treatment, counselling, social welfare services, and support peer group activities. The Paediatric Centre provides the services to children and adolescents and transfers them to the Adult Centre when they turn 16 years old. The Adult Centre provides continuous care and treatment service to the adolescents. Health care workers routinely offer information on SRH to all the adolescents aged 10 years or older when they attend their routine clinical reviews. For adolescents who reported risky sexual behaviors during a regular clinical review, health care workers provided counselling services on the details of SRH and family planning methods, gave them condoms, and suggested that they go for a free counselling and testing service for HIV with their partners.

Participants

The eligible study participants were adolescents aged 15–19 who were aware of their HIV status prior to the survey. Those aged 10–14 years were excluded from the study as SRH is a sensitive topic in Zambian culture, and it was deemed inappropriate to involve young adolescents in sexuality-related research.

We estimated a sample size of 165 to detect the association between educational experience and desire to have children based on a previous study that reported 55% prevalence of fertility intention among those with primary school education or higher and 32% among those with less than primary school education [25] using 5% of alpha, 80% of power, and 10% of potential missing data. However, we recruited 200 adolescents as the reference study used for the sample size estimation mainly targeted adults living with HIV. We did not use random sampling because reliable data of the target population and their contact information were not available during the study. We had a three-month data collection period to enroll at least 200 adolescents in the study as adolescent clients had review appointments every 3 months. We recruited the eligible adolescents when they came to the hospital for a clinical review appointment. Before recruiting adolescents, the research assistants asked health care workers or parents/primary caregivers to confirm the eligibility of the selected adolescents.

Data collection

We used a self-administered structured questionnaire for data collection. The questionnaire included basic characteristics of the participating adolescents, their sexual behavior, SRH issues, concerns about future marriage, and desire for having children, based on existing literature [14, 21, 22, 30, 31]. We developed the questionnaire in English because the study sample used English daily. Before the survey, we conducted a pre-test of the questionnaire to assess their English literacy, edited the questionnaire using simple English, and confirmed that the majority could self-administer the questionnaire. We trained research assistants who were peer educators working for adolescents' HIV care program at the study site. During the survey, respondents could ask the same-gender trained research assistants to help read-out in English or provide verbal translation into local language. Those who could not administer the questionnaire had an interview with the same-gender trained research assistants and responded everything except questions about sexual behavior.

Basic information included the adolescents' gender, age, level of education, survival statuses of parents, and status of taking ART. Regarding sexual behaviors, we first asked whether an adolescent had ever had sexual intercourse. For those who had experienced sexual intercourse, we asked for details about the first sexual intercourse including their age, the partners' age at that time, whether they had been aware of their HIV status, used a condom, and whether they were forced to have sexual intercourse. We also collected information on sexual experience in the preceding 12 months. For those who had had sexual intercourse during that period, we asked whether they disclosed their HIV status to their partner, knew their partners' HIV status before the intercourse, used a condom, and ever asked their partner to take an HIV test. We also asked for information about SRH including whether they had disclosed their HIV status to their intimate partners, who they were comfortable talking to about SRH issues, and whether they had learned about prevention of HIV infection with an intimate partner, the risk of infecting an intimate partner with HIV, how to disclose HIV status to others, and how to develop intimate relationships.

The study outcomes were having concerns (or anxieties) about marriage and a desire to have children in the future. First, we provided a structured question "Do you have any concerns about marriage?" in the questionnaire, and then asked to administer their specific concerns with a single English sentence. In the same way, we asked another structured question "Do you want to have children in the future?" followed by asking their reasons for wanting children.

Data analyses

For quantitative data, we first compared the distributions of background characteristics of the adolescents, their sexual behavior, and SRH issues using chi-square test. We then identified factors associated with having concerns about marriage and desire to have children by using the Generalized Linear Model. We included age, gender, education level, survival statuses of their parents, having someone to talk to about SRH issues, and having learned about four topics on SRH as independent variables of the models which were selected based on the existing literature [14, 23, 31, 33] and estimated crude and adjusted relative risks (RRs). We excluded missing data from the analyses and reported the number of respondents who declined to answer questions in the tables. We analyzed all the quantitative data using Stata (version 13.1).

For qualitative data, we performed thematic analysis to identify patterns of concerns about marriage and reasons they desired to have children. We followed the six phases in the data analysis process suggested by Braun [34]: (1) "familiarizing yourself with your data," (2) "generating initial codes," (3) "searching for themes," (4) "reviewing themes," (5) "defining and naming themes," and (6) "producing the report." Two authors (SO, KK) worked on Phases (1) and (2) independently and reviewed and discussed all codes to enhance reliability of the analyses. After that, the two authors conducted Phases (3), (4), and (5). Finally, SO conducted Phase (6). We manually analyzed all the qualitative data.

Ethical considerations

We obtained ethical approval from the Biomedical Research Ethics Committee of the University of Zambia and the Institutional Ethics Committee of National Center for Global Health and Medicine, Japan. We obtained written informed consent from all participants and written assent from parents or primary caregivers of adolescents aged 15, 16, and 17 years. We anticipated that adolescents may feel pressured to participate in the study as we recruited them at the hospital where they were receiving care. In addition, they may hesitate to respond about sexual behavior if they suspect the individual data could be shared with the hospital staff. To address these potential issues, we informed each adolescent about voluntary participation without any harm if they avail of care in the future and confidentiality in data management.

Results

We recruited 200 eligible adolescents in the study. We excluded two adolescents who withdrew during the survey and 15 adolescents who did not respond about their sexual behavior due to limited English literacy or voluntarily declined to answer. We excluded eight from the dataset because they were outside of the eligible criteria for age, although we asked their age at recruitment. Finally, we included the data of 175 adolescents in the analysis. Seventy-two (41.1%) were boys, and 103 (58.9%) were girls. Sixty-five percent had lost their fathers and/or mothers, and 94.3% were undergoing ART. No significant gender differences were found in the distributions of the basic characteristics (Table 1).

Table 2 shows the sexual behaviors of the adolescents. Thirty-six adolescents (20.6%) had ever experienced sexual intercourse with a mean age of 16.2 (SD 1.0) years among boys and 15.7 (SD 2.0) years among girls at the first intercourse ($p = .51$). Girls were more likely to have an older-aged partner than were boys ($p < .01$). Although 55.6% were already aware of their HIV status at the first intercourse, at least 33.3% did not use a condom. Only girls ($n = 4$) reported that their first sexual intercourse was forced. In the last 12 months prior to the survey, 22 adolescents (12.6%) reported having had sexual intercourse. Of the 22 adolescents, girls were more likely to disclose their HIV status to their partners ($p = .01$) and to know their partner's HIV status ($p = .05$) before engaging in the sexual relationship.

Table 3 shows the SRH issues of the adolescents. About half (48.8%) reported that they had concerns about marriage, and 87.4% desired to have children in the future with no significant gender differences. Twenty percent had disclosed their HIV status to their partners at least once. Higher proportions of the adolescents had learned about the prevention of HIV infection to a

Table 1 Basic characteristics of participants ($n = 175$)

	Total		Boys		Girls		
	$n = 175$		$n = 72$		$n = 103$		
	n	(%)	n	(%)	n	(%)	p
Age							
15 years	23	(13.1)	7	(9.7)	16	(15.5)	0.28
16 years	42	(24.0)	23	(31.9)	19	(18.5)	
17 years	38	(21.7)	13	(18.1)	25	(24.3)	
18 years	42	(24.0)	17	(23.6)	25	(24.3)	
19 years	30	(17.1)	12	(16.7)	18	(17.5)	
Educational experience							
Incomplete primary school	26	(14.9)	11	(15.3)	15	(14.6)	0.93
Completed primary school	88	(50.3)	35	(48.6)	53	(51.1)	
Completed secondary school or higher	61	(34.9)	26	(36.1)	35	(34.0)	
Parental survival status							
Both parents are alive	61	(34.9)	30	(41.7)	31	(30.1)	0.09
Mother was dead	34	(19.4)	13	(18.1)	21	(20.4)	
Father was dead	35	(20.0)	17	(23.6)	18	(17.5)	
Both parents were dead	45	(25.7)	12	(16.7)	33	(32.0)	
Currently taking ART							
Yes	165	(94.3)	70	(97.2)	95	(92.2)	0.16
No	10	(5.7)	2	(2.8)	8	(7.8)	

partner (82.9%) and the risk of HIV transmission to a partner (74.3%) compared with those who had learned about how to disclose their HIV status to others (58.9%) and how to develop intimate relationships (49.7%).

Table 4 shows the factors associated with having concerns about marriage ($n = 168$). Adolescents who wanted to have their own children were more likely to have concerns about their future marriage compared with those who did not desire to have children (Adjusted RR [ARR] = 2.51, 95% CI = 1.02 to 6.14). Table 5 shows the factors associated with desiring to have children ($n = 175$). The adolescents who had completed secondary school or higher were more likely to desire to have children than those who had not completed primary school (ARR = 1.35, 95% CI = 1.07 to 1.71). Adolescents whose parents were both dead were less likely to desire to have children compared with those whose parents were both alive (ARR = 0.80, 95% CI = 0.68 to 0.95).

Table 6 shows the adolescents' concerns or anxieties about future marriage. Out of 82 adolescents who reported that they were concerned about future marriage (Table 3), 63 (76.8%) described the specific concerns. The four major themes that emerged were: disclosing HIV status to partner, options in marriage, HIV transmission to partner and children. Adolescents were anxious about how to disclose HIV status to their intimate partners and their reactions afterwards: *"I wouldn't know how to tell him my HIV status if he is not HIV infected"* (Girl, age 15); *"If the person who will want to marry me finds out that I am HIV positive, he will change his mind about marrying me"* (Girl, age 17). Adolescents also worried about the risk of HIV transmission to their partners and children: *"Will I have to risk her health just for a child? If not, will she have to carry the burden with me?"* (Boy, age 19); *"Is there medicine that can reduce the risk of the baby contracting HIV from the mother?"* (Girl, age 17). To avoid infecting partner and children, some adolescents also considered remaining single or marrying a partner also living with HIV: *"I sometimes think it's better to remain single forever"* (Girl, age 18); *"I think I will have a wife who is (HIV) positive"* (Boy, age 17).

Table 7 shows the reasons why adolescents desired to have children. Out of 153 adolescents who showed the desires to have children in Tables 3, 102 (66.7%) explained the reasons. From the thematic analysis, four major reasons emerged: desire for parenting, children as family assets, positive perception on children, and natural matter. Some adolescents wished to become a parent: *"I want to know how it feels to be a mother"* (Girl, age 18). They expected to have children as household assets: *"I want them to help me when I get old"* (Girl, age 15); *"I want my family name to continue"* (Boy, age 17). Some adolescents showed their love for children and regarded children as sources of happiness

Table 2 Sexual behavior ($n = 175$)

	Total		Boys		Girls		
	n	(%)	n	(%)	n	(%)	p
First sexual experience							
Ever had sexual intercourse							
Yes	36	(20.6)	15	(20.8)	21	(20.4)	0.90
No	133	(76.0)	54	(75.0)	79	(76.7)	
Declined to answer	6	(3.4)	3	(4.2)	3	(2.9)	
Age at the first sexual intercourse ($n = 21$)	16.0	(1.6)	16.2	(1.0)	15.7	(2.0)	0.51
Partner's age at the first sexual intercourse ($n = 19$)	18.4	(3.0)	16.2	(2.6)	20.4	(1.8)	< 0.01
Already aware of HIV status ($n = 36$)							
Yes	20	(55.6)	6	(40.0)	14	(66.7)	0.19
No	11	(30.6)	7	(46.7)	4	(19.1)	
Declined to answer	5	(13.9)	2	(13.3)	3	(14.3)	
Used condom at first sexual intercourse ($n = 36$)							
Yes	16	(44.4)	6	(40.0)	10	(47.6)	0.77
No	12	(33.3)	6	(40.0)	6	(28.6)	
Declined to answer	8	(22.2)	3	(20.0)	5	(23.8)	
First sexual intercourse was forced ($n = 36$)							
Yes	4	(11.1)	0	(0.0)	4	(19.1)	0.17
No	25	(69.4)	11	(73.3)	14	(66.7)	
Declined to answer	7	(19.4)	4	(26.7)	3	(14.3)	
Sexual experience in the last 12 months							
Had sexual intercourse ($n = 175$)							
Yes	22	(12.6)	7	(9.7)	15	(14.6)	0.49
No	149	(85.1)	64	(88.9)	85	(82.5)	
Declined to answer	4	(2.3)	1	(1.4)	3	(2.9)	
Disclosed HIV status to partner in advance ($n = 22$)							
Yes	11	(50.0)	1	(14.3)	10	(66.7)	0.01
No	8	(36.4)	3	(42.9)	5	(33.3)	
Declined to answer	3	(13.6)	3	(42.9)	0	(0.0)	
Already knew partner's HIV status ($n = 22$)							
Yes	10	(45.5)	1	(14.3)	9	(60.0)	0.05
No	12	(54.6)	6	(85.7)	6	(40.0)	
Used condom ($n = 22$)							
Yes	12	(54.6)	5	(71.4)	7	(46.7)	0.53
No	6	(27.3)	1	(14.3)	5	(33.3)	
Declined to answer	4	(18.2)	1	(14.3)	3	(20.0)	
Asked partner for HIV testing ($n = 22$)							
Yes	7	(31.8)	1	(14.3)	6	(40.0)	0.38
No	9	(40.9)	3	(42.9)	6	(40.0)	
Declined to answer	6	(27.3)	3	(42.9)	3	(20.0)	

and joy in their lives: *"A child will bring happiness to me and my family"* (Girl, age 17). They also saw children as a blessing: *"Children all are wonderful gifts from God"* (Girl, age 19). Some adolescents stated that having children is a natural outcome of marriage and a human right: *"I am a human being and have the right to have a child. My (HIV-positive) status does not matter"* (Girl, age 17).

Table 3 Sexual and reproductive health needs

	Total		Boys		Girls		
	n	(%)	n	(%)	n	(%)	p
Have concerns about marriage (n = 168)							
Yes	82	(48.8)	31	(45.6)	51	(51.0)	0.49
No	86	(51.2)	37	(54.4)	49	(49.0)	
Desire to have children (n = 175)							
Yes	153	(87.4)	65	(90.3)	88	(85.4)	0.34
No	22	(12.6)	7	(9.7)	15	(14.6)	
Ever disclosed HIV status to an intimate partner (n = 172)							
Yes	35	(20.4)	14	(19.7)	21	(20.8)	0.48
No	71	(41.3)	33	(46.5)	38	(37.6)	
Never had an intimate partner	66	(38.4)	24	(33.8)	42	(41.6)	
Person to talk about SRH issues							
Friend	32	(18.3)	8	(11.1)	24	(23.3)	0.31
Mother	29	(16.6)	12	(16.7)	17	(16.5)	
Peers living with HIV	17	(9.7)	7	(9.7)	10	(9.7)	
Health care worker	7	(4.0)	2	(2.8)	5	(4.9)	
Other	64	(36.6)	32	(44.4)	32	(31.1)	
Nobody	26	(14.9)	11	(15.3)	15	(14.6)	
Education topics on HIV and SRH ever learned							
Preventing HIV transmission to partner							
Yes	145	(82.9)	60	(83.3)	85	(82.5)	0.89
No	30	(17.1)	12	(16.7)	18	(17.5)	
Risk of HIV transmission to partner							
Yes	130	(74.3)	52	(72.2)	78	(75.7)	0.60
No	45	(25.7)	20	(27.8)	25	(24.3)	
How to disclose HIV status to others							
Yes	103	(58.9)	40	(55.6)	63	(61.2)	0.46
No	72	(41.1)	32	(44.4)	40	(38.8)	
How to develop intimate relationships							
Yes	87	(49.7)	42	(58.3)	45	(43.7)	0.06
No	88	(50.3)	30	(41.7)	58	(56.3)	

Table 4 Factors associated with having concerns about marriage (n = 168)

	cRR	(95%CI)	aRR	(95%CI)
Age	0.99	(0.88–1.12)	1.11	(0.96–1.29)
Gender				
Boy	0.89	(0.65–1.24)	0.85	(0.62–1.15)
Girl	1.00		1.00	
Educational experience				
Incomplete primary school	1.00		1.00	
Completed primary school	1.55	(0.89–2.71)	1.50	(0.86–2.60)
Completed secondary school or higher	1.22	(0.67–2.23)	0.97	(0.51–1.83)
Parental survival status				
Both parents are alive	1.00		1.00	
Mother was dead	0.85	(0.55–1.32)	0.82	(0.53–1.27)
Father was dead	0.91	(0.60–1.37)	0.93	(0.64–1.35)
Both parents were dead	0.74	(0.48–1.13)	0.73	(0.48–1.12)
Have someone to talk about SRH issues				
Yes	1.20	(0.73–1.98)	1.25	(0.78–2.01)
No	1.00		1.00	
Learned about HIV and SRH				
0–3 items	1.00		1.00	
4 items	0.78	(0.55–1.12)	0.80	(0.55–1.17)
Want to have my children				
Yes	2.64	(1.08–6.43)	2.51	(1.02–6.14)
No	1.00		1.00	

Age is a continuous variable. cRR and aRR mean the crude and adjusted relative risk

Discussion

Twenty percent of the adolescents in our sample had experienced sexual intercourse, and at least 30% of them did not use a condom during the first intercourse. Nearly half of the adolescents expressed concerns about their future marriage. In contrast, the majority of them desired to have their own children in the future. Those who desired to have children were more likely to worry about their marriage. To the best of our knowledge, this is the first quantitative evidence built on the existing study findings in Zambia [30, 31].

Adolescents in the study were less likely to have had sexual intercourse (20.6%) compared with the adolescents (ages 15–19) in the national representative data (49.1% among girls and 47.7% among boys) [29]. Similarly, in the United States, perinatally HIV-infected youths were less likely to practice sexual intercourse compared with uninfected youths [35]. However, it should be highlighted that sexually active adolescents in this study engaged in risky sexual intercourse; nearly 30% did not use a condom during their first intercourse and recent intercourse. Moreover, sexual intercourse commonly took place without recognizing the HIV status, particularly among HIV-positive boys and their partners. In addition, girls had relatively older partners and tended to have forced intercourse. This indicates that girls could be particularly vulnerable to control by their partners' demands for unprotected intercourse. Both girls and boys were sexually active, but the

Table 5 Factors associated with desiring to have children (n = 175)

	cRR	95%CI	aRR	95%CI
Age	1.01	(0.97–1.05)	0.97	(0.92–1.03)
Gender				
Boy	1.06	(0.95–1.18)	1.02	(0.92–1.14)
Girl	1.00		1.00	
Educational experience				
Incomplete primary school	1.00		1.00	
Completed primary school	1.11	(0.88–1.39)	1.17	(0.94–1.45)
Completed secondary school or higher	1.24	(0.99–1.54)	1.35	(1.07–1.71)
Parental survival status				
Both parents are alive	1.00		1.00	
Mother was dead	0.90	(0.77–1.04)	0.88	(0.76–1.03)
Father was dead	0.93	(0.82–1.06)	0.92	(0.81–1.05)
Both parents were dead	0.82	(0.69–0.97)	0.80	(0.68–0.95)
Have someone to talk about SRH issues				
Yes	1.10	(0.90–1.34)	1.10	(0.90–1.34)
No	1.00		1.00	
Learned about HIV and SRH				
0–3 items	1.00		1.00	
4 items	1.02	(0.90–1.14)	1.00	(0.88–1.15)

Age is a continuous variable. cRR and aRR mean the crude and adjusted relative risk

Table 6 Concerns about future marriage

Main theme	Sub-theme
Disclosing HIV status to partner	Do not know how to disclose my HIV status to partner
	Concern about partner''s reaction after disclosing my HIV status
Options in marriage	Not getting married may be better
	HIV-positive partner may be suitable
HIV transmission to partner	Don''t know how to protect partner from HIV infection
	Concern about the risk of HIV transmission to partner
HIV transmission to children	Don''t know how to protect children from HIV infection
	Concern about the risk of HIV transmission to children

Out of 82 adolescents who had concerns about future marriage, 63 (76.8%) provided open-ended answers to explain the specific concerns or anxieties

Table 7 Reasons that adolescents desire to have children

Main theme	Sub-theme
Desire for parenting	Desire for becoming a parent
	Desire for taking care of children
Children as family assets	Children as my caretakers
	Children as the successors of family
Positive perception on children	Love for children
	Happiness brought by children
	Blessing from God
Natural matter	Natural outcome of marriage
	Human right

Out of 153 adolescents who desired to have children in the future, 102 (66.7%) explained the reasons

and the risk of HIV transmission. This indicates that adolescents were facing a dual pressure with rejection and infection in intimate relationships. Similar findings have been reported in Canada, the United States, and Rwanda [21, 22, 36]. Most adolescents in this study had learned about the risk of HIV transmission and the preventive methods, but they had limited information on the ways to develop intimate partnerships and disclose HIV status to others. In addition, health care workers were less utilized as primary counsellors or advisors for their SRH issues. Health care workers should make further effort to develop a better relationship with adolescents and provide them with comprehensive information on SRH.

Most of the adolescents expressed the desire to have children. They felt that having children has an important meaning in their adulthood. It means that they can achieve their dreams and happiness, secure family assets, and that it is human nature and their right. On the other hand, they were afraid of HIV transmission to their children and had insufficient knowledge about prevention of mother-to-child transmission. Similarly, in the United States and Rwanda, a strong fear of mother-to-child transmission was associated with lower intention to have children [14, 36]. In this study, adolescents who had lost both parents were less likely to desire to have their own children. Loss of parents is linked to multiple negative consequences: psychological distress, caretaking responsibility for younger siblings, dropping out of school, and vulnerability to sexually transmitted diseases and early pregnancy [33, 37, 38]. Due to such childhood experiences and uncertain life expectancy due to being affected by HIV, orphaned adolescents may have a lower motivation to have their own children. Adolescents who completed secondary education had a higher intention to have children. Educational experience is known as a protective factor against health risks in adolescence [39]. On the other hand, those who did not complete primary education had a passive desire for having children. This

process or context of engaging in sexual relationships was not the same.

Adolescents' concerns about marriage were not related only to marriage. Their concerns were widely associated with intimate relationships—namely, disclosing their HIV status to partners, potential rejection afterwards, may indicate that they had limited access to information and/or low literacy about SRH. Orphaned or low-educated adolescents need special support for their proactive choice of future pregnancy and childbirth.

Adolescents showed unmet SRH needs about intimate and sexual relationships, marriage, pregnancy, and childbirth. However, the current HIV care and treatment services for adolescents do not fully respond to their needs. The health care workers must make more efforts to reach all adolescents regardless of their gender, socio-economic status (e.g. family structure, educational level), and childhood background. Education and counselling should primarily emphasize basic prevention of HIV transmission for safe sexual relationships while considering gender sensitivity and vulnerability. In addition, information on the benefits and risks of disclosing HIV status to a partner should be provided. Follow-up counselling after self-disclosure is also essential for those in psychological distress facing negative outcomes of disclosure. To respond to the complicated SRH needs of adolescents, training on adolescent-centered SRH care should be offered to health care workers. In addition, many Zambians experience the first marriage and pregnancy in late adolescence or early adulthood. It will be beneficial for adolescents to discuss and prepare for safe pregnancy and childbirth in collaboration with family planning and prevention of mother-to-child transmission of HIV programs.

This study has several limitations. First, the generalizability of the study findings is limited as we conducted the study at a tertiary hospital in the national capital with no comparison groups. Second, convenience sampling for recruiting study participants at regular clinical reviews may have contributed to selection bias, because adolescents with no access or no compliance with care were not included in the study, but they would have different patterns of sexual behaviors and different needs regarding SRH. Third, we did not collect data on marital status or route of HIV transmission, which could influence to sexual behavior. Further studies at multiple sites with various target populations would be recommended, and sub-group analysis by geographical area, compliance with care, marital status, and the routes of HIV transmission could provide the study results more clearly. Third, we collected information on sensitive issues about sexual behaviors, which may lead to under-reporting and an increase in missing data. Thus, the study findings could be under-estimated and should not be simply compared with results in other settings. The future study needs to use anonymous survey methods, such as computer-assisted survey. Fourth, the small sample size may limit the power to identify significant associations between participants' characteristics and the study outcome. Despite the limitations, this study used quantitative and qualitative data and identified the knowledge gaps in how HIV infection affects current and future SRH and well-being among adolescents.

Conclusions

Zambian adolescents living with HIV were sexually active. In addition, they were highly concerned about future marriage and fertility opportunities due to potential refusal by their partners and the risks of HIV transmission to their partners and children. HIV care and treatment services should cover a wider area of SRH needs and reach all adolescents regardless of their socio-demographic and -economic backgrounds.

Abbreviations
ART: Antiretroviral therapy; HIV: Human immunodeficiency virus; SRH: Sexual and reproductive health; WHO: World Health Organization

Acknowledgements
The authors would like to thank all study participants, research assistants, and health care workers at University Teaching Hospital for supporting this study. We are grateful to Dr. Kenichi Komada for his technical assistance.

Funding
This work was supported by The Grant for National Center for Global Health and Medicine (26–2 and 28–1).

Authors' contributions
SO, NI, SMK, MM, and CK conceived and designed the study and implemented the survey. SO analyzed the quantitative and qualitative data and drafted the manuscript. KK analyzed the qualitative data. NI, SMK, and MJ critically reviewed the manuscript. All authors approved submission of the manuscript.

Competing interests
The authors declare that they have no competing interests.

Author details
[1]Department of Community and Global Health, Graduate School of Medicine, The University of Tokyo, Tokyo, Japan. [2]Department of Educational Psychology, Sociology, and Special Education, School of Education, University of Zambia, Lusaka, Zambia. [3]Paediatric HIV Centre of Excellence, University Teaching Hospital, Lusaka, Zambia. [4]Institute of Decision Science for a Sustainable Society, Kyushu University, Fukuoka, Japan. [5]Bureau of International Health Cooperation, National Center for Global Health and Medicine, Tokyo, Japan.

References
1. UNAIDS. The gap report. Geneva: UNAIDS; 2014.
2. WHO. HIV and adolescents: guidance for HIV testing and counselling and care for adolescents living with HIV: recommendations for a public health approach and considerations for policy-makers and managers. Geneva: WHO; 2013.

3. UNAIDS. AIDSinfo. No date. http://aidsinfo.unaids.org/#. Accessed 29 Sep 2017.
4. UNICEF. 2014 annual results report: HIV and AIDS. New York: UNICEF; 2014.
5. WHO. Health for the world's adolescents: a second chance in the second decade. Geneva: WHO; 2014.
6. Ferrand RA, Munaiwa L, Matsekete J, Bandason T, Nathoo K, Ndhlovu CE, et al. Undiagnosed HIV infection among adolescents seeking primary health care in Zimbabwe. Clin Infect Dis. 2010;51(7):844–51.
7. Mofenson LM, Cotton MF. The challenges of success: adolescents with perinatal HIV infection. J Int AIDS Soc. 2013;16:18650.
8. Gray GE. Adolescent HIV–cause for concern in southern Africa. PLoS Med. 2010;7(2):e1000227.
9. Koenig LJ, Nesheim S, Abramowitz S. Adolescents with perinatally acquired HIV: emerging behavioral and health needs for long-term survivors. Curr Opin Obstet Gynecol. 2011;23(5):321–7.
10. Agwu AL, Fairlie L. Antiretroviral treatment, management challenges and outcomes in perinatally HIV-infected adolescents. J Int AIDS Soc. 2013;16:18579.
11. Mellins CA, Malee KM. Understanding the mental health of youth living with perinatal HIV infection: lessons learned and current challenges. J Int AIDS Soc. 2013;16:18593.
12. Williams PL, Abzug MJ, Jacobson DL, Wang J, Van Dyke RB, Hazra R, et al. Pubertal onset in children with perinatal HIV infection in the era of combination antiretroviral treatment. AIDS. 2013;27(12):1959–70.
13. Koenig LJ, Pals SL, Chandwani S, Hodge K, Abramowitz S, Barnes W, et al. Sexual transmission risk behavior of adolescents with HIV acquired perinatally or through risky behaviors. J Acquir Immune Defic Syndr. 2010; 55(3):380–90.
14. Ezeanolue EE, Wodi AP, Patel R, Dieudonne A, Oleske JM. Sexual behaviors and procreational intentions of adolescents and young adults with perinatally acquired human immunodeficiency virus infection: experience of an urban tertiary center. J Adolesc Health. 2006;38:719–25.
15. Wiener LS, Battles HB, Wood LV. A longitudinal study of adolescents with perinatally or transfusion acquired HIV infection: sexual knowledge, risk reduction self-efficacy and sexual behavior. AIDS Behav. 2007;11(3):471–8.
16. Brogly SB, Watts DH, Ylitalo N, Franco EL, Seage GR 3rd, Oleske J, et al. Reproductive health of adolescent girls perinatally infected with HIV. Am J Public Health. 2007;97:1047–52.
17. Bakeera-Kitaka S, Nabukeera-Barungi N, Nostlinger C, Addy K, Colebunders R. Sexual risk reduction needs of adolescents living with HIV in a clinical care setting. AIDS Care. 2008;20(4):426–33.
18. Lolekha R, Boon-Yasidhi V, Leowsrisook P, Naiwatanakul T, Durier Y, Nuchanard W, et al. Knowledge, attitudes, and practices regarding antiretroviral management, reproductive health, sexually transmitted infections, and sexual risk behavior among perinatally HIV-infected youth in Thailand. AIDS Care. 2015;27(5):618–28.
19. WHO. Sexual health. 2017. http://www.who.int/topics/sexual_health/en/. Assessed 20 Dec 2017.
20. WHO. Reproductive health. 2017. http://www.who.int/topics/reproductive_health/en/. Accessed 20 Dec 2017.
21. Fernet M, Wong K, Richard ME, Otis J, Levy JJ, Lapointe N, et al. Romantic relationships and sexual activities of the first generation of youth living with HIV since birth. AIDS Care. 2011;23:393–400.
22. Fair C, Albright J. "Don't tell him you have HIV unless he's 'the one'": romantic relationships among adolescents and young adults with perinatal HIV infection. AIDS Patient Care STDs. 2012;26(12):746–54.
23. Cooper D, Moodley J, Zweigenthal V, Bekker LG, Shah I, Myer L. Fertility intentions and reproductive health care needs of people living with HIV in cape town, South Africa: implications for integrating reproductive health and HIV care services. AIDS Behav. 2009;13(Suppl 1):38–46.
24. Mmbaga EJ, Leyna GH, Ezekiel MJ, Kakoko DC. Fertility desire and intention of people living with HIV/AIDS in Tanzania: a call for restructuring care and treatment services. BMC Public HealthBMC Public Health. 2013;13:86.

25. Kawale P, Mindry D, Stramotas S, Chilikoh P, Phoya A, Henry K, et al. Factors associated with desire for children among HIV-infected women and men: a quantitative and qualitative analysis from Malawi and implications for the delivery of safer conception counseling. AIDS Care. 2014;26(6):769–76.
26. WHO. Consolidated guideline on sexual and reproductive health and rights of women living with HIV. Geneva: WHO; 2017.
27. Menon A, Glazebrook C, Campain N, Ngoma M. Mental health and disclosure of HIV status in Zambian adolescents with HIV infection: implications for peer-support programs. J Acquir Immune Defic Syndr. 2007;46(3):349–54.
28. National AIDS Council, Ministry of Health, Ministry of Community Development Mother and Child Health. Zambia country report: monitoring the declaration of commitment on HIV and AIDS and the Universal access: biennial report. Lusaka: National AIDS Council; 2014.
29. Central Statistical Office (CSO) [Zambia], Ministry of Health (MOH) [Zambia], ICF International. Zambia Demographic and Health Survey 2013--14. Rockville: Central Statistical Office, Ministry of Health, ICF-International; 2014.
30. Mburu G, Hodgson I, Kalibala S, Haamujompa C, Cataldo F, Lowenthal ED, et al. Adolescent HIV disclosure in Zambia: barriers, facilitators and outcomes. J Int AIDS Soc. 2014;17:18866.
31. Hodgson I, Ross J, Haamujompa C, Gitau-Mburu D. Living as an adolescent with HIV in Zambia – lived experiences, sexual health and reproductive needs. AIDS Care. 2012;24(10):1204–10.
32. National HIV, AIDS STI, TB Council. National HIV AIDS strategic framework 2017--2021. Lusaka: National HIV AIDS STI TB Council; 2017.
33. Cluver LD, Orkin M, Gardner F, Boyes ME. Persisting mental health problems among AIDS-orphaned children in South Africa. J Child Psychol Psychiatry. 2012;53(4):363–70.
34. Braun V, Clarke V. Using thematic analysis in Psychology. Qual Res Psychol. 2006;3(2):77–101.
35. Elkington KS, Bauermeister JA, Robbins RN, Gromadzka O, Abrams EJ, Wiznia A, et al. Individual and contextual factors of sexual risk behavior in youth perinatally infected with HIV. AIDS Patient Care STDS. 2012;26(7):411–22.
36. Van Nuil JI, Mutwa P, Asiimwe-Kateera B, Kestelyn E, Vyankandondera J, Pool R, et al. "Let's talk about sex": a qualitative study of Rwandan adolescents' views on sex and HIV. PLoS One. 2014;9(8):e102933.
37. Kang M, Dunbar M, Laver S, Padian N. Maternal versus paternal orphans and HIV/STI risk among adolescent girls in Zimbabwe. AIDS Care. 2008;20(2):214–7.
38. Bazile J, Rigodon J, Berman L, Boulanger VM, Maistrellis E, Kausiwa P, et al. Intergenerational impacts of maternal mortality: Qualitative findings from rural Malawi. Reprod Health. 2015;12(Suppl 1):S1.
39. Viner RM, Ozer EM, Denny S, Marmot M, Resnick M, Fatusi A, et al. Adolescence and the social determinants of health. Lancet. 2012;379(9826):1641–52.

9

Prevalence and associated factors of risky sexual behaviors among undergraduate students in state universities of Western Province in Sri Lanka

Upuli Amaranganie Pushpakumari Perera[1]* and Chrishantha Abeysena[2]

Abstract

Background: Risky sexual behaviors (RSB) are becoming an important problem all over the world. RSB are defined as behaviors leading to sexually transmitted diseases and unintended pregnancies. The objective of this study was to determine the prevalence and associated factors of RSB among undergraduate students in state universities of Western Province in Sri Lanka.

Methods: A descriptive cross sectional study was conducted on1575 second and third year undergraduates using stratified cluster sampling of the selected universities. A pretested self-administered questionnaire was used to assess socio-demographic, knowledge attitudes and behavior on reproductive health. RSB was defined as reporting of one or more following behavior/s; having more than one sexual partner, use of alcohol or inability to use condom or other contraceptive methods in sexual activities. The results were expressed as prevalence and its 95% confidence interval (CI) of RSB. Multiple logistic regression was performed ascertain the association between RSB and possible associated factors. The results were expressed as adjusted odds ratios (AOR).

Results: Prevalence of RSB in last 1 year and 3 months periods were 12.4%, (95% CI: 11.8–13.1) and 12.1% (95% CI: 11.5–12.7) respectively. The significantly associated risk factors for RSB were, attended night clubs in last month (AOR = 3.58, 95% CI: 1.29–9.88), alcohol consumption within last 3 months (AOR = 2.67, 95% CI: 1.87–3.80) and good knowledge on condoms (AOR = 2.82, 95% CI: 1.94–4.10). Those who thought religion was very important to their lives (AOR = 0.68, 95% CI: 0.48–0.95) was a protective factor.

Conclusions: Alcohol consumption and attending night clubs were associated with RSB. Necessary measures should be taken to reduce risk behaviors within university to reduce RSB.

Keywords: Attitudes, Knowledge, Reproductive, Sexual, Undergraduates

* Correspondence: tauapp100@gmail.com
[1]Postgraduate Institute of Medicine, University of Colombo, 36/1, Naiwala, Essalla, Veyangoda, Sri Lanka
Full list of author information is available at the end of the article

Plain English summary

Risky sexual behaviors (RSB) are defined as behaviors leading to sexually transmitted diseases and unintended pregnancies. Currently about 100,000 undergraduate students studying at state universities in Sri Lanka who may be at risk of practicing RSB. This study seeks to determine the prevalence of such behaviors among this group of students.

Data were collected from second and third year undergraduate students with a questionnaire on sexual behaviors, other risk behaviors, knowledge and attitudes on sexual and reproductive health. Of students surveyed 12.4% were found to practice RSB within the last 1 year period. Several other behaviors such as alcohol consumption within the last 3 months, attending night clubs in last month and those with good knowledge on condoms were associated with RSB. Those who thought religion was very important to their lives were less likely to practice RSB. Suggestions were made to take necessary steps to minimize alcohol consumption within university and outside, to discourage night clubs attendance by facilitating more recreational activities and to promote religious activities.

Background

Risky sexual behaviors (RSB) are becoming an important problem all over the world. The Centers for Disease Control and Prevention (CDC) defines RSB as Sexual behaviors leading to unintended pregnancies and sexually transmitted infections (STI) include Human immuno-deficiency Virus (HIV) and acquired immuno-deficiency syndrome (AIDS) [1]. It includes having multiple sexual partners, having sex without using a condom or other contraceptive method. In addition to that, several authors have included the following factors in to their definition of RSB: initiation of first sex at early age before 18 years [2, 3], sexual activity done under the influence of alcohol and anal intercourse [4], sexual violence and transactional sex [3] and paid sex [5].

There is limited literature on sexual practices among various population groups in Sri Lanka. The prevalence of risk behavior among adolescents and young adults was higher than the expected level by parents and teachers [6–8]. Global prevalence studies including other Asian countries would give a better estimate of considerably higher RSB in undergraduates [9, 10]. There is a vast amount of literature on undergraduates' RSB in African countries indicating that higher prevalence of RSB among them ranging from 7 to 47% [11–17].

Known socio-demographic and economic risk factors associated with RSB are male sex [11, 12, 18], smoking [8, 20], night club attendance [11] and alcohol use [8, 9, 19–21]. In contrast, having a good relationship with friends, peers and parents [9], as well as religiosity [12, 22] have been found to be a protective measure against RSB.

There are more than 105,000 youths studying in universities in Sri Lanka where the majority are not in a relationship [23]. University life is a shift towards greater freedom from family and school backgrounds for most of them. It provides an opportunity to practice new friendships, social mixing and consequently to engage in risky behaviors including RSB [9]. The findings of this study could potentially support to develop programs to reduce RSB and to improve the knowledge and practices via the existing system of tertiary education. Therefore we conducted this study to determine the prevalence and factors associated with RSB among undergraduates in the state universities of the Western Province in Sri Lanka.

Methods

Study design

An institution-based descriptive cross-sectional study was conducted in four state universities in the Western Province of Sri Lanka (Univeristy of Colombo, University of Sri Jayewardenepura, University of Kelaniya and University of Moratuwa), representing around 17% of total undergraduates enrolled in state universities in the country.

Study population

The study population was undergraduate students studying in second and third years which were 18,280 in number [23]. Undergraduates from foreign countries and clergymen undergraduates were excluded. First year students were excluded as they are new to the environment. So their risk behaviors may not be due to as the same factors as second and third year students. Fourth and fifth year students were excluded as these advanced years are not conducted in every course. Exclusion of foreign students was done due to their different socio-cultural background.

Sample size and sampling technique

Calculated sample size was 1314 with expected prevalence of 13% of heterosexual intercourse without condoms among unmarried, out of school adolescents [7], 1.96 Z value, 3% of precision and a correction for design effect of 2.45 [24, 25] and 10% of non-respondents.

A multistage cluster sampling technique with probability proportional to size (PPS) was used to select a representative sample of undergraduates (Fig. 1). A cluster was defined as a tutorial group or a whole batch according to the structure of the selected undergraduates group. The average cluster size was considered as 30.

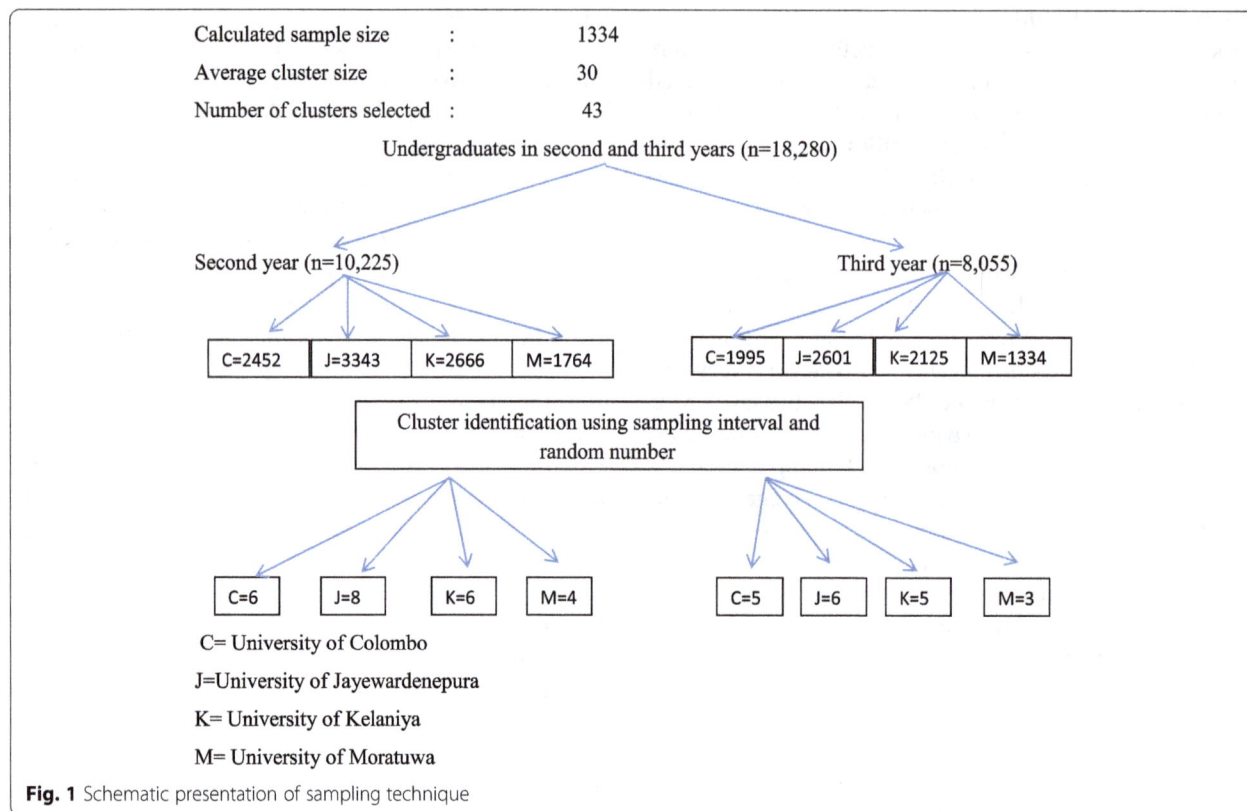

Calculated sample size	:	1334
Average cluster size	:	30
Number of clusters selected	:	43

Fig. 1 Schematic presentation of sampling technique

Then we allocated the clusters for each academic year and university according to the proportion of undergraduates. Undergraduates were stratified according to their respective university and academic years and academic streams. Finally clusters were identified within each stratum based on PPS according to the number of students in each university and academic year.

Data collection

Data were collected on socio-demographic factors, other risk behaviors including consumption of alcohol, smoking and using narcotic drugs, sexual behavior and knowledge and attitudes in selected aspects of reproductive health (RH) among undergraduates. Sri Lanka Behavioral Surveillance Survey questionnaire [26], Youth risk behavior surveillance questionnaire used by CDC [1] and Illustrative Questionnaire for Interview Surveys with Young People [27] were used as guides to develop the questionnaire.

The validity of the questionnaire was ensured by assessing the judgmental validity which included face, content and consensual validity. Validity was determined by assessing the agreement of the experts on whether or not the conceptual definition has been used appropriately in the tool. A multi-disciplinary panel of experts in the fields of public health,

reproductive health and language was used for assessment of validity. The questionnaire was forward-translated into Sinhala and back-translated to English. Data were collected using a pre-tested self-administrative questionnaire after obtaining permission. The filled questionnaires in an envelope were collected by trained research assistant. The data collection procedure was supervised by the first author. Informed written consent was obtained from the participants. Ethical clearance was taken from the Ethical Review Committee, Faculty of Medicine, University of Kelaniya.

Knowledge on some aspects of RH was measured with statements on unsafe abortions, contraceptives including condoms, STIs including HIV/AIDS and sexual and RH rights. Attitudes on RH was measured with statements on contraceptives, condoms and HIV/AIDS which contained five responses; strongly agree, agree, neutral, disagree and strongly disagree.

RSB was defined as reporting one or more following behavior/s; having more than one sexual partner, alcohol use with sexual activities, inability to use condom to prevent STI in sexual activities with commercial sex workers or non-commercial partners, unable to use contraceptive methods to prevent unintended pregnancy in sexual activities with commercial sex workers or non-commercial partners. RSB was defined as for the last 1 year and the last 3 months separately.

Data analysis

Data were analyzed with Statistical Package for Social Science (SPSS) (Version 16). Prevalence and 95% confidence interval (CI) of RSB were calculated for last 1 year and last 3 months periods separately. Sex specific RSB and university specific RSB was calculated for last 3 months period. To ascertain the association between RSB and other variables binary logistic regression was performed. Variables with p value less than or equal to 0.20 at binary were entered into multiple logistic regression analysis. Hosmer Lemshow goodness of fit with backward elimination was used to test for model fitness. Variables with p value of < 0.05 at multiple regression were considered as statistically significant. The results were expressed as Odds Ratio (OR) and adjusted odds ratios (AOR).

Results

Background information

The study sample consisted of 1575 undergraduates from four state universities in the Western Province. Majority of respondents were females ($n = 926$, 58.8%) and unmarried (98.5%, $n = 1551$). Mean age was 23 (SD = 0.9) years. The sample consisted more Sinhalese (94.1%, $n = 1480$) than non-Sinhalese and Buddhists (89.8%, $n = 1414$) than non-Buddhists. Socio-demographic factors are shown in Table 1.

The prevalence of RSB

The prevalence of RSB among undergraduates were 12.4% ($n = 196$;, 95% CI: 11.8–13.1) and 12.1% ($n = 190$, 95% CI: 11.5–12.7) for last 1 year and last 3 months respectively. The highest percentage (16.8%, $n = 57$) of undergraduates with RSB was in University of Kelaniya followed by University of Sri Jayewardenepura (12.5%, $n = 72$). Males (19.1, 95% CI 16.1–22.2) had more RSB than females (7.2, 95% CI 5.5–8.9) ($p < 0.001$).

Sexual behavior of the participants

In the study sample 21.2% ($n = 334$) reported ever having had sexual exposure. Males (32.7%, $n = 211$) had more ever sexual exposure than females (13.1%, $n = 122$) ($p < 0.001$). Majority of undergraduates (63.9%, $n = 205$) who ever had sexual exposure experienced their first intercourse after 20 years of age. More females (75%, $n = 87$) than males (57.8%, $n = 118$) had their first sexual exposure before the age of 20 years ($p = 0.002$). Out of 334 undergraduates had sexual exposure ever, 3.3% ($n = 11$) stated that their first sexual experience was a forced sex. Majority

(75.4%, $n = 252$) of the respondent's first sexual partner was a girl/boyfriend.

Out of 334 with had ever sexual exposure only 18% ($n = 60$) of the respondents had used condoms in first sexual intercourse while only 1.5% ($n = 5$) of the respondents had used alcohol in first sexual intercourse. Out of all undergraduates, 13.7% ($n = 216$) had more than one life time sexual partners.

Percentage of undergraduates who had sexual intercourse within last 1 year was 87.7% ($n = 293$) out of 334 respondents who ever had sex. Majority of them had one sexual partner irrespective of whether they have engaged in sexual intercourse in last 1 year or last 3 months. Ninety four (5.96%) and 79 (5.01%) respondents had multiple sexual partners within last 1 year and 3 months respectively. The majority (85.8%, $n = 176$) of undergraduates those who had sexual intercourse within last 1 year had not used condoms in their last sexual activity. Out of 17 undergraduates that had sexual intercourse with commercial sex worker, 58.8% ($n = 10$) had used condom at their last sexual activity. The percentage used condoms at last sex with non-commercial sex partners were 12.4% ($n = 24$).

Factors associated with RSB in bivariate analysis

Being a male undergraduate and belonging to Sinhala ethnicity showed significant association with RSB in bivariate analysis. As shown in Table 2, RSB for last 3 months was negatively associated with engaging more religious activities and considering religion as more important to their lives. Having to the opportunity to talk with parents and siblings regarding sexual problems showed negative association with RSB.

Further, RSB were significantly associated with undergraduates who attended nightclubs more than once within last month, those who had used internet facilities > 2 h per day, those who went to cinema ≥2 per months, who had taken alcohol within last 3 months, who had smoked within last 3 months, who had taken ganja (cannabis) within last 3 months and who had physical fight within last 1 year in university (Table 3).

Good knowledge on contraceptives, good knowledge on condoms, good knowledge on sexual and RH rights, good overall knowledge on RH, favorable attitudes on contraceptives, favorable attitudes on condoms and favorable overall attitudes on RH showed statistically significant associations in bivariate analysis with RSB (Table 4).

Factors associated with RSB in multivariate analysis

Multiple logistic regression model included 1575 participants. RSB during the last 3 months showed significant association with four factors. Those who had taken alcohol within last 3 months (AOR 2.59, 95% CI: 1.82–3.70),

Table 1 Socio-demographic characteristics among the undergraduates

Characteristics		Frequency	Percentage
Sex	Male	645	41.0
	Female	926	58.8
Age (in years)	21	20	1.3
	22	449	28.5
	23	696	44.2
	24	307	19.5
	25	83	5.3
	26	11	0.7
Academic year	Second	930	59.0
	Third	645	41.0
University	Kelaniya	339	21.5
	Sri Jayewardenepura	576	36.6
	Colombo	353	22.4
	Moratuwa	307	19.5
Nationality	Sinhalese	1480	94.1
	Tamil	58	3.7
	Muslims	33	2.1
	Other	1	0.1
Religion	Buddhism	1414	89.8
	Roman Catholic	65	4.1
	Non Roman Catholic Christian	6	0.4
	Islam	45	2.9
	Hindu	39	2.5
	Other	3	0.2
Residence	Own home	453	28.8
	Relative's house	36	2.3
	University hostel	411	26.1
	Boarding place	671	42.6
Academic streams	Art	516	32.8
	Commerce	424	26.9
	Bio Science	248	15.7
	Mathematics	387	24.6
Type of School	Boys'	262	21.0
	Girls'	345	27.6
	Mixed	642	51.4
Marital status	Single	1551	98.5
	Married	13	0.8
	Divorced	1	0.1
	Separated	1	0.1
	Living together	5	0.3

those who had attended nightclub more than once in last month (AOR 3.61; 95% CI: 1.31–9.97), and those who had good knowledge on condoms (AOR 2.91, 95% CI: 2.00–4.24), showed positive association with RSB. Those who considered the religion to be important to their lives (AOR 0.67, 95% CI: 0.48–0.95), showed negative association with RSB. (Table 5) Reanalysis of data excluding the variable 'use of alcohol within last three months' had not changed the results.

Discussion
In this study an attempt has been made to assess the prevalence of RSB and factors associated to RSB among undergraduate students in state universities of Western Province in Sri Lanka.

Prevalence of RSB
The prevalence of RSB was 12.4 and 12.1% for last 1 year period and for last 3 months period respectively. Prevalence among male and female undergraduates were 19.1 and 7.2% respectively. A study carried out among first year Agricultural undergraduates of University of Ruhuna, Sri Lanka reported that 2% had multiple sexual partners during last 3 months which was considered as a risk behavior [28]. In the present study, having multiple partners during last 3 months was 5% and the observed difference may be due to the difference of the sample selected i.e. second and third year representing all study streams from four universities. Another study carried out among Ethiopian undergraduates revealed that 18.6% of them had lifetime multiple sexual partners which was 13.7% in the present study [29]. Their use of condoms during first sexual intercourse was 11.2%, much lower than the present 18% figure. Their figure for not using condoms within the last 1 year period was 39.4% from those who had sex in last 1 year. In the present study, not using condoms in last sexual activity was 85.8% which was much higher. The figure may be due to the reason that our young people are having "somewhat mutually monogamous" relationships which they would think the need of condom use is unnecessary.

Factors associated with RSB
In the present study, those who had good knowledge on condoms showed a positive association with RSB. This finding was in line with a study carried out in Washington which discussed an association with knowledge on condoms and condom usage. Failure to use protective method in risk behavior may not be due to the ignorance but may be the inability of perceiving the risk [30]. Undergraduates who had experienced or are interested in sexual behaviors may be enthusiastic in finding more information on preventive measures of STI i.e. usage of

Table 2 Unadjusted odds ratios for association of risky sexual behavior with socio-demographic, social and economic factors

Factors	Risky sexual behavior		OR	p value
	Yes No (%)	No No (%)	(95%CI)	
Sex				
Male	123 (64.7)	522 (37.8)	3.02 (2.20–4.15)	< 0.001
Female	67 (35.3)	859 (62.2)	Reference	
Age				
≤ 22 yrs	55 (29.3)	414 (30.0)	1.04 (0.74–1.45)	0.83
> 23 yrs	133 (70.7)	964 (70.0)	Ref	
Residence				
Outside home	137 (72.1)	948 (68.5)	1.19 (0.85–1.66)	0.31
In home	53 (27.9)	436 (31.5)	Ref	
Religion				
Buddhist	176 (92.6)	1238 (89.4)	1.50 (0.84–2.64)	0.17
Non-Buddhists	14 (7.4)	147(10.6)	Ref	
Ethnicity				
Sinhala	188 (98.9)	1292 (93.3)	6.77 (1.65–27.69)	0.002
Non- Sinhala	2 (1.1)	93 (6.7)	Ref	
Income				
≤ 50,000 rupees	139 (77.2)	1055 (82.8)	0.70 (0.48–1.03)	0.07
> 50,000 rupees	41 (15.8)	219 (17.2)	Ref	
Financial support				
> 3000 Rs/month	13 (9.8)	81(7.8)	1.28 (0.69–2.37)	0.43
≤ 3000 Rs/month	119(90.2)	951 (92.2)	Ref	
Academic year				
Second	112 (58.9)	818 (59.1)	1.005(0.74–.37)	0.98
Third	78 (41.1)	567 (40.9)	Ref	
Academic stream				
Bio-Science	26 (13.7)	222 (16.0)	0.83 (0.54–1.29)	0.41
Non Bio-Science	164 (86.3)	1163 (84.0)	Ref	
School type				
Mixed	70 (49.0)	575 (51.8)	0.89 (0.63–1.26)	0.51
Non-mixed	73 (51.0)	534 (48.2)	Ref	
Religious activities				
More	58 (30.5)	615 (44.8)	0.54 (0.39–0.75)	< 0.001
Less	132 (69.5)	759 (55.2)	Ref	
Importance of religion				
More	118 (62.1)	1084 (78.3)	0.46 (0.33–0.63)	< 0.001
Less	72 (37.9)	301 (21.7)	Ref	
Access to talk with relative,				
Yes	110 (57.9)	969 (70.1)	0.59 (0.43–0.80)	0.001
No	80 (42.1)	416 (30.0)	Ref	
Access to talk with friends				
Yes	177 (93.2)	1231 (88.9)	1.70 (0.95–3.06)	0.07
No	13 (6.8)	154 (11.1)	Ref	

Table 3 Unadjusted odds ratio for association of risky sexual behaviors with other risk behaviors

Other risk behavior	Risky sexual behavior		OR	p value
	Yes No (%)	No No (%)	(95%CI)	
Attend night clubs in last month				
≥ once /month	9 (4.7)	8 (0.6)	8.56 (3.26–22.46)	
Not in last month	181 (95.3)	1377 (99.4)	Ref	< 0.001
Using Internet facilities				
≥ 2 h/day	88 (46.3)	526 (38.0)	1.41(1.04–1.91)	
< 1 h/day	102,953.7)	859 (62.0)	Ref	0.027
Monthly frequency of going to cinema halls				
≥ 2per month	34 (17.9)	134 (9.7)	2.03 (1.35–3.07)	0.001
< 1 per month	156 (82.1)	1251(90.3)	Ref	
Had taken alcohol in last three months				
Yes	79 (41.6)	195 (14.1)	4.34 (3.14–6.02)	< 0.001
No	111 (58.4)	1190 (85.9)	Ref	
Had smoked within last three months				
Yes	33 (17.4)	76 (5.5)	3.62 (2.33–5.63)	< 0.001
No	157 (82.6)	1309 (94.5)	Ref	
Had taken Marijuana within last three months				
Yes	15 (7.9)	32 (2.3)	3.62 (1.92–6.83)	
No	175 (92.1)	1353 (97.7)	Ref	< 0.001
Had physical fighting in last one year in university				
Yes	25 (13.2)	35 (2.5)	5.84 (3.41–10.01)	
No	165 (86.8)	1350 (97.5)	Ref	< 0.001

condoms. Peltzer has stated that those who had recent sexual exposures had correct knowledge on condoms [31].

The present study revealed that those who considered religion is more important to their lives were less likely to be associated with RSB than those who did not. Similar comparable results were also reported among adolescent and young adults in USA [22]. In contrast to the findings, a study done among undergraduates at the University of Kentucky revealed that students with higher religious beliefs but lower religious behaviors were at risk for risky sexual practices [32].

Frequently attending nightclubs showed significant positive association with RSB in the present study. In compatible with these findings, attending night clubs showed significant association with having sex ever, having multiple sexual partners and having sex with commercial sex workers in a study from Ethiopia [33]. The difference in the degree of association may be due to the different definitions of RSB in these two studies. Difference of academic year of selected study participants may have contributed to the observed dissimilarity. The Ethiopian study had selected undergraduates from all 5 years including 1st, 4th and 5th academic years which we have

excluded in the present study. Another study conducted among undergraduates had showed different degree of positive association between RSB and attending night clubs [11].

Present study showed a statistically significant positive association with alcohol consumption within the past 3 months' time. The results were compatible with few other studies [16, 25, 34, 35]. Alcohol use together with sexual activities itself are within the definition of RSB in our study, even though none of them had taken alcohol intake as a factor in their definition of RSB. The observed association may be due to an impaired decision making ability and dis-inhibition behavior due to alcohol consumption.

Kebede et al. revealed a positive association between unprotected sex and using alcohol daily [20]. Alcohol consumption has been measured for past 3 months' time while unprotected sex for the period of last 1 year. Undergraduates in England perceived that life style in university provided opportunities for risky sex via high level of alcohol consumption along with other factors like increased sexual opportunities [35]. As described by Cooper, drinking alcohol may have an association that could not be described easily [21]. Therefore there exists

Table 4 Unadjusted odds ratios for association of RSB with knowledge and attitudes on reproductive health

Knowledge and attitude aspect	Risky sexual behavior		OR	p value
	Yes No (%)	No No (%)	(95%CI)	
Knowledge on Unsafe abortions				
Good	109 (57.4)	730 (52.7)	1.21 (0.89–1.64)	
Average[a]	81 (42.6)	655 (47.3)	Ref	0.227
Knowledge on Contraceptives				
Good	71 (37.4)	376 (27.1)	1.60 (1.17–2.0)	
Average[a]	119 (62.6)	1009 (72.9)	Ref	0.003
Knowledge on Condoms				
Good	145 (76.3)	597 (43.1)	4.25 (3.00–6.04)	< 0.001
Average[a]	45 (23.7)	788 (56.9)	Ref	
Knowledge on Sexually Transmitted Infections				
Good	35,918.4)	227 (16.4)	1.15 (0.78–1.71)	0.481
Average[a]	155 (81.6)	1158 (83.6)	Ref	
Knowledge on HIV/AIDS				
Good	125 (66.8)	851(62.0)	1.23 (0.89–1.71)	0.201
Average[a]	62(33.2)	521 (38.0)	Ref	
Knowledge on Sexual and Reproductive health rights				
Good	58 (30.5)	327 (23.6)	1.42 (1.02–1.98)	
Average[a]	132 (69.5)	1058 (76.4)	Ref	0.038
Overall knowledge on Reproductive health				
Good	45 (23.7)	241 (17.4)	1.47 (1.03–2.12)	0.035
Average[a]	145(76.4)	1144 (82.6)	Ref	
Attitude on contraceptives				
Desirable	75 (39.5)	402 (29.2)	1.58 (1.15–2.16)	0.004
Undesirable	115 (60.5)	974 (70.8)	Ref	
Attitude on Condoms				
Desirable	121 (63.7)	487 (35.4)	3.20 (2.33–4.38)	< 0.001
Undesirable	69 (36.3)	888 (64.6)	Ref	
Attitude on HIV/AIDS				
Desirable	93 (49.5)	588 (42.7)	1.32 (0.97–1.78)	0.081
Undesirable	95 (50.5)	788 (57.3)	Ref	
Attitude on Overall Reproductive health				
Desirable	92 (48.4)	388 (38.0)	2.41 (1.77–3.28)	< 0.001
Undesirable	98 (51.6)	997 (72.0)	Ref	

[a]Satisfactory and poor knowledge were amalgamated as average knowledge
OR, odds ratio, CI, confidence interval

Table 5 Adjusted odds ratios for Risky Sexual Behavior among undergraduates within last three months

Variable	β co-efficient	SE	OR	95% CI	p value
Had taken alcohol within last three months	0.951	0.18	2.59	1.82–3.70	< 0.001
Attended night clubs more than once in last month	1.284	0.52	3.61	1.31–9.97	0.013
Good knowledge on condoms	1.069	0.19	2.91	2.00–4.24	< 0.001
Considered religion was more important to their lives	−0.399	0.175	0.67	0.48–0.95	0.022

Hosmer and Lemeshow Test Chi-square value 3.8, p value 0.43
SE, standard error, OR, odds ratio, CI, confidence interval

a definite need for further research, both quantitative and qualitative in order to describe relationship between alcohol consumption and RSB.

Given the cross sectional nature of the study design, it was difficult to identify cause and effect association between the variables. As the discussed topic was very sensitive and the information was self-reported, there may be possibility of deliberately hiding of information in relation to unacceptable behavior. The results could be generalized to all the universities in Western Province and all university students in Sri Lanka as participants for the study are from all over the country.

Conclusions
Risky sexual behavior was prevailing among undergraduates at a rate of 12.4%. Males had more RSB than females. Those who had taken alcohol within last 3 months, had attended night clubs more than once in the last month and had good knowledge on condoms were associated with higher risk of RSB Undergraduates' consideration of the religion as more important to their lives had lower risk with RSB.

Authorities of university and health care providers should consider the need and take necessary actions to establish accessible, affordable RH services within university. They should consider taking necessary steps to minimize alcohol consumption within university and outside society. Authorities within university and outside should discourage night clubs attendance among undergraduates by encouraging more recreational activities with the help of peer leaders, academic and non-academic staff members and other organizations. Religious activities should be promoted within universities and outside.

Abbreviations
AIDS: Acquired immuno deficiency syndrome; CDC: Centers for disease control and prevention; CI: Confidence interval; HIV : Human immunodeficiency virus; OR: Odds ratio; PPS: Probability proportionate to size; RH: Reproductive health; RSB: Risky sexual behaviors; SPSS: Statistical package for social science; STI: Sexually transmitted infections

Acknowledgements
All the undergraduates who participated for the study and the staff of the Universities, data collectors and the members of the Board of Study in Community Medicine, Postgraduate Institution of Medicine.

Funding
The Medical Research Institute of the Ministry of Health, Sri Lanka funded for the data collection of the study.

Authors' contributions
Both authors have contributed equally to the design the study. UP and CA analyzed and interpreted the data. UP was responsible for the conduct of the literature review and implementation of study and a major contributor in writing the manuscript. All authors read and approved the final manuscript.

Competing interests
The authors declare that they have no competing interests.

Author details
[1]Postgraduate Institute of Medicine, University of Colombo, 36/1, Naiwala, Essalla, Veyangoda, Sri Lanka. [2]Department of Public Health, Faculty of Medicine, University of Kelaniya, Kelaniya, Sri Lanka.

References
1. Brener ND, Kann L, Kinchen SA, Grunbaum JA, Whalen L, Eaton D, et al. Methodology of the youth risk behavior surveillance system. Morb Mortal Wkly Rep. 2004;53(RR-12):1–13.
2. Madise N, Zulu E, Ciera J. Is poverty a driver for risky sexual behavior? Evidence from National Surveys of adolescents in four African countries. Afr J Reprod Health. 2007;11(3):83–98.
3. Abels MD, Blignaut RJ. Sexual risk behavior among sexually active first year students at the University of the Western Cape, South Africa. Afr J AIDS Res. 2011;10(3):255–61.
4. Averett S, Corman H, Reichman NE. Effects of Overweight on Risky Sexual Behavior of Adolescent Girls. https://www.nber.org/papers/w16172. Accessed 24 Dec 2012.
5. Silas J. Poverty and Risky Sexual Behaviors: Evidence from Tanzania, ICF International Calverton, Maryland, USA. 2013. pubs/pdf/WP88/WP88.pdf. Accessed 10 Dec 2015.
6. Fernando NS. Sexual behavior and substance abuse among youth in the coastal region in Galle district. Thesis (MD in Community medicine, Postgraduate Institute of Medicine, University of Colombo). 2009.
7. Thalagala N, Rajapaksha L. National survey on emerging issues among adolescents in Sri Lanka. In: UNICEF; 2004.
8. Perera B, Reece M. Sexual behavior of young adults in Sri Lanka: implications for HIV prevention. AIDS Care. 2006;18(5):497–500.
9. Sujay R. Premarital Sexual Behavior among Unmarried College Students of Gujarat, India. In: Health and Population Innovation Fellowship Programme, Working paper. New Delhi: Population Council; 2009.
10. Raj RP, Padam S, Edwin RT. There are too many naked pictures found in papers and on the net : factors encouraging premarital sex among young people of Nepal. Health Sci J. 2010;4(3):162–74.
11. Dingeta T, Oljira L, Assefa N. Patterns of sexual risk behavior among undergraduate university students in Ethiopia: a cross-sectional study. Pan Afr Med J. 2012;12:33.
12. Tura G, Alemseged F, Dejene S. Risky sexual behavior and predisposing factors among students of Jimma University, Ethiopia. Ethiop J Heal Sci. 2012;22(3):170–80.
13. Musiime KE, Mugisha JF. Factors associated with sexual behaviour among students of Uganda martyrs university. Int J Public Health Res. 2015;3(1):1–9. www.openscienceonline.com/author/download?paperId=1347&stateId=8000. Accessed 10 Jan 2016.
14. Soboka B, Kejela G. Assessment of Risky Sexual Behaviors among Arba Minch University Students, Arba Minch Town, Snnpr, Ethiopia. J Child Adolesc Behav. 3(2). https://doi.org/10.4172/2375-4494.1000189. Accessed 17 Jan 2016.
15. Mavhandu-Mudzusi, AH, Asgedom T. The prevalence of risky sexual behaviours amongst undergraduate students in Jigjiga University, Ethiopia Health Sagesoheid. 2016;21 (17):179–86. www.scielo.org.za/pdf/hsa/v21n1/56.pdf. Accessed 31 Mar 2016.
16. Wordofa D, Shiferaw S. Sexual risk behaviors and its associated factors among undergraduate students in Madda Walabu university, Southeast Ethiopia: a facility based cross sectional study. Epidemiology. https://doi.org/10.4172/2161-1165.1000207. Accessed 30 Apr 2016.
17. Bayissa D, Mebrahtu G, Bayisa G, Mekuanint Y. Assessment of Early Sexual Initiation and Associated Factors among Ambo University Undergraduate Students, Ambo, Ethiopia. J Health Med Nurs. 2016;25:35-40.
18. Ruangkanchanasetr S, Plitponkarnpim A, Hetrakul P, Kongsakon R. Youth risk behavior survey: Bangkok, Thailand. J Adolesc Health. 2005;36:227–35.

19. Cooper ML. Alcohol use and risky sexual behavior among college students and youth: evaluating the evidence. J Stud Alcohol. 2002;14:101–17.
20. Kebede D, Alem A, Mitike G, Enquselassie F, Berhane F, Abebe Y, et al. Khat and alcohol use and risky sex behavior among in-school and out-of-school youth in Ethiopia. BMC Public Health. 2005;14(5):109.
21. Cooper ML. Does drinking promote risky sexual behavior? A Complex Answer to a Simple Question. Drinking Risk Sexual Behav. 2006;15(1):19–23.
22. Haglund KA, Fehring RJ. The Association of Religiosity, Sexual Education, and Parental Factors with Risky Sexual Behaviors among Adolescents and Young Adults, Nursing Faculty Research and Publications Nursing. https://epublications.marquette.edu/nursing_fac/3/. Accessed 16 Aug 2012.
23. http://www.ugc.ac.lk/en/statistics/university-statistics-2012.html. Accessed 17 Feb 2013.
24. Center for Research on Environment, Health and Population Activities. Determining an Effective and Replicable Communication Based Mechanism for Improving Young Couples' Access to and Use of Reproductive Health Information and Services in Nepal - An Operations Research Study. http://citeseerx.ist.psu.edu/viewdoc/download;jsessionid=9FE1397D0F6752DF473913172427D3A3?doi=10.1.1.175.7549&rep=rep1&type=pdf. Accessed 10 Dec 2015.
25. Martiniuk ALD, Steel O'Connor K, King WD. A cluster randomized trial of a sex education program in Belize, central America. Int J Epidemiol. 2003;32:131–6.
26. Rawstorne P, Worth H. Sri Lanka Behavioural Surveillance Survey: First Round Survey Results 2006–2007, Colombo Ministry of Healthcare and Nutrition, Sri Lanka. http://www.aidscontrol.gov.lk/images/pdfs/hiv_data/2006_2007_BSS_Report.pdf. Accessed 17 Feb 2013.
27. Cleland J. Illustrative Questionnaire for Interview-Surveys with Young People http://www.who.int/reproductivehealth/topics/adolescence/questionnaire. Accessed 21 Jan 2013.
28. Somaratna WA. Study on knowledge and attitudes on HIV/AIDS and current sexual practices among first year agriculture students of university of Ruhuna, Dissertation. 2010 (Diploma in Reprod Health, Postgraduate Institute of Medicine, University of Colombo).
29. Henok A, Kassa A, Lenda A, Nibret A, Lamaro T. Knowledge, attitude and practice of risky sexual behavior and condom utilization among regular students of Mizan-Tepi university, South West Ethiopia Journal of child and adolescent behavior https://doi.org/10.4172/2375-4494. Accessed 25 May 2016.
30. Morrison DM, Baker SA, Gillmore MR. Sexual risk behavior, knowledge and condom use among adolescents in juvenile detention. J Youth Adolescence. 1994;23(2):271–8.
31. Peltzer K. Knowledge and practice of condom use among first year students at University of the North. Curationis. 2001;24(1):53–7.
32. Prassel HB. The influence of religiosity on risky patterns of drug usage and sexual practices in underage undergraduate students. Theses and Dissertations–Psychology. 2016;102. https://uknowledge.uky.edu/psychology_etds/102.
33. Mulu W, Yimer M, Abera B. Sexual behaviors and associated factors among students at Bahir Dar University: a cross sectional study. Reprod Health. 2014;11(84). https://doi.org/10.1186/1742-4755-11-84.
34. Fentahum N, Mamo A. Risky sexual behaviors and associated factors among male and female students in Jimma zone preparatory schools, south West Ethiopia: comparative study. Ethiop J Health Sci. 2014;24(1):59–68.
35. Chanakira E, O'Cathain A, Goyder EC, Freeman JV. Factors perceived to influence risky sexual behaviours among university students in the United Kingdom: a qualitative telephone interview study. BMC Public Health. 2014. https://doi.org/10.1186/1471-2458-14-1055.

10

Odon device for instrumental vaginal deliveries: results of a medical device pilot clinical study

Javier A. Schvartzman[1], Hugo Krupitzki[1], Mario Merialdi[2,3], Ana Pilar Betrán[2], Jennifer Requejo[4], My Huong Nguyen[2], Effy Vayena[5], Angel E. Fiorillo[1], Enrique C. Gadow[1], Francisco M. Vizcaino[1], Felicitas von Petery[1], Victoria Marroquin[1], María Luisa Cafferata[6], Agustina Mazzoni[6], Valerie Vannevel[7], Robert C. Pattinson[7], A Metin Gülmezoglu[2], Fernando Althabe[6], Mercedes Bonet[2*] and for the World Health Organization Odon Device Research Group

Abstract

Background: A prolonged and complicated second stage of labour is associated with serious perinatal complications. The Odon device is an innovation intended to perform instrumental vaginal delivery presently under development. We present an evaluation of the feasibility and safety of delivery with early prototypes of this device from an early terminated clinical study.

Methods: Hospital-based, multi-phased, open-label, pilot clinical study with no control group in tertiary hospitals in Argentina and South Africa. Multiparous and nulliparous women, with uncomplicated singleton pregnancies, were enrolled during the third trimester of pregnancy. Delivery with Odon device was attempted under non-emergency conditions during the second stage of labour. The feasibility outcome was delivery with the Odon device defined as successful expulsion of the fetal head after one-time application of the device.

Results: Of the 49 women enrolled, the Odon device was inserted successfully in 46 (93%), and successful Odon device delivery as defined above was achieved in 35 (71%) women. Vaginal, first and second degree perineal tears occurred in 29 (59%) women. Four women had cervical tears. No third or fourth degree perineal tears were observed. All neonates were born alive and vigorous. No adverse maternal or infant outcomes were observed at 6-weeks follow-up for all dyads, and at 1 year for the first 30 dyads.

Conclusions: Delivery using the Odon device is feasible. Observed genital tears could be due to the device or the process of delivery and assessment bias. Evaluating the effectiveness and safety of the further developed prototype of the BD Odon Device™ will require a randomized-controlled trial.

Keywords: Instrumental vaginal delivery, Odon device, Second stage of labour

* Correspondence: bonetm@who.int
[2]UNDP/UNFPA/UNICEF/WHO/World Bank Special Programme of Research, Development and Research Training in Human Reproduction (HRP), Department of Reproductive Health and Research, World Health Organization, Avenue Appia 20, CH-1211 Geneva 27, Switzerland
Full list of author information is available at the end of the article

Plain English summary

The Odon device is an innovation, presently under development, intended to assist vaginal birth when second stage takes longer than what is considered safe or if complications arose (e.g. baby is large or distressed). The objective of the study was to find out whether this new device helps pushing out of the baby through the birth canal. The study included women at their first delivery and women who delivered before, with uncomplicated pregnancies and one fetus in two hospitals in Argentina and South Africa. Delivery with the Odon device was attempted in women undergoing normal, uncomplicated labour. The Odon device was inserted successfully in 46 of the 49 women included (93%), and successful delivery with expulsion of the fetal head after one-time application of the Odon device was achieved in 35 (71%) women. Genital tears occurred in 29 (59%) women. As the use in humans has been limited, increased risk of tears and other unknown risks cannot be ruled out. Four women had cervical tears but no women had severe perineal trauma. All babies were born alive and vigorous. No adverse maternal or infant outcomes were observed at 6-weeks follow-up, and at 1 year for the first 30 mothers and babies. Delivery using the Odon device is feasible. These findings suggest continuing evaluating the effectiveness and safety of new prototypes of the BD Odon Device™ in a clinical comparative trial with a standard device before introduction in clinical practice.

Background

Prolonged or complicated second stage of labour is associated with potentially serious maternal complications and deaths as well as stillbirths and neonatal morbidity and mortality [1].

Currently, the main options for managing prolonged/complicated second stage of labour are instrumental vaginal delivery (IVD) with forceps or vacuum extractor, and caesarean section. IVD is one of the six critical functions of basic emergency obstetric and neonatal care [2], but currently under-used, particularly in low-resource settings where rates are as low as 1-5% [3, 4]. In high-resource settings, IVD rates tend to be higher (up to 15%) [5, 6], but declining rates have been reported in several countries [4]. These trends are inversely correlated with the increasing rates of caesarean sections worldwide [7].

There are multiple factors associated with low or declining use of IVD. None of the available instruments are without risk for the mother or the baby. While use of forceps is associated with increased maternal perineal trauma, need for analgesia and neonatal facial injury, cephalhaematoma and subgaleal haemorrhage are associated with vacuum birth [8]. Failure rates are also reported to be relatively high, particularly with the use of

vacuum extractor at around 20% [8]. An additional barrier is the high level of skill and continuous training required to perform safe and effective IVD [9, 10]. This limits the use of IVD if birth attendants are not provided with sufficient resources to obtain and maintain the necessary skills.

The design and development of innovative IVD instruments that are safe for mothers and babies, easy for different cadres of skilled birth attendants to use, cost-effective, and affordable in low resource settings is a priority [11]. In this sense, the Odon device is a technological innovation intended to fulfil this gap, by improving outcomes associated with prolonged or complicated second stage of labour and reduce the skill level and equipment required to perform assisted vaginal deliveries.

We present results of an early terminated study designed to evaluate the feasibility and preliminary safety of delivery with early prototypes of the Odon device in singleton term pregnancies under non-emergency conditions.

Methods
Study design and participants

This was a hospital-based, multi-phased, open-label, medical device pilot clinical study without control group. The study methods were described in detail elsewhere [12].

The design of the study in phases included an evaluation of the first five multiparous women, the next 25 multiparous with 1 year follow-up, and then the inclusion of both multiparous and nulliparous women until completion of the sample size. Therefore, women were enrolled in three phases: 1) multiparous women with a previously successful spontaneous vaginal delivery with 1 year follow up (2011-2012); 2) multiparous and nulliparous with 6-weeks follow up (2014-2015) at a private not-for-profit tertiary hospital in Buenos Aires, Argentina. In 2013, Becton Dickinson and Company (BD) licensed the development rights of the Odon device. In consequence, the trial was paused in January 2015 for BD to conduct preclinical studies [13–15] and develop a new prototype. 3) The third phase included multiparous and nulliparous women with follow-up until discharge at a public tertiary hospital in Pretoria, South Africa (2017). The new BD Odon device was planned to be applied in additional women at public hospitals in Argentina (2 hospitals), Kenya (1) and South Africa (4) for completion of the sample size, before the study was prematurely terminated. After the 49th case, the company decided to end this pilot study in favour of a randomized pivotal clinical trial to be conducted in Europe and India.

Women were invited to participate if they were between 18 and 35 years old, had no pre-existing health conditions and uncomplicated singleton pregnancies in the third trimester in Argentina or while in the hospital admitted for induction of labour in South Africa. Written informed consent was obtained before labour during antenatal care in Argentina or at the hospital after admission for childbirth in South Africa. Women were eligible for application of the Odon device during the second stage if the following conditions were met:

- fetus was alive and had a normal fetal heart rate as assessed by continuous electronic fetal monitoring;
- fully dilated cervix;
- ruptured membranes;
- any anterior occiput position;
- station level equivalent to 2 cm or more below the spines (station + 2 or lower).

Women were excluded if they did not confirm consent to participate in the study verbally before application of the device, or if any maternal or fetal complication arose during labour.

All women and their infants were followed until discharge and at 6-weeks postpartum. The first 30 mother/infant dyads recruited were also followed up to one year, as per protocol. No mother/infant dyad was lost to follow-up.

All the applications of the device were supervised, and assisted as required, by another obstetrician trained in the use of the device. A training plan for obstetricians applying the device was developed for implementation of the last phase of the study.

The Department of Reproductive Health and Research from the World Health Organization (WHO) was the sponsor and performed overall coordination of the study. A Data and Safety Monitoring Board (DSMB) and an expert committee independently reviewed the study progress and all cases. Based on these assessments, the study governing bodies supported continuing the series of studies necessary to evaluate feasibility, effectiveness and safety of the new BD Odon Device.

The study was approved by the WHO Research Ethics Review Committee; the Ethics Committee in Research of CEMIC and the National Drugs, Food, and Technology Administration of Argentina (ANMAT) in Argentina; and the The Research Ethics Committee, Faculty Health Sciences, University of Pretoria and the Medicines Control Council in South Africa. This study was registered in the Australian New Zealand Clinical Trials Registry (registration number ACTRN12613000141741).

Intervention - the Odon device

The Odon Device (Fig. 1) is made of two main components: a plastic sleeve and an inserter (or applicator). The sleeve is made of flexible polyethylene, with an internal fold in contact with the fetal head and the

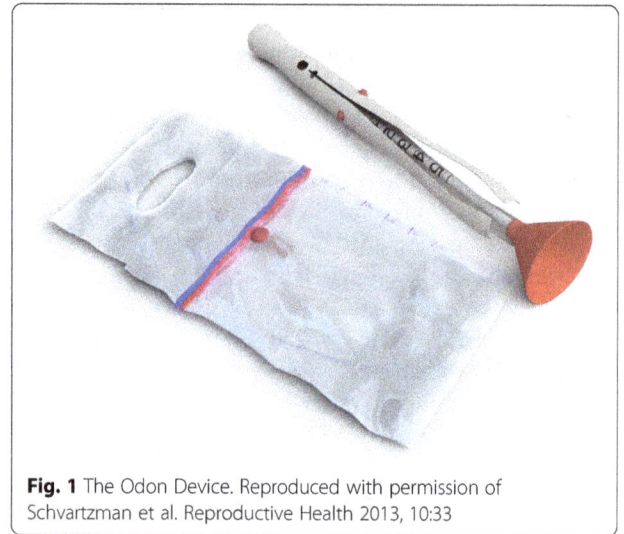

Fig. 1 The Odon Device. Reproduced with permission of Schvartzman et al. Reproductive Health 2013, 10:33

external fold in contact with the vaginal wall. The sleeve contains an air chamber (cuff) that is inflated around the fetal head by a manually operated bulb pump. The inserter consists of a handle with four pronged flexible spatulas that slide around the fetal head and help to position the sleeve. A plastic cup (plastic bell) at the tip of the inserter facilitates the application and protects the fetal head. The inserter has a progress indicator allowing the operator to check when the correct depth of insertion has been reached. The application technique of the Odon device is described in Fig. 2.

The devices used in Argentina were manufactured, and assembled by MDV (Muller, Dordoni, Visani) Srl in Buenos Aires, Argentina. The device used in South Africa was manufactured by BD in Singapore. During the study, design modifications, both to the inserter and the plastic sleeve, were introduced to improve usability, facilitate insertion and avoid loss of air pressure in the air cuff. Four slightly different prototypes of the device were used in Argentina. Device modifications were evaluated by the study DSMB and the Odon Device Research Group. These groups conferred that the modifications introduced potentially improved safety and usability and did not interfere with interpretation of the study results.

Outcome measures

The list of safety and feasibility outcomes is available elsewhere [12]. Feasibility was assessed as successful application of the device defined as (1) reaching number 4 or 5 in the reading window of the inserter (Fig. 2, image 3), (2) successful inflation of the device without air leaks after the expulsion, and (3) successful expulsion of the fetal head with the plastic sleeve around the head (Fig. 2, image 5) after one-time application of the Odon device. Cases in which the plastic sleeve detached at the moment of crowning were reported as "crowning with

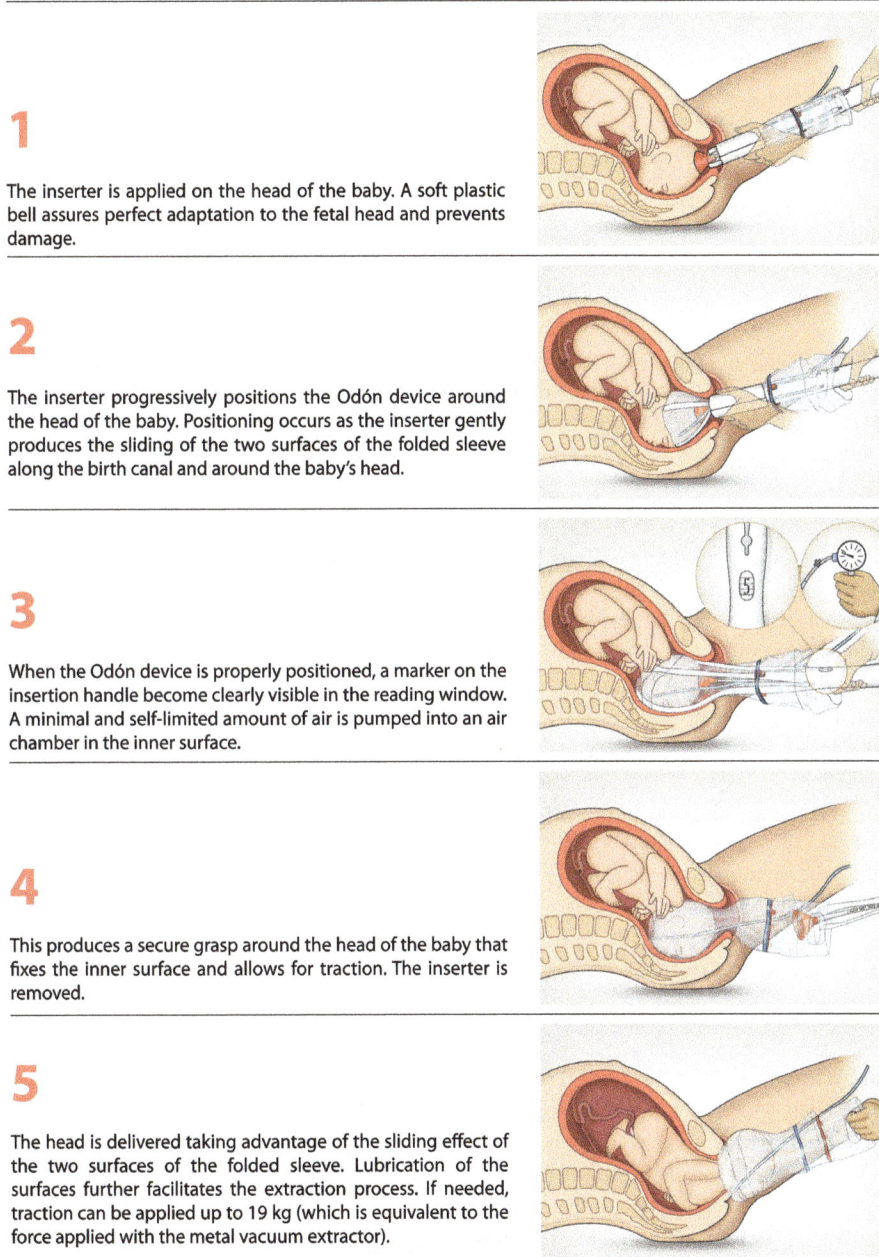

1

The inserter is applied on the head of the baby. A soft plastic bell assures perfect adaptation to the fetal head and prevents damage.

2

The inserter progressively positions the Odón device around the head of the baby. Positioning occurs as the inserter gently produces the sliding of the two surfaces of the folded sleeve along the birth canal and around the baby's head.

3

When the Odón device is properly positioned, a marker on the insertion handle become clearly visible in the reading window. A minimal and self-limited amount of air is pumped into an air chamber in the inner surface.

4

This produces a secure grasp around the head of the baby that fixes the inner surface and allows for traction. The inserter is removed.

5

The head is delivered taking advantage of the sliding effect of the two surfaces of the folded sleeve. Lubrication of the surfaces further facilitates the extraction process. If needed, traction can be applied up to 19 kg (which is equivalent to the force applied with the metal vacuum extractor).

Fig. 2 Visualization of the use of the Odon device. Reproduced with permission of Schvartzman et al. Reproductive Health 2013, 10:33

Odon". Insertion refers to the introduction and withdrawal of the inserter (Fig. 2, images 1 to 4).

Maternal and neonatal safety was assessed at labour, delivery and before discharge. Vaginal and cervical lacerations were evaluated by a systematic exploration of the birth canal and uterine cervix using vaginal spatulas after delivery. For the first 48 women/infant dyads the following safety outcomes were assessed at 6-weeks: perineal or vaginal haematoma, postpartum haemorrhage, infection, fever, blood transfusion, maternal or infant re-admission to hospital. For the first 30 dyads the following outcomes were assessed at the one-year follow-up: urinary incontinence, faecal/flat incontinence, perineal pain, dyspareunia, infant developmental impairment (assessed through maternal interview, contact with the paediatrician and review of medical record) and death.

Sample size

A total sample size of 130 was estimated to measure potential maternal and infant complications with a reasonable precision, allowing detection rates of adverse maternal or infant outcomes between 2% (0.4%-6.1%)

and 20% (13.5%-27.9%) with a 95% confidence interval width not larger than 15%. Details are published elsewhere [12]. The current study was terminated early in June 2017 in favour of a comparative trial. At that time, 48 women were recruited in Argentina and one woman in South Africa and results are presented in this manuscript.

Statistical analysis

This is a descriptive analysis and no statistical inferences were done. Continuous variables are reported in means and ranges; categorical variables in percentages, with exact binomial 95% confidence intervals (CI) computed for successful application of the device and genital lacerations in the total sample.

Results

Ninety women were invited to participate in the study during three study periods: between February 2011 and September 2012, March 2014 and January 2015, and May-June 2017. Exclusions included two women who did not fulfil eligibility criteria, 20 who did not provide written informed consent, and nine who were group B streptococcus (GBS) positive. At labour, one woman presented arrest of labour progress, one prolonged rupture of membranes, five had fetal complications and labour progressed too fast in one woman. Additionally, two women were excluded because their labours occurred during a study pause in recruitment in March 2014.

Forty-nine women were recruited, 30 multiparous women in the first phase, 18 in the second phase and one nulliparous woman in the third phase.

Characteristics of the women

Table 1 shows selected characteristics of the women at the time of labour and delivery. The average maternal age was 31 years. The onset of labour was spontaneous in 40 cases and induced in eight. Augmentation of labour, with oxytocin or artificial rupture of membranes, was performed in 47 women. In Argentina, all women were under epidural anaesthesia.

Feasibility outcomes

Table 2 shows feasibility and safety outcomes in all women and by parity. The Odon device was successfully inserted in all women but three. The insertion process took on average 1 min and 27 s, with 34/49 of the insertions taking less than 1 min and 30 s (data not shown). Thirty-five out of 49 delivered successfully with the Odon device (71%, 95% CI 57-83%), with similar rates between nulliparous and multiparous women. In Argentina, successful Odon device deliveries was achieved more frequently with the improved and more

Table 1 Characteristics of 49 women and their infants enrolled in the Odon device pilot study

	Mean or n (N = 49)	range or %
Maternal characteristics		
Maternal age (years)	31.2	(19-35)
Parity at eligibility		
Nulliparous	13	27%
Parity 1	21	43%
Parity 2 or more	15	30%
BMI at end of pregnancy	26.1	(22.7 – 40.8)
Labour and Delivery characteristics		
Spontaneous onset of labour	41	84%
Spontaneous rupture of membranes	14	29%
Augmentation of labour with oxytocin	39	76%
Vertex variety of position[a]		
Occiput anterior	36	73%
Left occiput anterior	10	20%
Right occiput anterior	3	6%
Epidural analgesia	48	98%

[a]One case was interpreted as anterior position at obstetrical examination but at delivery was occiput posterior position; *BMI* Body mass index

advanced prototypes (22/27, 81%) than with the earlier ones (13/21, 61%) (data not shown).

There were 14 non-successful applications according to the study predefined criteria. Two of failed insertions mentioned above were due to difficulties in positioning the device spatulas using the first prototype of the device, and the case in South Africa. The device slipped off in nine of the remaining cases and broke off (handle detached from the sleeve during traction) in two cases. Eleven of those women had a spontaneous delivery, and three had a forceps (two for maternal fatigue and one for fetal bradycardia).

Maternal and infant outcomes

After delivery, perineal or vaginal tears were observed in two-thirds of the women (29/49, 59%, 95% CI 44-73%) (Table 3). Most of the tears occurred in nulliparous and were vaginal. There were no third or fourth degree perineal tears. Overall, 28 women received sutures. All four cervical tears occurred in the lateral sides of the cervix. One showed mild bleeding and all four were sutured following the local protocol. No other adverse maternal outcomes were reported.

Before discharge from hospital, no serious maternal or neonatal adverse outcomes were reported. Two women received antibiotic treatment for foul smelling lochia with no fever, and one for urinary tract infection. One woman had hypoesthesia of the anterior region of the

Table 2 Feasibility of delivery with the Odon device in 49 women enrolled in the Odon device pilot study: All women and by parity

Indicators	Multiparous	Nulliparous	Total
	N = 36	N = 13	N = 49
	Mean or n (%)	Mean or n (%)	Mean or n (%)
Device application			
Fetal Station			
Station + 2/Hodge's 3rd	22 (61%)	10 (77%)	32(65%)
Station + 3/Hodge's 4th	14 (39%)	3 (23%)	17 (35%)
Vertex variety of position[a]			
Occiput anterior	26 (72%)	10[*] (77%)	36 (73%)
Left or right occiput anterior	10 (28%)	3 (13%)	13 (27%)
Mean time of insertion (minutes:seconds)	01:39	00:50	01:27
Successful application of the Odon device			
Yes[b]	26 (72%)	9 (69%)	35 (71%)
No	10 (28%)	4 (31%)	14 (29%)
Spontaneous delivery, failed insertion	2	1	3
Spontaneous delivery, fetal descent with Odon	2	0	2
Spontaneous delivery, crowning with Odon[c]	4	2	6
Forceps	2	1	3
Reasons of non-successful delivery with Odon device			
Device was difficult to place	2	1	3
Device broke off	1	1	2
Device slipped off, air leaks[d]	5	1	6
Device slipped off, no apparent cause	2	1	3

[a]One case was interpreted as anterior position at obstetrical examination but at delivery was occiput posterior position
[b]Successful application of the device was defined as: (1) reaching number 4 or 5 in the reading window of the inserter, (2) successful inflation of the device without leaks after the expulsion, and (3) successful expulsion of the fetal head with the plastic sleeve around the fetal head after one-time application of the Odon device
[c]Plastic sleeve detached at the moment of crowning
[d]Five cases were caused by air leaks in the air cuffs, as documented by post-application examination of the cuffs, and one was caused by an air leak in the bulb pump

right leg thigh due to epidural anaesthesia. All perineal repairs healed normally. Two neonates were admitted to the neonatal intensive care unit for less than 7 days with respiratory distress for causes that were thought unrelated to the device. No other neonatal complications (jaundice, infection, and need of phototherapy, fetal or neonatal death) were reported.

No adverse outcomes were recorded in the six-week or one-year follow-up visits (for the first 30 women/infant dyads only). No unexpected adverse events were reported. No substantial differences were observed in safety outcomes among the five prototypes used (data not shown).

Discussion

We evaluated feasibility and preliminary safety of application of the Odon device in 49 women with non-prolonged/non-complicated second stage of labour. The device was successfully inserted in 46 women, and successful delivery with the device was achieved in close to three-fourths of the women. Two-thirds of the women had vaginal, cervical or first/second degree perineal tears, but no third or fourth degree perineal tears were observed. No long-term maternal or neonatal adverse outcomes were observed.

Often new devices and procedures are introduced in medical practice without having been properly evaluated [16, 17], failing to provide adequate protection to patients and sufficient evidence on safety and to health care providers. However, the design of medical device studies requires specific approaches [18, 19]. This study was designed in phases to ensure safety by a periodic assessment of short- and long-term (one year) outcomes by an independent DSMB. For example, the design of the study included an evaluation of the first five cases and at one-year after delivery of the first 30 cases. As per protocol, upon conclusion of this follow-up period no further cases were recruited. This approach ensured that participants were not exposed to unnecessary risks and was also in line with requirements of the ethics committees. The design of the study in phases

Table 3 Maternal and neonatal outcomes during delivery and immediate postpartum (24-48 h) of 49 women enrolled in the Odon device pilot study: All women and by parity

Indicators	Multiparous N = 36 Mean (range) or n (%)	Nulliparous N = 13 Mean (range) or n (%)	Total N = 49 Mean (range) or n (%)
Maternal outcomes			
Any vaginal or perineal tears[a]	18 (50%)	11 (85%)	29 (59%)
Any vaginal or perineal tears[a] and/or episiotomy	23 (64%)	12 (92%)	35 (71%)
Vulvar tears	2 (5%)	0	2 (4%)
Vaginal lower half tears	9 (25%)	11 (85%)	20 (40%)
Vaginal upper half tears	0	0	0
Perineal 1st degree tear	8 (22%)	1 (8%)	9 (19%)
Perineal 2nd degree tears	1 (3%)	1 (8%)	2 (4%)
Perineal 3rd/4th degree tears	0	0	0
Episiotomy	7 (19%)	2 (15%)	9 (18%)
Cervical tears[b]	2 (5%)	2 (15%)	4 (8%)
Postpartum infection	1(3%)	1(8%)	2 (4%)
Infant outcomes			
Male	21 (58%)	9 (69%)	30 (61%)
Mean gestational age (weeks)	39.8 (37 - 41)	40.0 (38 - 41)	39.6 (37.0- 40.0)
Mean birth weight (grams)	3654 (2780 - 4560)	3488 (2880 - 4090)	3610 (2780 - 4560)
Apgar score at 5 min ≥ 7	36	13	49 (100%)
Caput succedaneum and moulding	3 (8%)	5 (38%)	8 (16%)
Cephalhematoma[c]	0	1 (8%)	1 (2%)
Admission to neonatal intensive care unit	1 (3%)	1 (8%)	2 (4%)

[a]Women may have more than one type of vaginal or perineal, excluding cervical tears
[b]Thirty-women had at least one type of vaginal, perineal or cervical tears
[c]One moderate

also allowed for introduction of modifications of the device during the study. The study DSMB and the Odon Device Research Group conferred that the modifications introduced potentially improved safety and usability and did not interfere with interpretation of the study results, as the principles of operation of the device did not change. While this is common in feasibility studies of new devices, and recognised by regulatory bodies [18], we acknowledge this may limit the interpretation of the results as a whole. Although the groups are small, no substantial differences were seen in terms of safety outcomes across the different prototypes used.

This study has several limitations. The study was carried out mainly at one hospital, and the majority of applications were performed by only two operators. If this facilitated acquisition of skills by the operators, feasibility still needs to be assessed with a larger number of operators and in different contexts. It was not possible to evaluate the level of discomfort and pain during application of the device, as all 48 enrolled women in Argentina were under epidural anaesthesia. It was planned to collect information on operator's impressions of use during

application of the device in the last phase of the study. However, this was not possible due to the early termination of the study. After the 49th case, the company decided to end this pilot study in favour of a randomized pivotal clinical study to be conducted in Europe and India. Ethical issues and consequences of premature discontinuation of studies have been extensively discussed in the literature [20–22].

It is difficult to compare the rates of vaginal/perineal tears in this study. While the overall rate of tears in the study (59%, $n = 29/49$) is comparable to rates associated with the hand held vacuum used in indicated cases: 45% of first or second degree tears; 68% of episiotomies; and 6% of third or fourth degree tears [8], which is the current available instrument associated with the lowest rate of perineal trauma. We acknowledge that the population in this study included women undergoing normal second stage of labour, while studies on the hand held vacuum [8] included a substantial proportion of women with prolonged second stage. Intact perineum in our sample compares to the 21 to 35% reported in the literature among low risk women (term, singleton, vertex presentation) [23]. It is notable that no intermediate or long-term adverse outcomes related to perineal trauma (e.g. perineal pain, incontinence, dyspareunia) were reported at the 6 week or 1 year follow-up.

We have observed four cervical tears in the lateral side of the cervix. The rate of clinically significant cervical tears after vaginal birth has been reported between 0.2 to 4.8% in different retrospective studies [24–27]. However, studies using routine colposcopy in consecutive cases of vaginal deliveries found much higher rates of any cervical injury, including erosion (79%), laceration (23% to 56%) and bruising (30%) without clinical signs [28–30]. One explanation of our findings is that the spatulas of the inserter may have caused harm by direct contact with the cervix. However, it is unlikely to be the only explanation, particularly with a fully dilated and effaced cervix and a fetus at station + 2 or lower. These findings may also be explained by observation bias. The fact that all women had a thorough vaginal examination may have prompted the diagnosis of an event that is underdiagnosed and underreported in routine practice [24].

At this stage, the increased risk of tears and other unknown risks cannot be ruled out. Also, it is not possible to know if women with indication for IVD could present higher rates of genital tears with Odon device compared to other instruments. Therefore, a fair assessment of the failures and complications commonly, such as birth canal tears, associated with IVD is not possible until a direct comparison between the Odon device and other existing instruments is conducted in a randomised clinical trial in the intended population. Further research is supported by results of preclinical studies showing that the Odon device was not associated with more perineal distension compared to forceps or vacuum [15]. Further improvements in the design of the device might also increase successful application in future research [31].

Conclusions

Our results suggest that delivery using the Odon device is feasible. However, observed genital tears could be due to the device or the process of delivery and assessment bias.

If proof of concept has been demonstrated, effectiveness and safety of the device remains to be assessed in a randomised trial, as the device in this study was applied under non-emergency conditions, in women with normal progress of labour and no indication of IVD. Efficacy, safety and feasibility remain also to be assessed in different facility-settings and countries. A regular risk-benefit assessment will be needed in order to mitigate risks arising from this kind of study, and clear stopping rules shall be developed, including discontinuation for reasons not related to efficacy, safety, or feasibility. Safety outcomes, including risk of genital tears, including cervical tears, and pain during application need to be carefully assessed in future research.

Abbreviations

BD: Becton Dickinson and Company; DSMB: Data and Safety Monitoring Board; GBS: Group B streptococcus; IVD: instrumental vaginal delivery; WHO: World Health Organization

Acknowledgements

We would like to thank Jorge Odon for his support to the study team. We would like to acknowledge Monica Lombardo and Rosa Garrido from Nobeltri SRL for their advice regarding regulatory approvals. We would like to thank Michael Boulvain for his comments on the manuscript. We thank Dr. Dalene Barnard and the staff of Kalafong Hospital for their support and participation in the study. Additional thanks for their preparatory activities are to investigators in Argentina (Roberto Casale, Lucio Rivola, Silvana Varela (Hospital Posadas, Buenos Aires); Gerardo Murga, Elena Hurtado (Maternidad de las Mercedes, Tucumán)), Kenya (Zahida Qureshi, Alfred Osoti (Kenyatta National Hospital, University of Nairobi, Nairobi)), and South Africa (Salome Maswime (Chris Hani Baragwanath Hospital, University of the Witwatersrand, Johannesburg); Professor Hennie Lombaard (Rahima Moosa Hospital, University of the Witwatersrand, Johannesburg); Stefan Gebhardt (Tygerberg Hospital, Faculty of Medicine and Health Sciences Stellenbosch University, Cape Town). We sincerely thank the women who participated in this study.

World Health Organization Odon Device Research Group (2010-2014) (names in alphabetical order): Hugo Krupitzki, Javier A Schvartzman (Centro de Educación Médica e Investigaciones Clínicas "Norberto Quirno" (CEMIC), Argentina); Fernando Althabe, José Belizán, Eduardo Bergel, (Institute for Clinical Effectiveness and Health Policy (IECS), Argentina); Franco Borruto, Alain Treisser (Centre Hospitalier Princesse Grace, Monaco); Michel Boulvain, (Hopitaux Universitaires de Geneve, Switzerland); Gian Carlo Di Renzo, (Santa Maria Della Misericordia University Hospital, Italy); Justus Hofmeyr (University of the Witwatersrand, University of Fort Hare, South Africa); Kevin Judge (Becton Dickinson (BD), USA); Tak Yeung Leung (The Chinese University of Hong Kong, Hong Kong); Ola Didrik Saugstad (Oslo University Hospital, Norway); Effy Vayena, (University of Zurich, Switzerland); Ana Pilar Betrán, A Metin Gülmezoglu, Mario Merialdi, My Huong Nguyen, Jennifer Requejo, Marleen Temmerman (World Health Organization, Switzerland).

World Health Organization Odon Device Research Group (from 2015) (names in alphabetical order): *Study Investigators*: Hugo Krupitzki, Javier A Schvartzman (Centro de Educación Médica e Investigaciones Clínicas "Norberto Quirno" (CEMIC), Argentina); Fernando Althabe, Maria Luisa Cafferata (Institute for Clinical Effectiveness and Health Policy (IECS), Argentina); Roberto Casale, Lucio Rivola, Silvana Varela (Hospital Posadas, Buenos Aires, Argentina); Gerardo Murga, Elena Hurtado (Maternidad de las Mercedes, Tucumán, Argentina);Alfred Osoti, Zahida Qureshi (University of Nairobi, Kenya); Dalene Barnard, Robert Pattinson, Valerie Vannevel (University of Pretoria, South Africa); Salome Maswime (Chris Hani Baragwanath Hospital, University of the Witwatersrand, Johannesburg, South Africa); Professor Hennie Lombaard (Rahima Moosa Hospital, University of the Witwatersrand, Johannesburg, South Africa); Stefan Gebhardt (Tygerberg Hospital, Faculty of Medicine and Health Sciences Stellenbosch University, Cape Town, South Africa). *Independent Scientific Advisory Committee*: Sabaratnam Arulkumaran (St George's, University of London, UK); Khalid Khan (Barts and The London School of Medicine and Dentistry, UK); Nina Kimmich (University Hospital Zurich, Switzerland); Tina Lavender (University of Manchester School of Nursing Midwifery & Social Work, UK); Pisake Lumbiganon (Khon Kaen University, Thailand); Nafissa Osman (Eduardo Mondlane University, Mozambique); Effy Vayena, (University of Zurich, Switzerland); Gijs Walraven (Aga Khan Development Network, France); Diane Whitham (Queen's Medical Centre, United Kingdom); Khaled Yunis (American University of Beirut Medical Center, Lebanon).*World Health Organization Secretariat*: (Switzerland) Mercedes Bonet, A Metin Gülmezoglu, Ndema Abu Habib, My Huong Nguyen.

Funding

This study is made possible through the generous support of the Saving Lives at Birth partners: the United States Agency for International Development (USAID), the Government of Norway, the Bill & Melinda Gates Foundation, Grand Challenges Canada, the UK Government, and the Korea International Cooperation Agency (KOICA). It was prepared by the authors and does not necessarily reflect the views of the Saving Lives at Birth partners.

Authors' contributions

JS, HK, APB, JR, EV, AEF, ECG and MM conceived the study and developed the study protocol. JS, HK, MB, VV, RP, and AMG developed the expanded protocol that was to be implemented in public hospitals in Argentina, Kenya and South Africa. APB, MB, MHN, VM, MLC, AM, AMG and FA contributed to data management and analysis. FMV and FvP contributed to the enrolment and follow up of subjects in Argentina. JS, HK and FA drafted the first version of the manuscript. All authors contributed to the manuscript, and read and approved the final manuscript.

Ethics approval and consent to participate

The study was approved by the Scientific and Ethical Review Group of the UNDP/UNFPA/UNICEF/ WHO/World Bank Special Programme of Research, Development and Research Training in Human Reproduction at the Department of Reproductive Health and Research of WHO, and the WHO Research Ethics Review Committee, Geneva, Switzerland, under reference number A65711 in September 2010, and continuing approvals in April 2013 and February 2017. The Ethics Committee in Research of CEMIC (reference number 529, in July 2009, and continuing approval in September 2010, October 2012, August 2013 and March 2017) and the National Drugs, Food, and Technology Administration of Argentina (ANMAT) (reference number 1-47-22,013/09-8 in December 2010, and continuing approval in October 2013 and August 2017) also approved the study in Argentina. The Research Ethics Committee, Faculty Health Sciences, University of Pretoria (reference number 222/2016 in September 2016 and march 2017) and the Medicines Control Council (February 2017) approved the study in South Africa. All women provided written consent for participation in the study.

Competing interests

M Merialdi was a WHO employee at the beginning of the study and until December 2013. Since February 2014, he is an employee of BD and provides scientific and technical advice on issues related to device development and evaluation. Since 2013, BD has a temporary exclusivity agreement with the inventor for the licensing of the BD Odon Device.
J Requejo is a member of the Becton Dickinson Odon Device Experts' Group and contributed to the conception and design of the clinical evidence generation plan for the BD Odon Device™. All other authors listed declared that they have no competing interest.

Author details

[1]Department of Obstetrics and Gynecology, Centro de Educación Médica e Investigaciones Clínicas "Norberto Quirno" (CEMIC-IUC - CONICET), University Hospital, Av. Galván 4102 1431FWO, Buenos Aires, Argentina. [2]UNDP/UNFPA/ UNICEF/WHO/World Bank Special Programme of Research, Development and Research Training in Human Reproduction (HRP), Department of Reproductive Health and Research, World Health Organization, Avenue Appia 20, CH-1211 Geneva 27, Switzerland. [3]Becton Dickinson and Company (BD), Franklin Lakes, NJ, USA. [4]Partnership for Maternal, Newborn and Child Health, World Health Organization, Avenue Appia 20, CH-1211 Geneva 27, Switzerland. [5]Department of Health Sciences and Technology, ETH Zurich, Auf der Mauer 17, 8092 Zurich, Switzerland. [6]Instituto de Efectividad Clínica y Sanitaria (IECS - CONICET), Dr Emilio Ravignani 2024, C1414CPV Buenos Aires, Argentina. [7]SAMRC Maternal and Infant Health Care Strategies, Department of Obstetrics and Gynaecology, University of Pretoria, Pretoria, South Africa.

References

1. Altman MR, Lydon-Rochelle MT. Prolonged second stage of labor and risk of adverse maternal and perinatal outcomes: a systematic review. Birth. 2006;33(4):315–22.
2. Monitoring emergency obstetric care. A handbook. Geneva: World Health Organization; 2009. Available at http://www.who.int/reproductivehealth/publications/monitoring/9789241547734/en/. Accessed 29 Nov 2017.
3. Ameh CA, Weeks AD. The role of instrumental vaginal delivery in low resource settings. BJOG. 2009;116(Suppl 1):22–5.
4. Bailey PE. The disappearing art of instrumental delivery: time to reverse the trend. Int J Gynaecol Obstet. 2005;91(1):89–96.
5. Euro-Peristat Project with SCPE and Eurocat, European Perinatal Health Report. The health and care of pregnant women and babies in Europe in 2010. Available at http://www.europeristat.com/reports/european-perinatal-health-report-2010.html. Accessed 29 Nov 2017.
6. Clark SL, Belfort MA, Hankins GD, Meyers JA, Houser FM. Variation in the rates of operative delivery in the United States. Am J Obstet Gynecol. 2007; 196(6):526.e1–5
7. Bailey PE, van Roosmalen J, Mola G, Evans C, de Bernis L, Dao B. Assisted vaginal delivery in low and middle income countries: an overview. BJOG. 2017;124(9):1335–44.
8. O'Mahony F, Hofmeyr GJ, Menon V. Choice of instruments for assisted vaginal delivery. Cochrane Database Syst Rev. 2010;11:Cd005455.
9. Cass GK, Crofts JF, Draycott TJ. The use of simulation to teach clinical skills in obstetrics. Semin Perinatol. 2011;35(2):68–73.
10. Cheong YC, Abdullahi H, Lashen H, Fairlie FM. Can formal education and training improve the outcome of instrumental delivery? Eur J Obstet Gynecol Reprod Biol. 2004;113(2):139–44.
11. Wall SN, Lee AC, Carlo W, Goldenberg R, Niermeyer S, Darmstadt GL, et al. Reducing intrapartum-related neonatal deaths in low- and middle-income countries-what works? Semin Perinatol. 2010;34(6):395–407.
12. World Health Organization Odon Device Research Group, Schvartzman JA, Krupitzki H, Betran AP, Requejo J, Bergel E, et al. Feasibility and safety study of a new device (Odon device) for assisted vaginal deliveries: study protocol. Reprod Health. 2013;10:33.
13. de Lange C, D Saugstad O, Solberg R. Assessment of cerebral perfusion with contrast-enhanced ultrasound during constriction of the neck mimicking malposition of the BD Odon device: a study in newborn piglets. BJOG. 2017;124(Suppl 4):26–34.
14. O'Brien SM, Winter C, Burden CA, Boulvain M, Draycott TJ, Crofts JF. Pressure and traction on a model fetal head and neck associated with the use of forceps, kiwi ventouse and the BD Odon device in operative vaginal birth: a simulation study. BJOG. 2017;124(Suppl 4):19–25.
15. O'Brien SM, Winter C, Burden CA, Boulvain M, Draycott TJ, Crofts JF. Fetal head position and perineal distension associated with the use of the BD Odon device in operative vaginal birth: a simulation study. BJOG. 2017; 124(Suppl 4):10–8.
16. Macklin R. Enrolling pregnant women in biomedical research. Lancet. 2010; 375(9715):632–3.
17. McCulloch P, Altman DG, Campbell WB, Flum DR, Glasziou P, Marshall JC, et al. No surgical innovation without evaluation: the IDEAL recommendations. Lancet. 2009;374(9695):1105–12.
18. Faris O, Shuren J. An FDA viewpoint on unique considerations for medical-device clinical trials. N Engl J Med. 2017;376(14):1350–7.
19. U.S. Department of Health and Human Services, Investigational device exceptions (IDEs) for early feasibility medical device clinical studies, including certain first in human (FIH) studies. Guidance for industry and Food and Drug Administration. 2013.
20. Lievre M, Ménard J, Bruckert E, Cogneau J, Delahaye F, Giral P, et al. Premature discontinuation of clinical trial for reasons not related to efficacy, safety, or feasibility. BMJ. 2001;322(7286):603–5.
21. Psaty B, Rennie D. Stopping medical research to save money: a broken pact with researchers and patients. JAMA. 2003;289(16):2128–31.
22. Ashcroft R. Responsibilities of sponsors are limited in premature discontinuation of trials. BMJ. 2001;323(7303):53.
23. Aasheim V, Nilsen ABV, Reinar LM, Lukasse M. Perineal techniques during the second stage of labour for reducing perineal trauma. Cochrane Database Syst Rev. 2017;6:CD006672. https://doi.org/10.1002/14651858. CD006672.pub3.
24. Melamed N, Ben-Haroush A, Chen R, Kaplan B, Yogev Y. Intrapartum cervical lacerations: characteristics, risk factors, and effects on subsequent pregnancies. Am J Obstet Gynecol. 2009;200(4):388.e1-4.

25. Landy HJ, Laughon SK, Bailit JL, Kominiarek MA, Gonzalez-Quintero VH, Ramirez M, et al. Characteristics associated with severe perineal and cervical lacerations during vaginal delivery. Obstet Gynecol. 2011;117(3):627–35.

26. Hopkins LM, Caughey AB, Glidden DV, Laros RK Jr. Racial/ethnic differences in perineal, vaginal and cervical lacerations. Am J Obstet Gynecol. 2005; 193(2):455–9.

27. Fahmy K, el-Gazar A, Sammour M, Nosair M, Salem A. Postpartum colposcopy of the cervix: injury and healing. Int J Gynaecol Obstet. 1991; 34(2):133–7.

28. Wilbanks GD, Richart RM. The puerperal cervix, injuries and healing. A colposcopic study. Am J Obstet Gynecol. 1967;97(8):1105–10.

29. Gainey HL, Keeler JE, Nicolay KS. Cervical damage in obstetrics. Part I. Cervical lacerations in primiparas. Obstet Gynecol. 1953;1(3):333–8.

30. Parikh R, Brotzman S, Anasti JN. Cervical lacerations: some surprising facts. Am J Obstet Gynecol. 2007;196(5):e17–8.

31. O'Brien SM, et al. Design and development of the BD Odon DeviceTM : a human factors evaluation process. BJOG. 2017;124(Suppl 4):35–43.

11

The no-go zone: a qualitative study of access to sexual and reproductive health services for sexual and gender minority adolescents in Southern Africa

Alex Müller[*] [ID], Sarah Spencer, Talia Meer and Kristen Daskilewicz

Abstract

Background: Adolescents have significant sexual and reproductive health needs. However, complex legal frameworks, and social attitudes about adolescent sexuality, including the values of healthcare providers, govern adolescent access to sexual and reproductive health services. These laws and social attitudes are often antipathetic to sexual and gender minorities. Existing literature assumes that adolescents identify as heterosexual, and exclusively engage in (heteronormative) sexual activity with partners of the opposite sex/gender, so little is known about if and how the needs of sexual and gender minority adolescents are met.

Methods: In this article, we have analysed data from fifty in-depth qualitative interviews with representatives of organisations working with adolescents, sexual and gender minorities, and/or sexual and reproductive health and rights in Malawi, Mozambique, Namibia, Zambia and Zimbabwe.

Results: Sexual and gender minority adolescents in these countries experience double-marginalisation in pursuit of sexual and reproductive health services: as adolescents, they experience barriers to accessing LGBT organisations, who fear being painted as "homosexuality recruiters," whilst they are simultaneously excluded from heteronormative adolescent sexual and reproductive health services. Such barriers to services are equally attributable to the real and perceived criminalisation of consensual sexual behaviours between partners of the same sex/gender, regardless of their age.

Discussion/ conclusion: The combination of laws which criminalise consensual same sex/gender activity and the social stigma towards sexual and gender minorities work to negate legal sexual and reproductive health services that may be provided. This is further compounded by age-related stigma regarding sexual activity amongst adolescents, effectively leaving sexual and gender minority adolescents without access to necessary information about their sexuality and sexual and reproductive health, and sexual and reproductive health services.

Keywords: Adolescents, Sexual and reproductive health and rights, Sexual and gender minorities, HIV, Service provision, Heteronormativity, Criminalisation, Stigma, Southern Africa, LGBT

* Correspondence: alex.muller@uct.ac.za
Gender, Health and Justice Research Unit, University of Cape Town,
Observatory, Cape Town, South Africa

Plain English summary

Little is known about how adolescents who are sexual or gender minorities (who may identify on the LGBT spectrum) access services for sexual and reproductive healthcare in Southern African countries This is because existing literature either assumes all adolescents are straight and cisgender or does not specifically ask about the sexual and gender identities of adolescents in their studies.

In order to find out about access to sexual and reproductive health services for sexual and gender minority adolescents, we conducted fifty interviews with people who provide sexual and reproductive health services, or who provide services to sexual and gender minority people (LGBT organisations) in Malawi, Mozambique, Namibia, Zambia and Zimbabwe.

We found that adolescents struggle to access services at LGBT organisations. This is because LGBT organisations mainly work with adults, because they fear being seen as promoting alternative sexuality to young people. Adolescents also struggle to access services at other organisations that specialise in sexual and reproductive health services, because these organisations do not cater to sexual and gender minorities, and may even be trans- or homophobic.

The combination of laws that criminalise consensual same sex/gender activity, and the social stigma towards sexual and gender minorities makes providing services to sexual and gender minority adolescents even more difficult. This is worsened by taboos against teenage sexuality as bad or immoral, and means that sexual and gender minority adolescents have little to no access to necessary information about their sexuality and sexual and reproductive health, and sexual and reproductive health services.

Background

Adolescents have significant needs related to HIV and sexual and reproductive health (SRH). Across Southern Africa, the birth rate amongst girls aged 15 to 19 years ranges from 8.2% in Malawi to 16.7% in Mozambique [1, 2]. Similarly, HIV/AIDS is now recognised as the primary reproductive health concern for teenagers, with young women (15 to 24 years of age) accounting for 26% of all new infections in the Eastern and Southern African region in 2016 [3, 4]. Given that adolescence is typically the period of sexual debut, good SRH services can significantly contribute to the prevention of unplanned pregnancy and HIV, as well as to limiting exposure to sexual violence and coercion [5]. Furthermore, with a generation of peri-natally HIV-infected adolescents now reaching sexual maturity due to increasing access to antiretroviral therapy, the integration of HIV and SRH services becomes even more important. Adolescents living

with HIV have health needs particular to their age demographic and context, and behavioural, medical, and social interventions and services must therefore be varied and specialised [3].

Legislative frameworks regulate adolescent sexuality and the provision of SRH services to adolescents. A number of 'ages' are legally determined: the most important in the context of SRH are the age at which adolescents can seek and consent to medical services without parental consent and the age at which adolescents are legally allowed to have sex. In many countries in Southern Africa, these ages are not aligned, leading to contradictions in the legal framework when, for example, a 15-year old teenager is not legally allowed to have sex, but is allowed to access contraception and HIV testing [6]. Further, these 'ages' not only determine what adolescents (legally) can and cannot do, but they also determine protective duties for healthcare providers, such as mandatory reporting requirements in cases where providers have knowledge of adolescent underage sex. In addition to the complex legal provisions, healthcare providers' own morals and values influence their service provision by determining when adolescents are 'worthy' or 'old enough' to access certain SRH services [7].

Most research evidence and policy responses on Southern African adolescents' HIV and SRH share one crucial shortcoming: they assume that adolescents identify as heterosexual, and exclusively engage in (penetrative, penis-vagina) sexual activity with partners of the opposite sex/gender.[1] Adolescents identifying as lesbian, gay or bisexual (sexual minority adolescents) and adolescents identifying as transgender or gender non-conforming (gender minority adolescents)[2] are often not recognised in SRH research and interventions, nor are their specific needs addressed (see, for example [5, 8–10]). An illustrative example is a report reviewing adolescents' sexual and reproductive health in Zimbabwe [11], which does not explicitly mention the sexual orientation or gender identities of the adolescents in question (and thus assumes them to be heterosexual and cisgender), nor whether health services address any non-normative SRH needs. This is common in programmes and research on adolescents. Articles that do mention sexual orientation simply list it as a factor that "marginalize[s] [adolescents] because of individual characteristics" but fail to outline or address substantial issues that pertain to the HIV and SRH needs of sexual and gender minority adolescents [12].

The underlying assumption of heterosexuality, and the subsequent omission of sexual and gender minority adolescents in research on adolescent SRH in Southern Africa, is indicative of wider societal heteronormativity [13], including in healthcare provision [14, 15] and research [16]. Heteronormativity is a social construct that assumes heterosexual identities and relationships are the norm, and thus makes sexual and gender minority identities invisible in all facets of social life, including in healthcare provision and research [13, 17]. Through its pervasive normative influence, it leads people, in and outside of the healthcare sector, to assume that every patient, healthcare provider, student, research participant, and researcher is heterosexual and cisgender. As a result, sexual and gender minority people's diverse health needs are not routinely recognized [18], documented [19], taught [20] or researched [21].

Despite advances in sexual orientation-related anti-discrimination laws globally, many countries still criminalise consensual same-sex activity [22]. In many Southern African countries, these laws originate from Victorian penal codes, introduced during British colonial rule, and offences are defined as 'sodomy' or 'carnal knowledge against the order of nature' [23]. The enforcement of such laws is inconsistent [24] and dependent on national political and social contexts. Regardless of enforcement, however, laws that criminalise same-sex behaviour effectively marginalise sexual and gender minority individuals. Although evidence from African countries is scant [25], public health research from other contexts shows that criminalisation and minority status lead to poorer health outcomes ranging from infectious disease to mental health [26]. Ironically, health policies in some of the same countries that criminalise same-sex activity categorise 'men who have sex with men' as 'key populations', indicating their necessity for health services due to their increased vulnerability to HIV resulting from social exclusion

and criminalising legal frameworks [27]. This vulnerability is confirmed by a study from South Africa (where there is no criminalisation) with both heterosexual and sexual minority teenagers: compared to heterosexual matched peers, sexual minority teenagers experienced higher levels of partner-perpetrated violence, and showed higher levels of depression, traumatic stress and substance use [28]. Whilst there is no current evidence, it is probable that these differences are even more pronounced in countries where same-sex activity is criminalised.

Given these restrictive legal frameworks around same-sex activity, as well as the invisibility of sexual orientation and gender identity in current adolescent sexual and reproductive health policies, our paper examines the current provision of SRH services, which include HIV-related services, to sexual and gender minority adolescents in five Southern African countries: Malawi, Mozambique, Namibia, Zambia, and Zimbabwe. Table 1 provides an overview of the current legal and policy framework related to same-sex activity in the five countries that our study was conducted. Included in this study is Mozambique, a country where consensual same-sex activity was decriminalised in 2014, as well as four countries with differing levels of criminalisation.

For the purposes of this research, adolescents were considered those aged 12 to 18. We argue that sexual and gender minority adolescents in these countries experience double-marginalisation due to their age and sexual and/or gender minority identity, and that they are routinely excluded from existing SRH services.

Table 1 Legal framework for sexual and gender minority adolescents in study countries

	Where in the law?	Male same sex activity criminalized	Female same sex activity criminalized	Enforced through arrests	'Promotion' or 'morality' law	Reporting duty for healthcare providers
Malawi	Penal Code Cap. 7:01, Sections 137A, 153, 154, 156	Yes "Against the order of nature", "Attempted unnatural offence", "Gross male indecency"	Yes "Gross female indecency"	Yes	No	No
Mozambique	No	No	No	No	No	No
Namibia	Roman Dutch common law (based on case law), no codified provision	Yes (not codified)	No	No	No	No
Zambia	The Penal Code Act (amended by Act 15 of 2005), Sections 155, 156, 15	Yes "Against the order of nature", "Attempted unnatural offence", "Gross indecency" Imprisonment of 7-14 years for adults, community service or counseling for children under the age of 18	Yes "Gross indecency" Imprisonment of 7-14 years for adults, community service or counseling for children under the age of 18	Yes	No	No
Zimbabwe	Criminal law (Codification and reform) Act Section 73	Yes "Sodomy" Fine and/ or imprisonment up to one year	No	Yes	No	No

Methods

Study design, sampling and recruitment

We conducted a qualitative interview-based study with representatives of organisations working with, or providing SRH services to adolescents in Malawi, Mozambique, Namibia, Zambia and Zimbabwe. These organisations do not have a specific focus on sexual and gender minority adolescents. In this paper, we refer to them as '(A)SRH organisations' – to signify provision of either specific adolescent sexual and reproductive health (ASRH) services, or general SRH services that are also open to adolescents. Additionally, in each of the five countries, we interviewed representatives of organisations focused on advocacy for, or services to, sexual and gender minority people – widely referred to as LGBT[3] (lesbian, gay, bisexual and transgender) organisations. Given that same-sex activity is criminalised in four out of the five countries in this research, all except Mozambique, and that, additionally, adolescent sexuality, homo- and bisexuality as well as gender non-conformity is heavily stigmatised in all five countries, we decided to interview these NGO representatives as proxies in order to protect sexual and gender minority adolescents from potential harms. Further, NGO representatives are in a better position to talk about pathways and barriers because they have the accumulated experiences of having worked across sectors at both service delivery and policy levels. Thus they are able to draw comparisons and better evaluate the impact of the law and policy framework on sexual and gender minority ASRH access. In order to gain better insight, where possible, we also interviewed government representatives involved in policymaking on issues of ASRH.

Potential participants were identified through three methods: (1) from a contact list of non-governmental organisations working with, or providing services to adolescents in each of the five countries that the researchers had compiled during the years of their work on SRH in Southern Africa; (2) by participants electing to be contacted for further research at the end of a related online survey of (A)SRH NGO workers, and (3) through referrals from the researchers' networks and participants themselves. We purposively sampled participants based on these three methods by contacting potential participants by email or phone and asking them to participate in the research.

Data collection

Qualitative interview data were collected from October 2015 to May 2016. In total, we conducted 50 interviews with 51 participants: seven participants in Malawi, nine in Mozambique, nine in Namibia (one interview had two participants), 13 in Zambia, and 13 in Zimbabwe (see Table 2 for more detail). Due to local proficiency and the pervasive use of English in the NGO sectors in

Table 2 Affiliation of participants, by country

Country	Adolescent/ SRH organisation	LGBT organisation	Policy maker	Total Participants
Malawi	4	2	1	7
Mozambique	8	1	–	9
Namibia	6	2	1	9
Zambia	11	1	1	13
Zimbabwe	10	1	2	13

Malawi, Namibia, Zambia, and Zimbabwe, researchers (AM, KD, TM and SS) interviewed participants in person in English. Two researchers were present for most interviews and all interviews were recorded and then transcribed. Additionally, the second researcher took notes during the interviews. One interview was conducted over the phone with a participant based in Malawi.

All interviews in Mozambique were conducted by an experienced research consultant through phone interviews in Portuguese which were recorded, transcribed and then translated into English.

Data analysis

All transcripts were imported to NVivo 11 for coding. A team of three researchers (AM, KD, SS) developed a coding framework based on the research questions, interview guide, and interview notes. Each researcher independently coded three transcripts using the coding framework. Afterward, the team discussed the coding process to identify any discrepancies in coding between the researchers and refined the codes. Thereafter, one researcher (AM) was responsible for coding the 50 transcripts for sexual orientation and gender identity-related codes. All coded data were read for similarities and the emergence of key themes, which then guided a further thematic analysis.

Research ethics

The University of Cape Town's Faculty of Health Sciences Human Research Ethics Committee approved this study (HREC reference number 683/2015). All participants understood that participation was voluntary, completed an informed consent process and signed an informed consent form prior to participating. For this paper, we use pseudonyms, and all responses have been anonymized.

Results

Attitudes towards sexual and gender minority adolescents

Participants from (A)SRH organisations were heterogeneous in their attitudes towards sexual and gender minority adolescents. Some affirmed sexual diversity and recognised that sexual and gender minority adolescents should receive SRH services without judgement. For example, Rutendo describes engaging with her colleagues during a training about providing services to minority adolescents:

... the question that kept coming throughout the training was, okay, a young person comes and asks a condom - "But what if I know that they're gay?" [laughter] and it's like, well, just give them the condom and, you know, they did not come to ask you "Should I be gay or not?", they've come to ask you for a condom. Deal with the issue at hand. And, you know, let them go. And, "Oh, so, what should I do if I find out someone's gay?" and I'm like "Just give the service that they've come for and let them go on their way." But I think there's that issue of interpretation of what does the law say, and what does it mean for services provision, and then you add on to that my own personal value system and what I think about those issues. (Rutendo, from an (A)SRH organisation in Zimbabwe)

Others, however, spoke about their own lack of knowledge on issues of sexual orientation and gender identity, calling homosexuality 'a new thing' and cited this as a reason for not bringing these issues up in their work with adolescents:

Even the NGOs that are operating in Malawi, not many of us know more about this issue. (Patience, from an (A)SRH organisation in Malawi)

Many participants like Patience had difficulty naming "this issue", suggesting an underlying discomfort. Rather than not knowing much about "this issue", participants may hold problematic or negative views about sexual and gender minority adolescents.

Other participants were more forthright in expressing their disapproval, arguing that same-sex activity was immoral, or that sexual and gender minority adolescents 'did not exist' in their country, or area. Caroline is emphatic about her perception of Zimbabwe as a heterosexual nation:

Discussing about lesbianism and preaching about it, you know, we can't do that here. We don't want to see all those young men and women that are into homosexuality. It's not a thing that we can discuss here in Zimbabwe. Here in Zimbabwe we've got a stance, we don't want it, people don't want it. (Caroline, from an (A)SRH organisation in Zimbabwe)

Similarly, Patrick, in Malawi sees same-sex activity as a product of the moral corruption of urban areas, which does not take place in modest rural areas:

These things are happening, more specially in towns. People, the very same sex, they are doing the sex. Women sleeping with women. Men sleeping with men. It happens all in town, not in the community areas, [which are] very modest areas, no. (Patrick, from an (A)SRH organisation in Malawi)

It was clear that the opinions of the participants reflect broader attitudes towards sexual orientation and gender identity in these countries. Many of the participants who were accepting of sexual and gender minority adolescents, both within LGBT organisations and in SRH organisations, spoke about how their environment was heavily infused with attitudes that discriminated against, and socially excluded adolescents based on their sexual orientation or gender identity:

There is nothing in the law that criminalises homosexuality in Mozambique or even same-sex relationships in Mozambique, legally there is nothing hampering it, but socially there is an immense barrier. (Victorino, from an (A)SRH organisation in Mozambique)

...what I've also found in this country is that it's the whole political rhetoric that then influences what happens on the ground. So, even our police find it easy to go and harass people and so forth because they know that, politically, no one is going to come down on them. Although, really, it's not legal. Yeah. (Rutendo, from an (A)SRH organisation in Zimbabwe)

In the professional experience of participants, such discrimination included bullying and violence at school and in other social spaces, the loss of friends and social networks, rejection by families and ejection from the family home, and experiencing discrimination when accessing public services, including healthcare.

(A)SRH services in public health facilities

While public health facilities technically provide ASRH services, these services are typically not accommodating for sexual and gender minority adolescents. Participants from LGBT organisations in all five countries described how heteronormative public health facilities were:

[LGBT adolescents] cannot even get the, even when we talk of the youth friendly facilities, even in those, they are not, they cannot, the people there, the training of the youth friendly facilities service providers does not include talking about sexual diversity, does not include the LGBTI people. It doesn't. And so, it falls through. (Munya, SRH consultant in Zimbabwe)

I don't want to have a broad brush that [...] healthcare [in Zambia] is homophobic – that's not the case – but how would youth know how to find that one practitioner that may, in fact, be sensitive and open to serving them? They wouldn't necessarily know that. And, so, it's very difficult but you could get shamed, shunned, reported; there's nothing to protect you. (George, a service provider in Zambia)

Consistently, participants attributed the deficiencies in service provision and the heteronormativity in public health facilities to health professionals' training, or lack thereof when it comes to sexual and gender minorities, and adolescents in particular:

We have nurses who complete the nursing program, but they do not have knowledge about issues related to gender identity and sexual orientation. Then appears someone in your office whose identity card has the name Antonio, however you see a transgender woman who is dressed differently from what the nurse expected for an Antonio to be dressed... We have cases of patients that have already been told that, 'I am here waiting for Antonio and not Mary.' The nurse just knows that Antonio has to dress as Antonio [...] So here starts the first hurdle, instead of the nurse offering to start health services, they judge that individual because of the way they dress, this is where the problems start. (Joao, from an LGBT organisation in Mozambique)

And, then, we don't really have, most of our medical personnel have not had the opportunity to be trained out of Zambia where you have the opportunity to interact with different kinds of patients. So, they don't really know how to treat a trans person when they come in for a service, for example. (Thandi, from an (A)SRH organisation in Zambia)

Furthermore, commodities for sexual and gender minority adolescents such as dental dams and lubricants were generally not available in public health facilities. Where private care exits, these may be available in a private pharmacy or a private clinic. Participants from LGBT organisations highlighted that the unavailability of commodities in public sector care was linked to the criminalisation of same-sex activity, and fears of 'promoting homosexuality':

Dental dams and finger cots are kind of illegal [...] because of its association with the LGBTI community. [...] So if you are providing dental dams, it's more like you're spearheading the act of homosexuality. So they are not usually accessible, you can't find them, because that would be seen as [...] trying to promote

homosexuality. So you'll never find it anywhere. (David, from an LGBT organisation in Zambia)

The need for parental consent to access SRH services and commodities in public health facilities is a barrier for all adolescents wanting to access these services. Participants from LGBT organisations highlighted how this can pose particular challenges for sexual and gender minority adolescents:

People have lost their family ties because they are homosexuals. And most of them are the youngsters that are not yet independent, who cannot stay on their own, who cannot pay for their own school fees, and some have even dropped out of school – we have so many people that have dropped out of school because their parents knew that they are homosexual and they say, 'no, we don't want a child like you.' So, it's a double dilemma that they can't go to health services so they can't access, let's say condoms for safer sex. They can't access condoms for safer sex at the health services, because they are underage and they can't go with parental permission. (Kennedy, from an LGBT organisation in Malawi)

As Kennedy explains, sexual and gender minority adolescents may be more likely to lose family support due to their disapproval of the adolescent's sexual orientation or gender identity. As a result, they may not access education and health services that require parental consent.

Heteronormativity in adolescent sexual and reproductive health services

Previous research has shown that confidentiality, youth-friendliness, a broad range of services, and affordable care are important factors in adolescents' preferences to access sexual and reproductive health services and information from private service providers, NGOs, or the public sector [29]. It is unsurprising that confidentiality and youth-friendliness are especially important for young people, as they are widely perceived as violating religious and moral norms by engaging in sexual activity [30]. Urban adolescents may have a stronger preference for private providers, which are perceived as more confidential, or NGO providers, which are perceived as youth-friendly [31]. This means that NGOs play a pivotal role in providing SRH services to adolescents, particularly in urban settings. This is arguably even more the case for sexual and gender minority adolescents, whose SRH concerns require practitioners to be direct and detailed in the information that they provide, as illustrated by Tafadzwa's description of the questions that practitioners should expect from sexual and gender minority youth:

What are the risks that are involved when it comes to SRH if you decide to engage in sexual activity? What does the law of Zimbabwe say if you have anal sex? What is sodomy? If you are caught, what does it mean? And then we also go, what are the risks that are involved in you having unprotected sex? And what can you do to prevent if you decide to? Where do I get the condoms? Where do I get the lubricants?
(Tafadzwa, from an LGBT organisation in Zimbabwe)

This quote explains the level of detail and reassurance sexual and gender minority adolescents need when deciding where to access SRH services. In our entire sample of NGOs, however, none provided services tailored to sexual and gender minority adolescents. Participants recognised that there are very few, if any, SRH education and services for sexual and gender minority teenagers:

[W]e do not have that system or recreational spaces where young people can go and speak or meet other young people to speak to about these things. So, it's really a struggle, there's not space for LGBT young people to get together, there's no environment created.
(Hilma, from an LGBT organisation in Namibia)

The reason for this gap in service provision among mainstream (A)SRH organisations is clear: pervasive heteronormativity in ASRH policy and provision. When we asked why they do not include sexual and gender minority teenagers in their service provision, Kelvin, from an SRH organisation in Zimbabwe, said: 'We're just taking them as a homogenous group, like they're all heterosexual'. That this is an erroneous assumption was clear to those working in the LGBT sector, as highlighted by Kennedy, a representative from an LGBT organisation in Malawi:

If you have the youth, the heterosexual youth that engage in the sex before the age of 18, why should we assume that we don't have adolescents who are homosexual who are also engaged in sex before the age of 18?

Heteronormativity creates a blind spot for sexual and gender minority adolescents, creating barriers to their ASRH access.

Sexual and gender minority stigma and criminalisation
Participants from (A)SRH organisations cited two major reasons upholding this heteronormative approach to ASRH services: the social stigma attached to homosexuality, and the criminalisation of same-sex activity. Stanley, who works at an (A)SRH organisation in Malawi, describes how these two issues converge to determine the content of SRH education and information materials for adolescents:

[The penal code] has impacted that people don't want to talk about these things and, also, we don't have sufficient communication, IEC [information, education, communication] material to use in terms of disseminating this. Of course, physically, these IEC materials are produced by the government and, you know, proofread by the National AIDS Commission, so we don't really have much of this information. So, they have an impact because no one wants to talk about it and we don't have sufficient IEC materials in terms of doing, you know, anal safer sex.

For Stanley, criminalisation in Malawi generates and compounds social stigma, and also means that the actual resources produced are subject to censorship – as they are produced by the state.

This was not the case in Malawi only. A number of participants across the five countries spoke about the challenges of including information about sexual orientation and gender identity into information materials. In Zambia, the control that government has in determining the content of SRH materials, including comprehensive sexuality education curricula, was evident:

We were directed to [...] remove those aspects that have got to do with lesbians and gays and so on from the peer education manual. So, we haven't completed it yet, it's still in the process of development, but we are warned to be [...] cautious in terms of how we include it in the manual because the government will not sign it off if it finds that there are these issues that are included there. (Cynthia, from an (A)SRH organisation in Zambia)

Beyond criminalisation (in four countries) and social stigma, discriminatory and judgmental attitudes of service providers in adolescent SRH organisations, as already described above, emerged as a third reason for not providing services to sexual and gender minority adolescents.

"Recruitment" panic: A barrier to LGBT organisations' service provision
As a further complication, participants from LGBT organisations in countries where same sex activity was criminalised (Malawi, Namibia, Zambia and Zimbabwe) very firmly stated that they were governed by the legal age of majority (18 in all focus countries) in determining who they can serve. This is different from the age at which adolescents can legally access SRH services: age 16 in Zambia and Zimbabwe, but not specifically defined in Malawi and Namibia [6].

In contrast to (A)SRH organisations, LGBT organisations did not provide services because they were afraid that work with adolescents would lead to increased public scrutiny and opposition, and moral backlash to their overall work:

As an organisation, we see the great need to do work on [ASRH]. [...] But still, as a director, I feel completely uncomfortable when I see a child in school uniform in the office. [...] The risk is quite high. [W]e would be attacked [for] the issue of 'recruiting and promotion'. [... A]lso the fact that it can taint our mandate as an organisation and [...] that religious groups shall attack and bring it down as a movement. (Hilma, from an LGBT advocacy organisation in Namibia)

It's like a no-go zone [...] during our meetings that we have with MSM clients, if we find that there is somebody who is below the age of 18, we ask them to [...] leave. (Blessing, from an LGBT advocacy organisation in Malawi)

'Recruitment and promotion of homosexuality' is not a criminal offence in any of the focus countries. Despite this, many participants were afraid of being accused of "recruit[ing] the youngsters into homosexuality" (Blessing, Malawi), of "initiating something" (David, Zambia), and thus of being "put in trouble" (Tafadzwa, Zimbabwe). While none of the relevant laws on same-sex activity actually outlaw work with adolescents, it was clear that LGBT organisations elected to only work with adults to avoid accusations that could damage their reputation or jeopardise their overall programmatic work.

Where organisations did provide education or services to teenagers, the interpretation of 'recruitment and promotion' also meant that they had to be careful in how SRHR education messages were framed:

It's just the language. We all know for a fact, when you write language like you're 'promoting the advancement and well-being of LGBT people'. But we now know, we don't use the term 'promotion', we just 'advance the well-being'. So, it's all about playing with language. (Hilma, from an LGBT organisation in Namibia)

Hence, the universally accepted terminology of 'health promotion' is eschewed in order to avoid any potential association with notions of 'promoting homosexuality'.

Mozambique, the only country in this research where same-sex activity is not criminalised, was the only country where the LGBT organisation representative did not mention the age of legal majority as defining access to services. However, even in this decriminalised context, sexual and gender minority youth are still highly stigmatised. Joao, a participant from a LGBT organisation in Mozambique, shared an experience that led them to determine that they will not work with teens younger than 15 years old.

Despite the relative legal freedom, Joao describes how fear of being seen to recruit young people to homosexuality shapes LGBT organisations' work:

[A boy] posted a photo on Facebook in one of our programs. It was a social program, he took a picture and he had our t-shirt and posted the photo on Facebook and someone from his family saw the photo and [said] that [organisation's name] was pushing it, and was promoting homosexuality to their child. As if their son's sexual orientation was the product of him participating in our programmes. We have had several situations like these, it is why strategically, the organisation decided that we will reduce our involvement with younger beneficiaries, taking into account that individuals older than 15 years are more aware of what they are and what they do.

This instance clearly describes how stigma can continue to impact sexual and gender minority adolescents' access to services, even in a decriminalised setting.

Resultantly, educational material tailored to sexual and gender minority adolescents on ASRH, including sexuality, did not exist in any of the countries in this study. This means that sexual and gender minority adolescents in these countries have hardly any access to information about safer sex, or to resources that could help them develop a healthy relationship to their sexuality:

[Sex between two men is] mentioned as something that happens, but [...] there is no special mention of specific HIV prevention strategies for that group like, you know, use of lubricants or anything like that, no. It's just mentioned that this can be there and, in the school material, it's then mentioned that [...] it is criminalised. (Rutendo, from an (A)SRH organisation in Zimbabwe)

Also as a result of being unable to provide services to teenagers themselves, LGBT organisations started organising referral networks to adolescent SRH organisations. Often, this involved careful vetting of potential referral organisations, and required substantial education on issues of sexual orientation and gender identity for the service providers of these organisations before referrals could take place. Hilma and Tafadzwa described how such referral systems worked in Namibia and Zimbabwe, respectively:

We are only since last year getting into the SRHR agenda because they excluded us for so long. [Adolescent SRH organisation] is the one that is working closely with us in the regions because they are the main service providers for young people, from 12 till 18 or above. Because at [adolescent SRH organisation], you can go in there and get your young child serviced with confidentiality guaranteed. [Adolescent SRH organisation] is also one of the friendliest partners that we have, that we always pick up the phone and say 'we are dropping ten people now'. The director will leave whatever he is [doing and] attend to our needs. So, [adolescent SRH organisation] is the only enabling clinic in this country for young [LGBT] people. (Hilma, from an LGBT organisation in Namibia)

What we do is, [...] if there are people from the LGBTI community that are under 18, we do have partners that we work with where we are able to refer them for specific services. If it's, for instance, they want counselling because a lot of young adults, they struggle with understanding their sexuality, we make sure that we do it with the [counselling service...] If they feel that they need somebody from the [LGBTI] community to provide the counselling, we do have people that have been trained to also have skills in family therapy [...] So sometimes we go in and actually do the counselling there because it's an established entity and also for safety reasons. (Tafadzwa, from an LGBT organisation in Zimbabwe)

These referrals appear to work for adolescents because (A)SRH organisations are perceived differently to LGBT organisations. Importantly, (A)SRH organisations are able to frame SRH services to sexual and gender minority adolescents within a public health approach rather than an advocacy approach, and thus provide them services without the risk of being perceived to 'promote and recruit', as illustrated here:

Because of the fact that our emphasis is on health, we are very comfortable to defend that approach [...]. And nobody can argue that [...] we are an advocate for the LGBT sector. We accept [LGBT adolescents] from a health perspective and we provide the service to the young person, to the LGBTI person on the basis of HIV prevention. We'd rather help this person, empower this person to help him or herself and therefore in the process reduce [HIV risk]." (Charles, from an (A)SRH organisation in Namibia)

However, this referral strategy is not sufficient to ensure access to SRH services for all sexual and gender minority adolescents. The referral networks between LGBT and (A)SRH organisations that our participants spoke about were based on individual relationships and networks. Without agreed-upon institutional commitments, access to SRH services for sexual and gender minority

adolescents is dependent not only on the brokerage of the LGBT organisation, but also on individual providers within the (A)SRH organisation. While this approach might work well when the individuals are sympathetic, it raises questions about the sustainability and longevity when (A)SRH organisations experience personnel changes – especially given the existing discriminatory attitudes of some adolescent organisations' staff.

The impact of criminalising laws on access to services

Participants spoke at length about how the current criminalisation of same-sex activity in four of the study countries impacts access to SRH services for sexual and gender minority adolescents. While none of the laws pose a direct legal barrier to services, the legal framework contributed to an environment of state-endorsed homophobia, in which public healthcare providers, and at times even private or NGO service providers, could refuse to provide services to sexual and gender minority adolescents. There were five distinct ways in which criminalising laws contributed to the barriers to sexual and reproductive health services that sexual and gender minority adolescents face.

First, Kennedy from Malawi (LGBT organisation) recounted that healthcare providers had reported sexual and gender minority patients who had sought SRH services to the police, because healthcare providers were under the (erroneous) impression that they had a duty to report:

We've had a report where some medical providers have reported the patient to the police. You see, you get to the confidential room, you tell them your problem and you open up because you expect the doctor to be confidential about issues, so you open up with them to say 'ok, I'm gay, and I have sex with several guys, and I have this problem,' and then there was a situation where the medical person said 'ok, fine, just wait for me here' and then went out, made a phone call to the police: 'I have a homosexual here.' Something like that. It happened in Malawi. And you can imagine that such a thing went all over the MSM networks, telling themselves, 'Guys, don't you ever go to such-such a hospital; they are going to arrest you; this is what happened to me.'

Second, as Kennedy's quote highlights, the fear of potentially being reported prevents sexual and gender minority adolescents from seeking services. This reluctance compounds with other reasons for which adolescents might not want to seek services, such as fear of age-related judgmental attitudes from healthcare and other service providers. Kennedy elaborated:

Despite the fact that [...] Malawi's trying [...] to promote the youth friendly services, the laws [criminalising same-sex activity] have been there before and they are still at the back of so many of our minds, including the service providers. So, you find out that even when the youth go there and go to places which are termed to be 'youth friendly service providers,' they still find some other service providers who [...] say 'How could you do that as young as you?' So, at the same time, even if we, the young MSM, were to access the services at the youth friendly service centres, they will also experience something similar to that, to say, 'How do you manage to be having sex through your anus?'

Third, criminalising laws contribute to and validate social stigma related to non-heteronormative sexual orientation and gender identity. Whether or not these laws are enforced, the fact that they exist is often used to justify discriminatory, harmful and exclusionary practices against sexual and gender minority adolescents. Shelton, who works for an LGBT organisation, explains how this played out prior to decriminalisation in Mozambique:

I would just say that there has never been a habit [...] of arresting people because they have sex with a same-sex partner. The point is that there was a law [that criminalised same-sex activity], if someone wanted to they could use the law, but in reality it was not used, it was not a real prison or a real penalty because of this, however Mozambique has a context with stigma for those who have sex with someone of the same sex.

Fourth, misinterpretation of criminalising laws perpetuates false perceptions that justify discriminatory practices. For example, some participants from (A)SRH organisations were under the impression that they could not talk about sexual orientation or gender identity during comprehensive sex education because they would be 'promoting' criminalised behaviour. Evelyn, who works at an (A)SRH organisation in Zimbabwe, was even under the impression that some HIV prevention commodities (dental dams and lubricants) were also criminalised:

You don't have commodities for young people who have got a different sexual orientation in Zimbabwe; you cannot come through our borders with that kind of material.

This is actually not true – Tafadzwa, from a Zimbabwean LGBT organisation, told us that the organisation had received a shipment of condoms and lubricant, paid for by the Ministry of Health under a Global Fund-funded 'key

population' programme. Thus, Evelyn's erroneous perception illustrates how social stigma and criminalising laws collide and lead to misinformation. This is also illustrated in an anecdote that Kennedy from Malawi (LGBT organization) shared about healthcare providers refusing to provide services to sexual and gender minority adolescents:

Sometimes even the service providers themselves feel like, 'Ok, if I'm going to provide the services to a homosexual, it means I'm condoning homosexuality and therefore I may be arrested as well,' for helping someone to be a homosexual or to stay a homosexual, something like that.

If and when such cases of discrimination come to the attention of an LGBT organisation, the organisation, acting on behalf of their client, often directly challenges the individual healthcare provider's refusal to provide services. However, in cases where the patient is an adolescent, organisations are limited in their response due to the concerns around perceptions of 'recruitment' and 'promotion of homosexuality' discussed in earlier sections.

Fifth, criminalisation contributes to confusion and misconceptions regarding healthcare professionals' duties given the contradictions between laws which criminalise same-sex behaviours and policies which promote HIV service provision to 'key populations,' including sexual and gender minorities. Evelyn from Zimbabwe said that this "discrepancy" means that, against what the law says, "we are giving [LGBT people] whatever they want, we are giving them access". Thandi, from a Zambian (A)SRH organisation, summarised her perception of the conflicting obligations of Zambian healthcare providers, echoing once more the need for trained, sensitive providers:

We should be having focused programming on health for this group but, like always, there was the push back to say, 'there's this law that does not allow.' So, if you're creating health programs for this group, you are in essence going against what the law provides for, because that then becomes an illegal service. But, also, the fact that who will be able to provide those services, because you need someone that understands but also that is non-judgemental to be able to provide the services.

Kennedy, from an LGBT organisation, observed the same impediment in Malawi:

[...] even the health service provider, themselves, [...] the legal framework has affected what is contained in their training [...] So you find out that they come back

from the training institutions without knowing how they are going to attend to the needs of the 'vilest' people, including MSM [men who have sex with men] or including LGBTI.

While this conflict between law and policy can be problematic, it can also serve as an opportunity to provide sexual and gender minority adolescents with SRH care:

I think if we were to smoothen things on the legal side, I think it would be easier for the service provider on the health side to then work with the adolescent. Sometimes, you want to engage them which is something that I think is something that really should be done, so you want to engage them and put in place certain intervention because of the legal issue behind the scenes, you may engage them but you may not be able to provide their service. So, yeah, that's a serious challenge. (Elvis, Zimbabwean policy maker)

According to this policymaker, public health framing is a potential loophole to ensure SRH service provision to sexual and gender minority people, further arguing that law reform should be considered in order to harmonise law and public health policy.

Discussion

In this paper, we presented data from in-depth interviews with 51 participants working in (A)SRH and LGBT organisations from five countries in Southern Africa. Our findings highlight the double-marginalisation of sexual and gender minority adolescents: they are excluded from LGBT-specific services aimed at adults, and at the same time, they are excluded from heteronormative (A)SRH services. This double-marginalisation is in large part due to, and reinforced by, laws that criminalise consensual sexual behaviour between partners of the same sex/gender, regardless of their age. However, the findings also reveal the role that homophobia and stigma play in these processes, including in Mozambique where same-sex/gender sexual behaviours have been decriminalised.

Our findings are subject to a number of limitations. First, we did not speak to sexual and gender minority adolescents themselves, to avoid placing them in a more vulnerable position. It is important to bear in mind that our findings are based on the perspective of service providers. However, we believe that service providers might actually have been better able to provide insight into pathways and policy-related barriers, as their work allows them to compare and collect individuals' experiences. Second, we focused our work on urban areas, as this was where most NGOs were located. Our findings might therefore neglect the specific barriers related to

geographical location that sexual and gender adolescents in rural areas face. Based on the literature, it can be assumed that attitudes around sexuality might be even more conservative [30], and access to ASRH services even more sporadic [32] in areas far from urban centres. Third, we did not speak to healthcare providers, which limits our insight into healthcare providers' attitudes and knowledge on sexual and gender minority adolescents. The impression that our participants gave of conservative and judgmental healthcare provider attitudes is confirmed by literature [14, 33], but further research will need to explore the relationship between provider attitude, knowledge, and socio-legal context.

Despite these limitations, our findings resonate with the literature. Other authors have recently pointed to the erroneous assumption of heteronormative homogeneity of adolescents in SRH policy: Judhistari and colleagues [34] critique the narrow view that such policies take, and Hindin and Fatusi [35] show how narrow ideas of who adolescents are fail to recognise the diverse needs within adolescent populations (due to, among others, dis/ability, sexuality and socio-economic status). Our findings highlight the consequences of heteronormative policies, which result in a complete lack of sexual and reproductive healthcare services for sexual and gender minority adolescents.

There are compelling arguments that show why sexual and gender minority adolescents in particular need access to such services: research from South Africa shows that HIV prevalence is higher among adult men who have sex with men than in the general population [36], and that 10% of adult women who have sex with women self-report that they are living with HIV [37]. Given that, in Southern Africa, 15-24 year olds currently have the highest HIV prevalence [3], this means that in all likelihood, sexual and gender minority adolescents carry a significant burden of HIV infection. Equally crucial is the mental health and well-being of sexual and gender minority adolescents, which is included in comprehensive definitions of sexual health [38]: international studies show that sexual and gender minority adolescents tend to have higher rates of depression and suicidal ideation and attempts, often because of their experiences of social exclusion and marginalisation due to their sexual orientation and gender identity [39]. A South African study evidences that sexual minority youth have higher levels of partner-perpetrated violence, and higher levels of depression, traumatic stress and substance use when compared to heterosexual matched peers [28]. Research further shows that structural stigma, including through criminalising laws, leads to worse mental health outcomes among sexual minority groups [26]. In brief, this means that sexual and gender minority adolescents in countries with criminalising laws might be in dire need of the services that are denied to them.

When the law criminalises consensual same-sex/gender sexual activity, our findings have shown that conversations with sexual and gender minority adolescents seeking SRH services, if and when they happen, tend to focus on the legal provisions and potential punishments. This has important implications for how sexual and gender minority adolescents can, or cannot, conceptualise consensual sex. If all sex they have is illegal and no SRH educational material targeting sexual and gender minority adolescents exists, these adolescents are not provided with vital information about sexual violence within same sex/gender sexual encounters and relationships. Research points to the importance of nuanced, detailed conversations about the nature and context of consent with adolescents in order to develop healthy ideas about sex and sexuality, and to prevent sexual and other forms of violence [40]. For sexual and gender minority adolescents, then, the illegality of any sex that they may engage in complicates these conversations and runs the risk of shifting the focus of the conversation on the legal parameters of sexuality rather than on nuanced discussions of mutual consent.

Further, due to the fluidity of punitive and stigmatising discourses such as those about 'recruitment and promotion of homosexuality', in countries where same-sex behaviours are criminalised, and even those where they are not, working with adolescents takes on an added dimension of risk for LGBT organisations. While not a law in the five study countries, the offence of 'recruitment' does exist in other African countries (for example, Uganda [41, 42]). This speaks to both the ability of homophobic legal discourses to travel on the continent and embed itself within and perpetuate societal homophobia, and the way in which they may override enabling local legal frameworks in the provision of ASRH services. Thus, LGBT organisations are wary of accusations of recruitment of minors due to societal homophobia and not because of, but despite, the legal framework.

Over the past 10 years, advocacy for better healthcare services and against the criminalisation of LGBT populations have been more successful when they were framed as public health arguments [43]. In other words, governments were more likely to concede some rights to sexual and gender minority people if these rights were linked to health concerns. For example, men who have sex with men and transgender individuals are now recognised as 'key populations' in many African countries, even if same-sex activity remains outlawed. In these countries, MSM and transgender people are explicitly mentioned in national policy documents by Ministries of Health, usually related to HIV prevention, and, with financial support from international funding sources such as the Global Fund, these Ministries of Health provide services for 'key populations'. As Epprecht [43] shows, the careful, nuanced argument that was successful in these cases

focused on public health rather than 'LGBT rights', and thus allowed governments to provide services to 'key populations' without requiring a public declaration that they support rights for sexual and gender minority people. Our findings caution, however, that these 'key populations' are usually conceptualised only as adults, and that sexual and gender minority adolescents are thus not included in programming and service provision. Our findings underscore the need to acknowledge adolescents as part of key populations [44], with special emphasis on young people's heterogeneity and particular vulnerabilities that Baggaley et al. [45] recently articulated.

Policy development, however, will need to be accompanied by mandatory education and training for healthcare and other service providers on serving sexual and gender minority adolescents, in order to ensure that key population policies are actually implemented for adolescents. Our findings highlight the sexual orientation- and/or gender identity-related barriers that sexual and gender minority adolescents face when accessing SRH services. These barriers compound age-related barriers that are already reported in the literature: nurses' judgment about sexuality at young ages [30], and discretionary service provision based on nurses' perceptions of an adolescent patient's 'worth' [7]. There is a clear need for policymakers and service providers to be aware of, and sensitive to, the double-marginalisation experienced by sexual and gender minority adolescents, based on both their age and sexual orientation and/or gender identity.

Conclusion

The African Commission on Human and People's Rights, in its resolution 275 [46] and a recent report [47], has emphasised the need to protect people against violence and other human rights violations on the basis of their real or imputed sexual orientation or gender identity [46, 47]. The report included a call for states to revise legislative frameworks that criminalise consensual same-sex/gender sexual behaviour. Our findings provide further evidence for the need for legislative reform by highlighting the deleterious consequences of denying SRH service provision to sexual and gender minority adolescents, particularly in countries with criminalising frameworks. The combination of laws that criminalise same-sex/gender sexual activity and societal homophobia effectively exclude sexual and gender minority adolescents from existing (A)SRH services, leaving this vulnerable group without access to information about their sexuality, about sexual health, and about how to protect themselves from HIV.

Endnotes

[1]In an attempt to be precise about what the existing laws criminalise, activists and scholars specify that it is 'same-sex activity' that is contentious, rather than gay/

lesbian/ bisexual or transgender identity. We agree, and at the same time are aware that the term 'sex' (denoting physical attributes) is inappropriate to refer to gender diversity and gender non-conformity, and therefore also include the term 'gender' (denoting people's identity, rather than their bodily characteristics).

[2]While LGBT (lesbian, gay, bisexual, transgender) holds a lot of recognition value in Southern Africa, we consciously decided to rather use the term 'sexual and gender minority adolescents'. This is not to assume that the experiences of people who identify as lesbian, gay, bisexual or transgender are the same – in fact, we are mindful of the heterogeneity, and the various, intersecting ways in which people who identify as LGBT are marginalized. Rather, we use this descriptor to highlight the commonalities of the source of this marginalization: heteronormative norms that result in the marginalization of all people whose identities or practices defy these norms.

[3]We decided to retain the terminology used by organisations themselves, and employed by our participants, and thus use the term 'LGBT' when referring to organisations, or when it is used in direct quotes.

Abbreviations

(A)SRH organisation: Organisations either providing specific adolescent sexual and reproductive health (ASRH) services, or general sexual and reproductive health services that are also open to adolescents; AIDS: Acquired immune deficiency syndrome; ART: Antiretroviral therapy; ASRH: Adolescent sexual and reproductive health services; HIV: Human Immunodeficiency Virus; IEC: Information, education, communication; LGBT(I): Lesbian, gay, bisexual and transgender (and intersex); MSM: Men who have sex with men; NGO: Non-governmental organisation; SADC: Southern African Development Community; SRH(R): Sexual and reproductive health (and rights)

Acknowledgements

We would like to thank all participants for being so generous with their time and insights, especially where pressing service needs meant that talking to us added additional hours to already long days. We also thank Dr. Solange Rocha for her assistance with interviews in Mozambique.

Funding

This study was funded by Ford Foundation.

Authors' contributions

AM conceptualised the study; AM, KD, TM and SS conducted interviews and developed initial themes during the interview process; AM, KD and SS analysed the data; AM drafted the manuscript; KD, TM and SS provided critical feedback and revisions to the manuscript. All authors read and approved the final manuscript.

Authors' information

AM is an Associate Professor at the Gender, Health and Justice Research Unit (GHJRU) at the University of Cape Town. TM and KD are both researchers at the same research unit. SS worked as a research fellow at the GHJRU.

Competing interests

The authors declare that they have no competing interests.

References

1. Magnani RJ, Karim AM, Weiss LA, Bond KC, Lemba M, Morgan GT. Reproductive health risk and protective factors among youth in Lusaka. Zambia J Adolesc Heal. 2002;30:76–86.
2. United Nations Population Fund. State of the world population 2017: worlds apart - reproductive health and rights in an age of inequality. New York; 2017. http://www.unfpa.org/sites/default/files/sowp/downloads/UNFPA_PUB_2017_EN_SWOP.pdf. Accessed 30 Oct 2017
3. Gray GE. Adolescent HIV–cause for concern in southern Africa. PLoS Med. 2010;7:e1000227. https://doi.org/10.1371/journal.pmed.1000178.
4. Joint United Nations Programme on HIV/AIDS. UNAIDS DATA 2017. Geneva; 2017. http://www.unaids.org/sites/default/files/media_asset/20170720_Data_book_2017_en.pdf. Accessed 1 Nov 2017
5. Bearinger LH, Sieving RE, Ferguson J, Sharma V. Global perspectives on the sexual and reproductive health of adolescents: patterns, prevention, and potential. Lancet. 2007;369:1220–31.
6. United Nations Population Fund. Harmonizing the legal environment for adolescent sexual and reproductive health and right – a review of 23 countries in east and southern Africa. 2017.
7. Müller A, Röhrs S, Hoffman-Wanderer Y, Moult K. 'You have to make a judgment call'. - morals, judgments and the provision of quality sexual and reproductive health services for adolescents in South Africa. Soc Sci Med. 2016;148:71–8.
8. Amuyunzu-Nyamongo M, Biddlecom A, Ouedraogo C, Woog V. Qualitative evidence on adolescents' views of sexual and reproductive health in sub-Saharan Africa. 2005.
9. Morris JL, Rushwan H. Adolescent sexual and reproductive health: the global challenges. Int J Gynecol Obstet. 2015;131:S40–2.
10. Capurchande R, Coene G, Schockaert I, Macia M, Meulemans H. 'It is challenging… oh, nobody likes it!': A qualitative study exploring Mozambican adolescents' and young adults' experiences with contraception. BMC Womens Health. 2016;16:48. https://doi.org/10.1186/s12905-016-0326-2.
11. Remez L, Woog V, Mhloyi M. Sexual and reproductive health needs of adolescents in Zimbabwe. Issues brief (Alan Guttmacher inst); 2014. p. 1–8. http://ovidsp.ovid.com/ovidweb.cgi?T=JS&PAGE=reference&D=prem&NEWS=N&AN=26159001%5Cnhttp://www.ncbi.nlm.nih.gov/pubmed/26159001
12. Chandra-Mouli V, Svanemyr J, Amin A, Fogstad H, Say L, Girard F, et al. Twenty years after international conference on population and development: where are we with adolescent sexual and reproductive health and rights? J Adolesc Health. 2015;56:S1–6.
13. Butler J. Gender trouble: feminism and the subversion of identity. London: Routledge; 1990.
14. Müller A. Beyond 'invisibility': queer intelligibility and symbolic annihilation in healthcare. Culture, health and sexuality; 2017. p. 1–14.
15. Meer T, Müller A. 'They treat us like we're not there': queer bodies and the social production of healthcare spaces. Heal Place. 2017;45:92–8.
16. Semp D. Questioning heteronormativity: using queer theory to inform research and practice within public mental health services. Psychol Sex. 2011;2:69–86.
17. Warner M. Introduction : fear of a queer planet. Soc Text. 1991;29:3–17. https://doi.org/10.1017/CBO9781107415324.004.
18. Makadon HJ. Ending LGBT invisibility in health care: the first step in ensuring equitable care. Cleve Clin J Med. 2011;78:220–4.
19. Haas AP, Lane A. Collecting sexual orientation and gender identity data in suicide and other violent deaths: a step towards identifying and addressing LGBT mortality disparities. LGBT Heal. 2015;2:84–7. https://doi.org/10.1089/lgbt.2014.0083.
20. Obedin-Maliver J, Goldsmith ES, Stewart L, White W, Tran E, Brenman S, et al. Lesbian, gay, bisexual, and transgender–related content in undergraduate medical education. JAMA. 2011;306:971–7.
21. Coulter RWS, Kenst KS, Bowen DJ. Scout. Research funded by the National Institutes of Health on the health of lesbian, gay, bisexual, and transgender populations. Am J Public Health. 2014;104:e105–12. https://doi.org/10.2105/AJPH.2013.301501.
22. Itaborahy LP, Zhu J. State-sponsored homophobia: a world survey of laws. 2014.
23. Epprecht M. Hetero sexual Africa?: the history of an idea from the age of exploration to the age of AIDS. Athens, Ohio: Ohio University Press; 2008. https://www.scopus.com/inward/record.uri?eid=2-s2.0-84899371121&partnerID=40&md5=46f9413b29e10553b2e2c6c7475ad725

24. Meer T, Lunau M, Oberth G, Daskilewicz K, Müller A. Lesbian, gay, bisexual, trans- gender and intersex human rights in southern Africa : a contemporary literature review 2012-2016. Johannesburg: HIVOS; 2017.

25. Muller A, Hughes TL. Making the invisible visible: a systematic review of sexual minority women's health in southern Africa. BMC Public Health. 2016; 16:307. https://doi.org/10.1186/s12889-016-2980-6.

26. Hatzenbuehler ML, Bellatorre A, Lee Y, Finch BK, Muennig P, Fiscella K. Structural stigma and all-cause mortality in sexual minority populations. Soc Sci Med. 2014;103:33–41.

27. Nalá R, Cummings B, Horth R, Inguane C, Benedetti M, Chissano M, et al. Men who have sex with men in Mozambique: identifying a hidden population at high-risk for HIV. AIDS Behav. 2015;19:393–404.

28. Thurston IB, Dietrich J, Bogart LM, Otwombe KN, Sikkema KJ, Nkala B, et al. Correlates of sexual risk among sexual minority and heterosexual south African youths. Am J Public Health. 2014;104:1265–9.

29. Michaels-Igbokwe C, Terris-Prestholt F, Lagarde M, Chipeta E, Cairns J, Integra Initiative. Young People's preferences for Family planning service providers in Rural Malawi: a discrete choice experiment. PLoS One. 2015;10:e0143287.

30. Wood K, Jewkes R. Blood blockages and scolding nurses: barriers to adolescent contraceptive use in South Africa. Reprod Health Matters. 2006;14:109–18.

31. Newton-Levinson A, Leichliter JS, Chandra-Mouli V. Help and care seeking for sexually transmitted infections among youth in low-and middle-income countries. Sex Transm Dis. 2017;44:319.

32. Yao J, Murray AT, Agadjanian V. A geographical perspective on access to sexual and reproductive health care for women in rural Africa. Soc Sci Med. 2013;96:60–8. https://doi.org/10.1016/j.socscimed.2013.07.025.

33. Meer T, Müller A. 'They treat us like we're not there': queer bodies and the social production of healthcare spaces. Health Place. 2017;45:92–8. https://doi.org/10.1016/j.healthplace.2017.03.010.

34. Judhistari RA, Kayastha S, Jahanath S. Young people and the Post-2015 development agenda: a critical look at youth SRHR movement building and agenda setting. arrow Chang. 2012;18:3.

35. Hindin MJ, Fatusi AO. Adolescent sexual and reproductive health in developing countries: an overview of trends and interventions. Int Perspect Sex Reprod Health. 2009;35:58–62.

36. Rispel LC, Metcalf CA, Cloete A, Reddy V, Lombard C. HIV prevalence and risk practices among men who have sex with men in two south African cities. J Acquir Immune Defic Syndr. 2011;57:69–76. https://doi.org/10.1097/QAI.0b013e318211b40a.

37. Sandfort TGM, Baumann LRM, Matebeni Z, Reddy V, Southey-Swartz I. Forced sexual experiences as risk factor for self-reported HIV infection among southern African lesbian and bisexual women. PLoS One. 2013;8(1):e53552.

38. Edwards WM, Div M, Coleman E, Ph D. Defining Sexual Health : A Descriptive Overview. Arch Sex Behav. 2004;33:189–95.

39. Russell ST, Joyner K. Adolescent sexual orientation and suicide risk: evidence from a National Study. Am J Public Heal J Public Heal. 2001;9191:1276–81.

40. Flood M. Changing men: best practice in sexual violence education. Women Against Violence. An Aust Fem J. 2006(18):26-36.

41. Carroll A, Mendos LR. State-sponsored homophobia: a world survey of sexual orientation Laws. Geneva; 2017. http://ilga.org/what-we-do/state-sponsored-homophobia-report/. Accessed 27 Oct 2017

42. Müller A. Transnational moralities and invisible sexual minorities: human rights discourse and religion in Uganda. In: Beckmann N, Gusman A, and Shroff C (eds). Strings Attached: AIDS and the Rise of Transnational Connections in Africa. Oxford: Oxford University Press; 2014. p. 289–310.

43. Epprecht M. Sexual minorities, human rights and public health strategies in Africa. Afr Aff (Lond). 2012;111:223–43. https://doi.org/10.1093/afraf/ads019.

44. World Health Organization. Consolidated guidelines on HIV prevention, diagnosis, treatment and care for key populations. Geneva; 2014.

45. Baggaley R, Armstrong A, Dodd Z, Ngoksin E, Krug A. Young key populations and HIV: a special emphasis and consideration in the new WHO consolidated guidelines on HIV prevention, diagnosis, treatment and Care for key Populations. J Int AIDS Soc. 2015;18:85–8.

46. African Commission on Human and Peoples' Rights. 275: resolution on protection against violence and other human rights violations against persons on the basis of their real or imputed sexual orientation or gender identity / resolutions / 55th ordinary session / ACHPR. 2014. http://www.achpr.org/sessions/55th/resolutions/275/. Accessed 27 Oct 2017.

47. African Commission on Human and Peoples' Rights. Ending violence and other human rights violations based on sexual orientation and gender identity: a joint dialogue of the African commission on human and peoples' rights, inter-American commission on human rights and United Nations. Pretoria; 2016.

12

Barriers and facilitators to institutional delivery in rural areas of Chitwan district, Nepal

Rajani Shah[1,2*], Eva A. Rehfuess[2,3], Deepak Paudel[2,4], Mahesh K. Maskey[1] and Maria Delius[2,5]

Abstract

Background: Giving birth assisted by skilled care in a health facility plays a vital role in preventing maternal deaths. In Nepal, delivery services are free and a cash incentive is provided to women giving birth at a health facility. Nevertheless, about half of women still deliver at home. This study explores socio-cultural and health service-related barriers to and facilitators of institutional delivery.

Methods: Six village development committees in hill and plain areas were selected in Chitwan district. We conducted a total of 10 focus group discussions and 12 in-depth-interviews with relevant stakeholder groups, including mothers, husbands, mothers-in-law, traditional birth attendants, female community health volunteers, health service providers and district health managers. Data were analyzed inductively using thematic analysis.

Results: Three main themes played a role in deciding the place of delivery, i.e. socio-cultural norms and values; access to birthing facilities; and perceptions regarding the quality of health services. Factors encouraging an institutional delivery included complications during labour, supportive husbands and mothers-in-law, the availability of an ambulance, having birthing centres nearby, locally sufficient financial incentives and/or material incentives, the 24-h availability of midwives and friendly health service providers. Socio-cultural barriers to institutional deliveries were deeply held beliefs about childbirth being a normal life event, the wish to be cared for by family members, greater freedom of movement at home, a warm environment, the possibility to obtain appropriate "hot" foods, and shyness of young women and their position in the family hierarchy. Accessibility and quality of health services also presented barriers, including lack of road and transportation, insufficient financial incentives, poor infrastructure and equipment at birthing centres and the young age and perceived incompetence of midwives.

Conclusion: Despite much progress in recent years, this study revealed some important barriers to the utilization of health services. It suggests that a combination of upgrading birthing centres and strengthening the competencies of health personnel while embracing and addressing deeply rooted family values and traditions can improve existing programmes and further increase institutional delivery rates.

Keywords: Qualitative study, Focus group discussion, Qualitative interview, Maternal health, Child birth, Nepal, Access to health services, Quality of health services, Cultural concepts

* Correspondence: rajani_shah89@yahoo.com
[1]Nepal Public Health Foundation, Kathmandu, Nepal
[2]Center for International Health, Ludwig-Maximilians-University, Munich, Germany
Full list of author information is available at the end of the article

Plain English summary

Giving birth at a health facility plays an important role in preventing maternal deaths. Although child birth services are free and women receive a cash incentive for giving birth at a health facility in Nepal, about half of women give birth at home. This study was conducted to identify the socio-cultural and health service factors influencing birth at health facility. Altogether, 10 group discussions and 12 interviews were conducted in plain and hill areas of Chitwan district of Nepal to collect data from mothers, their husbands and mothers-in-law, community members, service providers and health managers.

The factors that encouraged birth at a health facility were danger signs in giving birth, supportive husbands and mothers-in-law, availability of transport, a birthing facility located close to home, a sufficient cash incentive, as well as the availability and friendliness of health workers. The socio-cultural factors hindering birth at a health facility were the fact that child birth is perceived as a normal event, care available from family members, freedom of movement and a warm environment and appropriate foods being available at home, pregnant women's shyness and position in the family, the lack of roads and appropriate transportation, an insufficient cash incentive, the poor condition of birthing centres, including lack of equipment, and the young age and perceived lack of competence of health service provider and viewing service provider not competent.

Making improvements to birthing centres, enhancing the skills of service providers, and addressing family values and traditions are necessary to increase births at health facilities in Chitwan district.

Background

The maternal mortality ratio (MMR) in Nepal has decreased by 71% between the years 1990 and 2015 compared with an average reduction of 67% in Southern Asian countries during the same period. Nevertheless, the MMR (258 deaths per 100,000 live births) in Nepal remains higher than in all other Southern Asian countries except for Afghanistan [1].

Giving birth assisted by a skilled birth attendant in a health facility plays a vital role in preventing maternal deaths [2, 3]. Fifteen percent of pregnancies are associated with critical complications and unpredictable consequences and thus require access to emergency obstetric care [4]. Even an uncomplicated childbirth requires skilled care and the continuous presence of a health professional [5].

To encourage institutional delivery in Nepal, delivery services have been provided free of charge at government health facilities as well as selected private facilities [6] since 2009. To help overcome the country-specific transportation challenges and associated transportation

costs – Nepal is characterized by three distinct geographical terrains, i.e. plain areas, hill areas and mountain areas –a cash incentive for institutional deliveries was introduced by the national maternal healthcare programme called Aama in 2005 [7]. This amounts to Nepali Rupees (NRs) 500 ($5), 1000 ($10) and 1500 ($15) in plain, hill and mountain districts respectively. Since 2012, an additional NRs 400 ($4) has been provided for completing four antenatal care (ANC) visits according to schedule to pregnant mothers across all of the country [8].

Nevertheless, only 57% of births take place in a health facility [9]. Several studies have quantitatively examined the factors contributing to the low institutional delivery rate in Nepal and have provided useful insight [10–17]. A few qualitative studies have also been published in the Nepalese context [18, 19]. However, a more comprehensive understanding of the problem, which takes into account the perspectives of all those directly involved with the decision regarding the place of delivery and associated care, is much needed. By employing a qualitative research design, using both focus group discussions (FGDs) and in-depth interviews (IDIs), the present study attempts to achieve deeper insights into the problem and to identify useful pointers to solutions. It aims to obtain in-depth information on socio-cultural and health service-related barriers to and facilitators of institutional delivery from the perspectives of family and community members as well as health service providers at community level, and district health managers.

Methods

Study setting

Nepal is characterized by plain, hill and mountain ecological regions. As per the new constitution of Nepal issued in 2015, Nepal has been administratively restructured into 7 provinces and 77 districts; the latter are further divided into urban and rural municipalities [20]. Before restructuring, each of the 75 districts comprised rural village development committees (VDCs) and urban municipalities. Each VDC and municipality was further divided into smaller administrative units called wards [21]. The rural municipalities have been established through merging the previously existent VDCs.

Chitwan district is classified as a plain district but consists of both hill and plain areas. At the time of data collection, Chitwan had a population of approximately 580,000 [22]. It is among the six districts with the highest (> 0.550) human development index [23] One third of males in the district do not live with their families as they work elsewhere. Around 73% of females are married by 19 years of age and then live with their husbands' family [24].

In Chitwan, there are three major referral hospitals in the district headquarter, Bharatpur, among several other private hospitals with birthing facilities. Health services in rural areas are provided through one hospital, three primary health care centers, 38 health posts and two community health units (District Public Health Office: Birthing centres in Chitwan district 2017, unpublished data). At the time of data collection, a total of 14 birthing centres operated 24 h 365 days a year in 14 VDCs. Birthing centres are established at health facilities by assigning a midwife – i.e. an auxiliary nurse midwife (ANM) with 18-months of midwifery training – that can assist uncomplicated births [25]. In addition, each ward has at least one female community health volunteer (FCHV) to promote the utilization of maternal, child and reproductive health services [8]. While official reports show that 83% of deliveries in Chitwan district take place in health facilities, this masks a difference between rural and urban areas, with several rural areas, in both plain and hill regions showing much lower institutional delivery rates [26]. The geographically relatively advantaged situation of Chitwan, where most inhabitants live within reach of a health institution suggests that access to health services is not the predominant reason for choosing to deliver at home. Therefore, the district is particularly well-suited to explore the range of factors influencing the choice of place of delivery because women, in principle, have the opportunity to give birth at a health facility.

For this study, we purposively selected VDCs where the percentage of institutional deliveries was below the average for the district, including three VDCs in hill areas, i.e. Chandivanjyang (15%), Kabilas (41%)

and Kaule (7%), and three VDCs in plain areas, i.e. Padampur (78%), Piple (67%) and Ayodhyapuri (68%) (District Public Health Office: Data on maternal health in Chitwan 2010/2011, unpublished data); four of these VDCs had a birthing centre (Table 1). The population in these VDCs comprises 67% Janajatis, 25% Brahmans/Chhetris, 8% Dalits and less than 1% Muslims [27].

Study design and study participants

Mothers who had given birth between May 2011 and April 2012 were the focus of this study. We conducted 10 focus group discussions (FGDs) and 12 in-depth-interviews (IDIs) [28, 29] with relevant stakeholder groups (Table 1). For the FGDs we purposively selected – with the help of FCHVs – mothers who delivered at home, mothers who delivered at a health institution and their mothers-in-law. Participants for FGDs were identified according to the following criteria: mothers who had given birth in the year preceding the survey, residency in the study area during the time of delivery and willingness to take part in the study. In addition, we conducted IDIs with husbands, traditional birth attendants (TBAs), FCHVs and health workers (service providers), i.e. the in-charge and the ANM of the local health post. Moreover, we interviewed two district health managers: the district public health officer (DPHO) and the focal person for safe motherhood. Data triangulation by comparing and contrasting the perspectives of different groups of study participants as well as involving different approaches to data collection – i.e. FGDs as well as in-depth interviews helped to

Table 1 Data collection through focus group discussions and in-depth interviews

	Plain areas			Hill areas			Total
	Ayodhyapuri*	Piple*	Padampur	Chandi Vanjyang*	Kaule*	Kabilas	
Focus group discussions							
Mothers with home delivery		1	1	1		1	4
Mothers with institutional delivery		1	1		1	1	4
Mothers-in-law	1				1		2
In-depth interviews							
Husbands		1			1		2
TBAs	1				1		2
FCHVs	1			1			2
Service providers							
- In-charge of health post		1			1		2
- ANM	1			1			2
District health managers							
- DPHO	1						
- Safe motherhood focal person	1						

*with birthing centre

TBA Traditional birth attendant; FCHV Female community health volunteer; ANM Auxiliary nurse midwife; DPHO District public health officer consolidate the findings on enabling factors for and barriers to institutional delivery [30].

Data collection

Data collection was carried out between May and August 2012. The FGDs were conducted in a classroom of the local school during holidays or in a room inside a community building; the IDIs variably took place in a closed room inside a health facility, district health office, community building or the home of participants. The duration of FGDs ranged from 65 to 90 min, while the IDIs ranged from 45 to 75 min.

FGD and IDI guides, available upon request, were prepared on the basis of available literature [31–36]; their structure is depicted in Table 2. Probing questions were also formulated. After pre-testing the guides [37] with three FGDs in Piple VDC in areas that were not part of this study, minor modifications were made, such as changing the order of questions and rewording selected questions.

Data collection was carried out by RS in the Nepali language. All FGDs and IDIs were audio taped. Two Bachelor of Public Health students were trained and then, one at a time, helped with taking notes. All the data were transcribed from the audio recordings and notes. The transcripts were subsequently translated by RS into English.

Data analysis

Data were analyzed manually using thematic analysis [38]. Initially, the transcripts were read multiple times for familiarization with the data. Coding was done by RS and Jukki Chaudhary - a public health lecturer. Both coded the same two FGDs and three IDIs independently. The codes identified from the texts were then discussed and final codes decided, with input from MD. Using the final codes, RS then coded all the remaining transcripts [39], starting off with the FGDs with the mothers, followed by analysis of the FGDs with mothers-in-law and IDIs with husbands, community informants and service providers; the IDIs with the district level managers were analysed at the end. Following line-by-line coding, codes with similar meanings were grouped together to form a common theme. The themes were then reviewed by both researchers and some themes combined into a broader single theme with relevant sub-themes. Similarities or contrasting views of study

Table 2 Overall structure of the FGD and IDI guides

- Status of maternal health
- Trends in maternal care seeking behaviours
- Common practices before delivery and underlying reasons
- Common practices during delivery and underlying reasons
- Enabling factors contributing to institutional delivery
- Barriers to institutional delivery
- Roles of family members
- Roles of community members, i.e. TBAs, FCHVs, neighbours
- Opinions about birthing centres available in the community
- Suggestions to increase institutional delivery

participants were compared. Finally, the connections or relations between different themes as well as sub-themes were explained to identify the factors influencing institutional delivery in positive or negative ways. This last stage of the process was completed in an iterative manner through regular discussions between all members of the research team.

Ethical consideration

Ethical approval for the study was obtained from the Nepal Health Research Council (registration number 21/2012). Permission to conduct the study was obtained from the district public health office, Chitwan. Informed consent was obtained from the participants themselves or their parents, guardians or next of kin for participating mothers below the legal age; as many participants were illiterate, in particular mothers, informed consent was often obtained verbally rather than in writing. Voluntary participation was ensured throughout the study. All information collected was kept confidential. Personal identifiers were removed from the records after data analysis, and the analysis did not contain any identifying information.

Results

Socio-demographic characteristics differed between women who had given birth at home and women who had delivered in a health institution. Women who had delivered at home were older and of higher parity; all of them were from disadvantaged castes and the majority had only primary level education or no schooling at all (Table 3). Almost all mothers-in-law were illiterate; the majority belonged to a disadvantaged caste. The participating husbands were also from disadvantaged caste and were involved in both agriculture and labour work. The TBAs and FCHVs belonged to both disadvantaged and advantaged castes. The remaining six IDIs were conducted with ANMs and in-charge of the local health facility and district level managers.

During analysis, three major themes influencing the place of delivery emerged: socio-cultural norms and values, comprising traditional care during birth and the post-partum period and family hierarchy and social norms as important sub-themes; access to birthing facilities; and perceptions regarding the quality of health services. For each of these major themes, the arguments in favour or against institutional delivery varied according to people's background and where they live. Table 4 provides an overview of the insights gained regarding facilitators and barriers to institutional delivery. More detailed insights are provided in the following sections.

Socio-cultural norms and values
Traditional care during birth and the post-partum period
Many women considered giving birth to be a normal life event and believed that in the absence of complications

Table 3 Socio-demographic characteristics of mothers participating in FGDs

	Plain VDCs		Hill VDCs		Total
Place of delivery	Institutional delivery (n = 12)	Home Delivery (n = 12)	Institutional delivery (n = 12)	Home Delivery (n = 14)	
Age					
Up to 19 years	3	2	3	3	11
20–29 years	9	9	8	9	35
30 and above	0	1	1	2	4
Parity					
1st	7	5	7	5	24
2nd or more	5	7	5	9	26
Caste / ethnicity					
Disadvantaged*	11	12	8	13	44
Advantaged**	1	0	4	1	6
Educational status					
None or primary	5	6	4	12	27
Secondary or higher	7	6	8	2	23

*Disadvantaged: Dalits and disadvantaged Janjati (Chepang, Rai, Magar, Tamang, Darai, Chaudhary)
**Advantaged: Gurung, Newar, Brahman, Chhetri

there is no need for an institutional delivery. Even those living very close to a health post did not consider institutional delivery necessary, as they felt that they could easily obtain help at home in case of complications. In some plain areas, where TBAs were still active, some mothers and family members indicated that they preferred to be assisted by a TBA. Consulting a traditional healer for delivery was, however, not usually practiced. Very few trusted the traditional healers' estimates of birthing time and sought their help for identifying whether the pain was due to supernatural evil forces or not. Generally, in hill and plain areas, most of the mothers, family members and

TBAs believed that women should be taken to a birthing facility in case of complications, such as heavy bleeding, or after prolonged labour, which was described as continuous labour lasting for 24 h in plain areas and lasting for 72 h in hill areas.

"I think the main reason for not going to a health facility is that women think delivery is a normal event. Women hear mothers-in-law and mothers saying – 'we delivered more than 12 babies while cutting grass, cut the cord with sickle and put baby on lap'." (FCHV, hill VDC).

Table 4 Facilitators of and barriers to institutional delivery

Themes	Sub-themes	Facilitators	Barriers
Socio-cultural norms and values	Traditional care during birth and the post-partum period	• Institutional delivery in case of complications	• Childbirth as a normal life event • Care by family members, neighbours and TBAs • Freedom of movement during birth • Warm environment after birth • Food choices and practices
	Family hierarchy and social norms	• Husbands and parents-in-law supportive of institutional delivery	• Shyness • Low caste, poor education, early marriage • Husbands and parents-in-law not supportive of institutional delivery
Access to birthing facilities		• Ambulance available • Birthing centre nearby • Sufficient financial incentives • Material incentives: clothes for mother and baby	• Lack of roads (hill areas) or good roads • Distance from health institution (especially in hill areas) • Ambulance not always available • Insufficient incentives
Perceptions regarding the quality of health services		• 24-h availability of midwives • Friendliness of health workers	• Perceived incompetence of midwives • Young age of midwives • Poor infrastructure and lack of equipment at birthing centres • Low budget allocated to birthing centres

TBA Traditional birth attendant

"My wife had no complication to go to the health post. Even in case of complications, we have health workers of the health post always available to assist in home deliveries." (Husband, home delivery, hill VDC).

"If TBA can assist the birth, she says it will happen after some time. Then we don't need to take her (the mother) to the health institution. If she cannot conduct delivery, she would ask to take her to the health institution as soon as possible." (Mother-in-law, home delivery, plain VDC).

"If a woman cannot give birth even after two to three days, then we must take her to a health institution. Yesterday the woman who went to the health post for delivery was also suffering from labour for three days." (Mother, home delivery, hill VDC).

Mothers as well as their husbands reported that the care received from family members and neighbours during child birth was an important reason for their preference to deliver at home. The mothers – and, after birth, the children, too – were massaged with mustard oil. The possibility of free movement during birth was also seen as a clear advantage.

"At home, we have people holding our hands, legs and body, doing massage on them, and encouraging and giving comfort during labour and childbirth. In the hospital, no-one cares at all. Doctors come only at the time of delivery, they don't come earlier to listen to our problems." (Mother, home delivery, plain VDC).

"Women's movement and position during labour is restricted at health institutions. Women must keep sitting or lying in bed at the health facility. There are more difficulties at a health institution than at home." (Husband, home delivery, hill VDC).

After birth, the mother and her baby traditionally rest in a corner of the house. Since post-partum women are considered to be in a "cold" state, "hot" foods (where hot does not necessarily refer to temperature or spices) and a warm environment (usually a fire) are believed to be necessary to maintain health and regain strength. Consequently, food practices dictate that the mother is given special nutritious food that is categorized as hot and soft. Many mothers who gave birth at home mentioned that the opportunities to have hot foods immediately after birth and to keep the mother and newborn in a warm environment motivated them to give birth at home.

"After delivery women should stay in the health post until the bleeding stops. It is cold in the health post

and the baby can die due to hypothermia. They have the culture of staying in a corner of their house for many days after childbirth." (FCHV, hill VDC).

"There are no warm beds/clothes for mothers and no room with warm environment such as a heating facility to keep the baby warm after birth." (Husband, home delivery, hill VDC).

"Hot foods are available at home immediately after birth, at the hospital who would give us? People do not have money to buy food at a hotel." (Mother, home delivery, plain VDC).

"The expenses to take a woman to hospital could be used for her foods for postpartum period." (Mother, home delivery, plain VDC).

Family hierarchy and social norms

Shyness emerged as an important theme. Many mothers stated clearly that an important reason for not wanting to deliver at a health institution was their being shy to show their genitals to others, in particular to male doctors. Chepang mothers- a disad

taged Janajati caste- were reported to be even more timid than women belonging to other castes.

"I feel shy to show my genitals to others, and even to a female nurse." (Mother, home delivery, plain VDC).

"Chepang women are very shy, even some mothers-in-law are shy. They say that they will not show their genitals to anyone. … And women would prefer to deliver in the corner of their house." (Mother-in-law, institutional delivery, hill VDC).

Some mothers and FCHVs indicated that the mothers did not dare to talk with their family members about the option of institutional delivery. This perspective was shared by mothers-in-law, some of whom stated that there was a lack of communication between them and their daughters-in-law. A midwife attributed women's hesitation to speak openly to early marriage and low education.

"Pregnant women want to come to the health post, but they cannot say this to their family members. They feel shy and awkward to talk to family members about the place of delivery. They say it at the last stage, if they are unable to deliver the baby." (Mother, home delivery, hill VDC).

"My daughters-in-law didn't give any information about their labour. How would I know their

condition unless they tell me?"
(Mother-in-law, home delivery, hill VDC).

Within the family hierarchy, decisions are made by or in accordance with the husband and the parents-in-law. Some women reported that mothers-in-law were the decision makers in the family and that fathers-in-law generally supported their views. Often this led to an institutional delivery, although at times it could be the opposite, depending on the experiences and beliefs of different family members. Nevertheless, most of the women who delivered at home indicated that they had chosen to do so themselves rather than being persuaded by family members. Most women who had given birth at a health institution stated that their husbands had encouraged and supported their choice.

"We didn't go because of our confidence in being able to give birth at home, not due to pressure of our family members" (Mother, home delivery, plain VDC).

"My husband was willing to take me to the hospital, but my mother-in-law said it can be done at home. My husband was very afraid at first." (Mother, home delivery, plain VDC).

Access to birthing facilities
Despite the relatively large number of birthing centres in Chitwan district, physical access is still a challenge in some areas, especially where birthing centres are located far from a pregnant woman's home. Mothers living in hill areas faced greater difficulties in reaching a health facility than women living in the plain due to lack of roads and transportation. In fact, in a few places, women had to be carried in a bamboo basket, hammock or stretcher; when husbands were not at home and other men not available this constituted an important barrier. Some respondents were afraid of having an accident on the way to the health facility.

"We have taken a bamboo basket from the health post. It's difficult to carry a woman alone in a bamboo basket. We had kept a stretcher too, but a pregnant woman nearly died falling out of a stretcher. Roads are narrow, sloppy and steep." (FCHV, hill VDC).

"Men cannot be found in the village to carry a pregnant woman to the health facility. They are in other districts for work" (Mother, home delivery, hill VDC).

In contrast, in the plain, the ambulance was often readily available; however, some mothers reported that it

can take a long time for the ambulance to arrive. Difficulty in travelling due to poor road condition was also reported by some of the mothers living in plain areas.

"Ambulance comes immediately after we call. Other public vehicles are available in five minutes." (Mother, institutional delivery, plain VDC).

"When we called the ambulance, it had gone to drop another patient, so it was late. Labour pain occurred only for three hours. Delivery happened before the arrival of the ambulance." (Mother, home delivery, plain VDC).

"If we go to hospital, there would be jerking in the bus because of poor roads, our body shakes and blood moves. It's convenient to give birth at home." (Mother, home delivery, plain VDC).

Almost all participants were aware of the cash incentives for institutional delivery provided by the government. Some mothers and their family members reported that relatively little money was required for delivery at the nearest birthing centre. Many others, however, indicated that the incentive provided was not sufficient to meet all of the expenses related to an institutional delivery, such as transportation fare, cost of food during the stay at the health facility and additional food costs for those carrying the woman to the health facility in hill areas.

"As foods can also be taken from home, a lot of money is saved if we go to the nearest birthing centre. NRs. 100 is enough for delivery here. People with low economic status are going to the local birthing centre." (Mother, institutional delivery, plain VDC).

"Community people ask to go to health facility but a lot of money is necessary for hiring the ambulance, food in hospital, providing food to the people who carry the mothers, etc.; a small sum of incentive provided is like a drop in the ocean." (Mother, institutional delivery, hill VDC).

"Many people are required to carry a woman to a health facility. Those who carry need to be provided with alcohol and other snacks in the hotel. Postpartum mothers need 'Jaulo'- a soft food made from rice and pulse, soon after birth. About NRs. 2000 is needed. So, they don't care about NRs. 900 provided by the health facility." (FCHV, hill VDC).

"We would expect hot soup and nutritious food provided to the mother after birth, in addition to the cash being provided." (Mother, institutional delivery, hill VDC).

However, FCHVs of both hill and plain areas believed that the lack of money was not the main reason for delivering at home. In fact, some respondents suggested that a material incentive was valued more than a monetary incentive because the gifts could be used by the mother and the newborn themselves.

"Money is not the reason for not going to health institution. When a traditional healer comes they immediately sacrifice rooster to serve him and give him at least NRs. 500 for helping them."
(FCHV, hill VDC).

"The money we give may not reach the hand of the mother, the husband may spend it on drinking or the mother-in-law may use it for smoking. A blanket for the mother and clothes for the newborn provided by a non-governmental organization have impressed the mothers more. The number of health facility deliveries has increased significantly in the last two months since provision with the clothes started" (Service provider at a health post, hill VDC).

Perceptions regarding the quality of health services

Supported by recent government programmes many new birthing centres have been set up over a relatively short period of time. The quality of the infrastructure, including the lack of a warm environment, and the availability of the necessary equipment, especially in relation to complicated deliveries, as well as the competence of health personnel were put into question by many local people. Family members, FCHVs and health workers also reported that there was a problem in accommodating mothers and their accompanying family members. Consequently, women able to access health facilities, tended to prefer hospitals in the district headquarter Bharatpur to local birthing centres. One of the district health managers attributed these infrastructure problems to the low budget allocated by the government.

"There is no waiting room, there is a problem in maintaining privacy due to lack of partition of the room, the delivery bed is inappropriate, and the available one is not in good condition." (Service provider at a health post, hill VDC).

"If women need to do surgery, they don't have the required equipment and instruments at the health post. So, people are not assured of the service provided from the health post." (Mother, home delivery, hill VDC).

"Those of higher economic status go to a hospital. Some of them don't have trust in the services of the health post. Middle and lower class women visit the local health facility for delivery." (Service provider at a health post, plain VDC).

"NRs. 100000 ($1000) is provided for the opening of two birthing centres per year. Managing the infrastructure, beds, and other materials with fifty thousand is very difficult. Only a delivery bed costs thirty to forty thousand rupees." (District health manager).

Concern was also expressed about the competence of the midwives at the new birthing centres. Most of the mothers and family members who had not visited the nearest birthing facility justified this by considering the midwives at the facility as not sufficiently competent to deliver care or manage referrals appropriately. Their opinion was shared by FCHVs, who added that these concerns were largely attributable to the midwives being very young. In fact, many of the midwives themselves felt uncertain about their competence due to their lack of skilled birth attendant training and unavailability of materials.

"Some people say that ANMs are young and are here to learn. Small girls cannot perform well." (FCHV, plain VDC).

"We have not received SBA training, so, we lack skills to manage complicated cases. We lack materials even like epi set, placenta bowel, hand washing pot, etc." (Service provider at a health post, plain VDC).

On the other hand, some mothers and FCHVs praised the fact that midwives were available day and night, and regarded midwives to be both friendly and caring. This positive behaviour by health personnel towards patients and visitors was reported to encourage use of health facilities.

"Midwives at nearby birthing centre do not get angry and teach good things." (Mother, institutional delivery, plain VDC).

"People might have heard about better services being provided by the health facilities than before, and the people might have gone to the facilities due to the love/affection, proper care and good behavior of the health workers towards the people." (FCHV, plain VDC).

Discussion

This qualitative study identified a broad range of issues that influence place of delivery. Three major themes –

socio-cultural norms and values (with the sub-themes traditional care during birth and the post-partum period and family hierarchy and social norms), access to birthing facilities, and perceptions regarding the quality of health services – emerged. Importantly, the analysis combined insights obtained through FGDs and IDIs conducted with mothers who had recently given birth, different family members and distinct health personnel involved with care during pregnancy, childbirth and the post-partum period offering overlapping and at times contrasting perspectives. In the following sections, findings and perspectives identified through the present study are compared with those already available in the literature for Nepal and other low- and middle-income countries.

In contrast to several previously undertaken quantitative studies in Nepal, we believe that this qualitative study adds value by providing in-depth insights into issues that local people care about deeply. Such issues, in particular socio-cultural aspects that vary much across cultures, cannot be easily assessed through a quantitative survey. In addition, such issues can easily be dismissed as they are perceived to be "normal" within a society and thus may not be articulated. Since this study was carried out in an area with relatively good access to health facilities and a relatively high institutional delivery rate it is especially suited to explore underlying reasons other than infrastructural problems, which still constitute a main reason for not using health facilities in many other parts of Nepal.

Socio-cultural norms and values
Traditional care during birth and the post-partum period
In this study, most of the mothers and their family members believed that an institutional delivery was necessary if complications occurred during childbirth. In contrast, with uncomplicated cases, some mothers considered it to be unnecessary, having seen their own mothers and mothers-in-law give birth at home. This is consistent with the findings of a community-based study in Nepal where about one third of mothers did object to the necessity of an institutional delivery [11]. In another study in Nepal, having experienced or witnessed an uncomplicated home delivery was a major reason for rejecting institutional delivery [40]. Similarly, in two studies from Indonesia and Ethiopia childbirth was perceived as a natural phenomenon. Seeking help from a health service provider rather than a TBA was only considered necessary in complicated cases [35, 41].

In addition, this study found that Nepali cultural practices during and after childbirth, such as being able to move freely during labour, staying in a warm environment, having special foods and enjoying traditional massages, were important reasons for giving birth at home. Freedom of movement and care by family members

during delivery were previously articulated as reasons for home delivery in Nepal [18]. A more in-depth study of cultural practices and beliefs about childbirth and the post-partum period in Nepal identified rituals regarding the delivery of the placenta and cord cutting, seclusion of and care for women after birth, purification and naming ceremonies and food practices, and stressed that these rituals influence the use of health services [42]. In rural Laos home deliveries were preferred for the emotional and physical care provided by husbands and other family members during labour, including back massages and gentle touching of the belly [43]. Similarly, providing warmth to mothers by locating them close to a coal fire was cited as one of the reasons for choosing home deliveries in Ethiopia [44]. Many different rituals in the post-partum period are found around the globe. The mother is often confined to a specific place, sometimes because she is considered to be impure. Food rules and taboos, while varying greatly between regions, appear to be universally important [45].

Family hierarchy and social norms
In the patrilocal system of Nepal, after marriage women move to the home of their husbands' family; many of them are very young when giving birth to their first child. Within the traditional family hierarchy young mothers have a subordinate position, they tend to be very shy and usually follow the decisions made by other family members [18, 33, 46].

In our study, most mothers reported that their husbands generally supported an institutional delivery but many women were only taken to a birthing facility when complications occurred. Similar findings were obtained in a quantitative study undertaken in the same area [13]. A previous study in Nepal reported that husbands played a cardinal role in the decision to give birth at a health facility [47]. Similarly, in rural Bangladesh, those women delivering at a health institution had husbands who had set aside money and arranged for transportation [48]. Several factors prevented husbands in Nepal from supporting their wives during pregnancy, birth and the post-partum period: lack of knowledge about their role in childbirth, social stigma, embarrassment and job responsibilities [49]. In Uganda, husbands accompanying their wives in cases of severe obstetric complications reported that they lacked information about their role during childbirth; unfriendly health personnel further confused them [50].

In the current study, most mothers-in-law supported an institutional delivery, while some were opposed to it, mainly because they did not consider it essential; shyness in communication between pregnant women and their mothers-in-law may have contributed to this. Another study conducted in Nepal estimated that in 13% of pregnancies the mother-in-law forbade an institutional delivery, because she considered it to be unnecessary and too expensive [11]. Similar reasons were described when ANC use was not supported by mothers-in-law [51]. In addition to feeling shy in communicating with other family members, pregnant women consulted in our study hesitated to go to a health facility because they feared lack of privacy, coupled with a feeling of timidity. Shyness and fear of institutional delivery were also cited in another study in Nepal [11] as well as in a study in rural Laos [43].

Access to birthing facilities

Physical access to a birthing facility is determined by a combination of distance from the health facility and availability of transport. In the current study, many participants indicated that due to the establishment of birthing centres at health posts in remote areas and the reliable availability of an ambulance, access had improved, even for poor and disadvantaged women. In another study in the hill areas of Nepal the lack of roads was shown to be an important barrier to reaching the birthing facility [18]. Other studies in Nepal indicated that women who could reach a birthing facility within one hour were more likely to have an institutional delivery than those who took longer to get there [10–13, 15]. Consistent results were observed in rural Zambia [52], Indonesia [35] and rural Laos [43].

Although the significance assigned to an institutional delivery (or lack thereof) played a greater role than financial means, money was nevertheless of concern for many people, especially in hill areas. The government incentive was reported to be inadequate to cover the full range of expenses incurred as a result of an institutional delivery, including the cost of transportation and food. Related to this, another study undertaken in Nepal showed that women did not dare demand an institutional delivery because of worries about the associated financial burden [18]. Similarly, significant out-of-pocket expenses for transportation and food for women and their accompanying persons were of concern in Laos [53].

Perceptions regarding the quality of health services

In our study, a woman's decision to give birth in a health facility was positively influenced by the 24-h availability of a midwife and the friendly and caring behaviour of health workers. In contrast, women, their family members and FCHVs were all concerned about the perceived limited competence of the midwives. Consistently, a study in Nepal reported locally voiced doubt about the ability of the midwives in managing deliveries [54]. Lack of confidence in midwives working in rural health facilities has also been reported by studies in Ethiopia [41] and Indonesia [35], where village midwives were

perceived to be young and inexperienced whereas TBAs were considered to be more mature and caring.

Moreover, some participants in the present study were concerned about the state of the infrastructure and available equipment at birthing centres; they also specifically worried about the lack of a heating system, suitable accommodation and appropriate foods. Lack of medication and inadequate equipment at the health facility along with the absence of an operating theatre, X-ray machines and laboratories for blood testing were identified as reasons for bypassing nearer birthing centres in a quantitative study among mothers in the same area of Nepal [55]. Similarly, in another study in Nepal, the lack of competent health workers and equipment in rural birthing centres discouraged women from using these facilities [56].

Strengths and limitations of the study

Unlike a facility-based study, this community-based study included mothers who had given birth at home, in local birthing centres, at more remote health facilities across the Chitwan district as well as at hospitals at the district headquarter. VDCs and participants in FGDs and IDIs were selected purposively to capture views across the full caste and socio-economic spectrum. The insights gained therefore reflect a broad range of experiences of women during pregnancy, birth and the post-partum period. Importantly, the study's findings apply to Chitwan district, in particular more remote plain and hill areas; they cannot be taken to apply to other districts of Nepal that may be characterized by a different geographical terrain as well as different ethnic, socio-cultural and socio-economic conditions.

This study has attempted to capture the views and experiences of women, their family members and other community members including FCHVs, as well as the views and experiences of health professionals at different levels of the health system. The triangulation of these multiple perspectives helped to tease out enablers and barriers to institutional delivery, which may be used as a starting point for strengthening enablers and overcoming barriers. As has become apparent during the analysis, even within a defined geographical area, there is much heterogeneity in the experiences and views between locations and in relation to personal and family backgrounds.

All data collection and transcription was undertaken in the local language by RS, who is a native Nepali speaker from Chitwan district, with the help of Nepali students who were trained in taking notes. Translations from Nepali into English were undertaken by RS with the help of competent local colleagues. The coding frame was developed by two independent coders, and all stages of the analysis involved several researchers to limit subjective interpretation. Since identification of codes was done on few FDGs and IDIs, it is possible that some information has been missed. Data analysis was undertaken in English, which may have distorted some of the more nuanced statements; where necessary, RS did go back to the original recordings to ensure that participants' views were adequately captured.

Conclusion

In the recent past, Nepal has paid increasing attention to the need to raise institutional delivery rates. Notably, in Chitwan district, the health system has made much progress in terms of providing physical and financial access to birthing centres and other health facilities offering relevant care during pregnancy, childbirth and the post-partum period. At community level, people increasingly recognize the importance of institutional delivery, especially in relation to complicated obstetrical situations. Yet, the findings of this study have provided some insights into the reasons why many women and their families in rural areas of Chitwan still reject giving birth at health facilities with some concrete implications for policy and practice. Importantly, they suggest that there is a need to strengthen the infrastructure of birthing centres in terms of heating equipment and accommodation, as well as to improve delivery of care through SBA training of midwives and sufficient availability of medical equipment and supplies. Similarly, at least in hill areas, access to suitable transportation must be improved and may require additional financial incentives. Moreover, focusing only on the biomedical aspects of a safe delivery is insufficient in overcoming existing socio-cultural barriers. This study has provided deep insights into some of the values and traditions that shape expectations with respect to the time around birth. For example, ensuring a warm environment at the birthing centre is critical, and families should be able to obtain or prepare culturally appropriate "hot" foods for women who recently delivered a baby. Also, husbands and mothers-in-law should be involved in programmes to increase uptake of institutional delivery.

National incentive programmes should consider local facilitators for and barriers to institutional delivery and enhance demand as well as improve quality of services such as friendly and culturally sensitive care. The successes or failures of the attempts to overcome the barriers that currently discourage women from making use of health facilities for giving birth should be carefully researched to enable learning over time.

Abbreviations

ANC: Antenatal care; ANM: Auxiliary nurse midwife; DPHO: District public health officer; FCHV: Female community health volunteer; FGD: Focus group discussion; IDI: In-depth interview; MMR: Maternal mortality ratio; NRs: Nepali rupees; TBA: Traditional birth attendant; VDC: Village development committee

Acknowledgements

Rajani Shah is thankful to the Farrar Foundation, UK for its financial support to the field study. She is grateful to Tania Gavidia and Nawaraj Upadhaya for their help in qualitative report writing of the PhD thesis, of which the current paper is a part. Thanks to Dinesh Kumar Malla for his help in organizing field work of the study. The authors are grateful to Jukki Chaudhary for her help in coding the transcripts, as well as to the District Public Health Office, Chitwan, female community health volunteers, note-takers during data collection, participants of the study, and translators of Nepali transcripts to English for their support and contributions.

Funding

The study was funded with the award received for the study from The Farrar Foundation, UK. The funding body did not have any role in the design of the study, in collection, analysis and interpretation of data or in preparation of the manuscript.

Authors' contributions

RS designed the study, developed the tools, undertook data collection and analysis and wrote the manuscript. MD and ER participated in the design of the study, and contributed to all other phases; MD was also closely involved with data analysis. DP supported the development of tools. MKM guided the design of the study. All authors commented on previous versions of the manuscript and approved the final manuscript.

Authors' information

RS is a Founding Member of the Nepal Public Health Foundation, Kathmandu, Nepal and Associate Professor at Shree Medical and Technical College, Bharatpur, Chitwan, Nepal. MKM is Executive Chair at the Nepal Public Health Foundation, Kathmandu, Nepal. DP is Health Director at Save the Children, Kathmandu, Nepal. ER is a Senior Scientist at the Institute of Medical Informatics, Biometry and Epidemiology, Pettenkofer School of Public Health, LMU, Munich, Germany. MD is a senior consultant in Obstetrics and Gynecology at LMU, Munich University, Germany.

Competing interests

The authors declare that they have no competing interests.

Author details

[1]Nepal Public Health Foundation, Kathmandu, Nepal. [2]Center for International Health, Ludwig-Maximilians-University, Munich, Germany. [3]Institute for Medical Information Processing, Biometry and Epidemiology, Pettenkofer School of Public Health, Ludwig-Maximilians-University, Munich, Germany. [4]Save the Children, Kathmandu, Nepal. [5]Department of Obstetrics and Gynecology – Campus Grosshadern, Ludwig-Maximilians-University, Munich, Germany.

References

1. WHO. Trends in maternal mortality: 1990–2015: estimates from WHO, UNICEF, UNFPA, World Bank Group and the United Nations Population Division. Geneva: World Health Organization; 2015.
2. Campbell OM, Graham WJ. Strategies for reducing maternal mortality: getting on with what works. Lancet. 2006;368(9543):1284–99.

3.   Bhutta ZA, et al. Can available interventions end preventable deaths in mothers, newborn babies, and stillbirths, and at what cost? Lancet. 2014; 384(9940):347–70.

4.   UNFPA. Saving mothers' lives, the challenge continues. 2004. Available from: https://www.unfpa.org/sites/default/files/pub-pdf/savingmotherslives.pdf. Accessed 20 Dec 2013].

5.   Kerber KJ, et al. Continuum of care for maternal, newborn, and child health: from slogan to service delivery. Lancet. 2007;370(9595):1358–69.

6.   FHD. Safer Mother Programme Working Guideline- 2065/2009. Government of Nepal: Kathmandu: Family Health Division, Ministry of Health and Population; 2009.

7.   GoN. Operational guidelines on incentives for safe delivery services. Government of Nepal: Ministry of Health and population; 2005.

8.   DoHS. Annual Report 2072/73 (2015/2016). Kathmandu, Nepal: Department of Health Services, Ministry of Health, Government of Nepal; 2017.

9.   MoH. Nepal Demographic and Health Survey 2016. Kathmandu, Nepal: Ministry of Health, Nepal; new ERA; and ICF; 2017.

10. Wagle RR, Sabroe S, Nielsen BB. Socioeconomic and physical distance to the maternity hospital as predictors for place of delivery: an observation study from Nepal. BMC Pregnancy Childbirth. 2004;4(1):8.

11. Shrestha SK, et al. Changing trends on the place of delivery: why do Nepali women give birth at home? Reprod Health. 2012;9:25.

12. Karkee R, Binns CW, Lee AH. Determinants of facility delivery after implementation of safer mother programme in Nepal: a prospective cohort study. BMC Pregnancy Childbirth. 2013;13(1):193.

13. Shah R, et al. Factors affecting institutional delivery in rural Chitwan district of Nepal: a community-based cross-sectional study. BMC Pregnancy Childbirth. 2015;15(1):27.

14. Shahabuddin A, et al. Determinants of institutional delivery among young married women in Nepal: evidence from the Nepal demographic and health survey, 2011. BMJ Open. 2017;7(4):e012446.

15. Sharma SR, et al. Factors associated with place of delivery in rural Nepal. BMC Public Health. 2014;14(1):306.

16. Choulagai B, et al. Barriers to using skilled birth attendants' services in mid- and far-western Nepal: a cross-sectional study. BMC Int Health Human Rights. 2013;13(1):49.

17. Choulagai BP, et al. A cluster-randomized evaluation of an intervention to increase skilled birth attendant utilization in mid-and far-western Nepal. Health Policy Plan. 2017;32(8):1092–101.

18. Morrison J, et al. Exploring the first delay: a qualitative study of home deliveries in Makwanpur district Nepal. BMC Pregnancy Childbirth. 2014; 14(1):89.

19. Onta S, et al. Perceptions of users and providers on barriers to utilizing skilled birth care in mid-and far-western Nepal: a qualitative study. Glob Health Action. 2014;7(1):24580.

20. GoN. Ministry of Federal Affairs and Local Development *Available from* www.mofald.gov.np. Accessed 20 Jan 2018].

21. CBS. Nepal in figures. Kathmandu: National Planning Commission Secretariat, Central Bureau of Statistics; 2012a.

22. CBS. National Population and Housing Census 2011. Village Development Committee/Municipality. Kathmandu: National Planning Commission Secretariat, Central Bureau of Statistics; 2012b.

23. UNDP. Nepal Human Development Report 2014: Beyond Geography, Unlocking Human Potential. Kathmandu, Nepal: Government of Nepal, National Planning Commission; United Nations Development Programme; 2014.

24. CBS. National Population and Housing Census 2011, (National Report). Kathmandu: National Planning Commission Secretariat, Central Bureau of Statistics; 2012c.

25. Mahato PK, et al. Birthing centres in Nepal: recent developments, obstacles and opportunities. J Asian Midwives. 2016;3(1):18–30.

26. DPHO. Annual Health Report of Chitwan. Chitwan: District Public Health Office, Ministry of Health and Population, Government of Nepal; 2013.

27. CBS. National Population and Housing Census 2011 (Village Development Committee/Municipality), Chitwan. Kathmandu, Nepal: National Planning Commission Secretariat, Central Bureau of Statistics, Government of Nepal; 2014.

28. Boyce, C. and Neale, P., Conducting in-depth interviews: a guide for designing and conducting in-depth interviews for evaluation input. 2006.

29. Gill P, et al. Methods of data collection in qualitative research: interviews and focus groups. Br Dent J. 2008;204(6):291–5.

30. Farmer T, et al. Developing and implementing a triangulation protocol for qualitative health research. Qual Health Res. 2006;16(3):377–94.

31. Devkota, M.D., Utilization of rural maternity delivery services in six districts of Nepal: a qualitative study. 2006.

32. Simkhada B, Porter MA, Van Teijlingen ER. The role of mothers-in-law in antenatal care decision-making in Nepal: a qualitative study. BMC Pregnancy Childbirth. 2010;10(1):34.

33. Furuta M, Salway S. Women's position within the household as a determinant of maternal health care use in Nepal. Int Fam Plan Perspect. 2006;32:17–27.

34. Gabrysch S, Campbell OM. Still too far to walk: literature review of the determinants of delivery service use. BMC Pregnancy Childbirth. 2009;9(1):34.

35. Titaley CR, et al. Why do some women still prefer traditional birth attendants and home delivery?: a qualitative study on delivery care services in west Java Province, Indonesia. BMC Pregnancy Childbirth. 2010;10(1):43.

36. Mrisho M, et al. Factors affecting home delivery in rural Tanzania. Tropical Med Int Health. 2007;12(7):862–72.

37. Van Teijlingen ER, Hundley V. The importance of pilot studies 2001. Social Research Update, issue 35. Available from: http://sru.soc.surrey.ac.uk/SRU35. html. Accessed 25 Dec 2013.

38. Braun V, Clarke V. Using thematic analysis in psychology. Qual Res Psychol. 2006;3(2):77–101.

39. Bradley EH, Curry LA, Devers KJ. Qualitative data analysis for health services research: developing taxonomy, themes, and theory. Health Serv Res. 2007; 42(4):1758–72.

40. Dahal RK. Factors influencing the choice of place of delivery among women in eastern rural Nepal. IJMCH. 2013;1(2):30–7.

41. Shiferaw S, et al. Why do women prefer home births in Ethiopia? BMC pregnancy and childbirth. 2013;13(1):5.

42. Sharma S, et al. Dirty and 40 days in the wilderness: eliciting childbirth and postnatal cultural practices and beliefs in Nepal. BMC pregnancy and childbirth. 2016;16(1):147.

43. Sychareun V, et al. Reasons rural Laotians choose home deliveries over delivery at health facilities: a qualitative study. BMC pregnancy and childbirth. 2012;12(1):86.

44. Gebrehiwot T, et al. Health workers' perceptions of facilitators of and barriers to institutional delivery in Tigray, northern Ethiopia. BMC pregnancy and childbirth. 2014;14(1):137.

45. Dennis C-L, et al. Traditional postpartum practices and rituals: a qualitative systematic review. Women's Health. 2007;3(4):487–502.

46. Maru S, et al. Determinants of institutional birth among women in rural Nepal: a mixed-methods cross-sectional study. BMC pregnancy and childbirth. 2016;16(1):252.

47. Upadhyay P, et al. Influence of family members on utilization of maternal health care services among teen and adult pregnant women in Kathmandu, Nepal: a cross sectional study. Reprod Health. 2014;11(1):92.

48. Story WT, et al. Husbands' involvement in delivery care utilization in rural Bangladesh: a qualitative study. BMC Pregnancy Childbirth. 2012;12:28.

49. Mullany BC, Hindin MJ, Becker S. Can women's autonomy impede male involvement in pregnancy health in Katmandu, Nepal? Soc Sci Med. 2005; 61(9):1993–2006.

50. Kaye DK, et al. Male involvement during pregnancy and childbirth: men's perceptions, practices and experiences during the care for women who developed childbirth complications in Mulago hospital, Uganda. BMC pregnancy and childbirth. 2014;14(1):54.

51. Simkhada B, Porter MA, Van Teijlingen ER. The role of mothers-in-law in antenatal care decision-making in Nepal: a qualitative study. BMC pregnancy and childbirth. 2010;10(1):34.

52. Gabrysch S, et al. The influence of distance and level of care on delivery place in rural Zambia: a study of linked national data in a geographic information system. PLoS Med. 2011;8(1):150.

53. Sychareun V, et al. Provider perspectives on constraints in providing maternal, neonatal and child health services in the Lao People's democratic republic: a qualitative study. BMC pregnancy and childbirth. 2013;13(1):243.

54. Khatri RB, et al. Barriers to utilization of childbirth services of a rural birthing center in Nepal: a qualitative study. PLoS One. 2017;12(5):e0177602.

55. Shah R. Bypassing birthing centres for child birth: a community-based study in rural Chitwan Nepal. BMC Health Serv Res. 2016;16(1):597.

56. Karkee R, Lee AH, Pokharel PK. Women's perception of quality of maternity services: a longitudinal survey in Nepal. BMC Pregnancy Childbirth. 2014;14:45.

13

Patient and provider determinants for receipt of three dimensions of respectful maternity care in Kigoma Region, Tanzania-April-July, 2016

M. M. Dynes[1][*] [iD], E. Twentyman[1], L. Kelly[1], G. Maro[2], A. A. Msuya[3], S. Dominico[4], P. Chaote[5], R. Rusibamayila[6] and F. Serbanescu[1]

Abstract

Background: Lack of respectful maternity care (RMC) is increasingly recognized as a human rights issue and a key deterrent to women seeking facility-based deliveries. Ensuring facility-based RMC is essential for improving maternal and neonatal health, especially in sub-Saharan African countries where mortality and non-skilled delivery care remain high.

Few studies have attempted to quantitatively identify patient and delivery factors associated with RMC, and none has modeled the influence of provider characteristics on RMC. This study aims to help fill these gaps through collection and analysis of interviews linked between clients and providers, allowing for description of both patient and provider characteristics and their association with receipt of RMC.

Methods: We conducted cross-sectional surveys across 61 facilities in Kigoma Region, Tanzania, from April to July 2016. Measures of RMC were developed using 21-items in a Principal Components Analysis (PCA). We conducted multilevel, mixed effects generalized linear regression analyses on matched data from 249 providers and 935 post-delivery clients. The outcomes of interest included three dimensions of RMC—*Friendliness/Comfort/Attention*; *Information/Consent*; and *Non-abuse/Kindness*—developed from the first three components of PCA. Significance level was set at $p < 0.05$.

Results: Significant client-level determinants for perceived *Friendliness/Comfort/Attention* RMC included age (30–39 versus 15–19 years: Coefficient [Coef] 0.63; 40–49 versus 15–19 years: Coef 0.79) and self-reported complications (reported complications versus did not: Coef − 0.41). Significant provider-level determinants included perception of fair pay (Perceives fair pay versus unfair pay: Coef 0.46), cadre (Nurses/midwives versus Clinicians: Coef − 0.46), and number of deliveries in the last month (11–20 versus < 11 deliveries: Coef − 0.35). Significant client-level determinants for *Information/Consent* RMC included labor companionship (Companion versus none: Coef 0.37) and religiosity (Attends services at least weekly versus less often: Coef − 0.31). Significant provider-level determinants included perception of fair pay (Perceives fair pay versus unfair: Coef 0.37), weekly work hours (Coef 0.01), and age (30–39 versus 20–29 years: Coef − 0.34; 40–49 versus 20–29 years: Coef − 0.58).

Significant provider-level determinants for *Non-abuse/Kindness* RMC included the predictors of age (age 50+ versus 20–29 years: Coef 0.34) and access to electronic mentoring (Access to two mentoring types versus none: Coef 0.37).

(Continued on next page)

* Correspondence: mdynes@cdc.gov
[1]Centers for Disease Control and Prevention, Division of Reproductive Health, Atlanta, Georgia
Full list of author information is available at the end of the article

(Continued from previous page)

Conclusions: These findings illustrate the value of including both client and provider information in the analysis of RMC. Strategies that address provider-level determinants of RMC (such as equitable pay, work environment, access to mentoring platforms) may improve RMC and subsequently address uptake of facility delivery.

Keywords: Respectful maternity care (RMC), Disrespect and abuse (D&A), Maternal health, Maternal mortality, Multilevel modeling, Tanzania

Plain English summary

Lack of respectful maternity care (RMC) discourages women from seeking facility-based deliveries. RMC is essential for improving maternal and newborn health in sub-Saharan African countries where rates of maternal deaths and non-skilled delivery care are high. We conducted surveys in 61 facilities in Kigoma Region, Tanzania from April to July 2016. Principal components analysis was used to identify three dimensions of RMC. Multilevel regression analyses were conducted on matched data from 249 providers and 935 post-delivery clients. Our outcomes of interest included three dimensions of RMC: 1) *Friendliness, Comfort, and Attention*, 2) *Information and Consent*, and 3) *Non-abuse and Kindness*. Client age, self-reported delivery complications, provider perception of fair pay, cadre, and number of deliveries attended were important factors for receipt of RMC related to *Friendliness, Comfort, and Attention*. Having a birth companion, client religiosity, provider perception of fair pay, and provider age were important factors for receipt of RMC related to *Information/Consent*. Provider age and access to electronic mentoring were important factors for receipt of RMC related to *Non-abusive/Kindness*. Strategies that promote equitable pay, give providers short-term respite away from maternity care, and increase access to mentoring opportunities may improve RMC and uptake of facility delivery.

Background

Worldwide maternal deaths remain common, with approximately 830 women dying each day from known and largely preventable causes [1]. Access to and use of skilled birth attendance is key to prevention of maternal mortality [2]. Approximately 75–80% [3–7] of maternal deaths worldwide result from obstetric complications and are preventable given access to appropriate interventions. Maternal mortality remains a particularly formidable challenge in Tanzania, where the maternal mortality ratio (556 maternal deaths per 100,000 live births) has demonstrated no detectable reduction over the past 10 years [8]. The percentage of women delivering at a health facility (63%) remains low despite ongoing efforts to increase facility-based delivery [8].

Lack of respectful maternity care (RMC), which includes disrespect and abuse (D&A), has been increasingly recognized [9–14] and demonstrably identified as a key deterrent for women seeking facility-based deliveries [2, 9, 10, 15–28]. Lack of RMC decreases patient satisfaction with services and mediates lack of access to skilled maternity care by reducing the likelihood that patients will return to skilled care for future deliveries [13, 26–28], and by building distrust of facility-based delivery at the community level [29, 30]. Furthermore, lack of RMC may reduce access to appropriate intervention even among patients already within a facility for delivery care by reducing patient-provider communication [31].

The presence of provider-client interpersonal barriers is increasingly suspected to interfere with attempts to increase skilled birth attendance. Bowser and Hill's review describes seven manifestations of D&A which constitute the current typology in the D&A literature: physical abuse, non-consented care, non-dignified care (including verbal abuse), discrimination, abandonment, and detainment in facilities [11]. Such behaviors are widely recognized to violate patients' basic human rights. The White Ribbon Alliance (WRA) completed a review of international and multinational human rights instruments related to maternal health rights and the domains of D&A. The resulting Respectful Maternity Care Charter defined seven rights of childbearing women [32] (Table 1): Freedom from harm and ill treatment; Right to information, informed consent and refusal, and respect for choices and preferences, including the right to companionship of choice whenever possible; Confidentiality, privacy; Dignity, respect; Equality, freedom from discrimination, equitable care; Right to timely health care and to the highest attainable level of health; and Liberty, autonomy, self-determination, and freedom from coercion.

Worldwide, an alarmingly high prevalence of women have reported mistreatment according to these typologies of D&A, with reports ranging from 20 to 78% [12, 13, 22, 31, 33]. Understanding facilitators of and barriers to RMC is critical to the design of interventions to promote RMC in these contexts.

Qualitative studies have identified several potential patient factors associated with lack of RMC. These

Table 1 Survey questions and variable names included in the respectful maternity care analyses categorized by White Ribbon Alliance Respectful Maternity Care Charter Article—Kigoma Region, Tanzania, April–July 2016

White Ribbon Alliance Respectful Maternity Care Charter	Survey Question	Corresponding Variable Name
Article I: Every woman has the right to be free from harm and ill treatment	Did any of the health facility staff ever physically abuse you during your visit? By physical abuse, we mean, did they hit, slap, push, kick you, or use any other type of physical force against you.	*Absence of physical abuse*
Article II: Every woman has the right to information, informed consent and refusal, and respect for her choices and preferences, including the right to her choice of companionship during maternity care, whenever possible	Did the staff explain what will happen during your labor and delivery?	*Explain what will happen*
	Did the staff get your consent before proceeding with procedures and exams?	*Consent before procedures/exams*
	Did the staff explain procedures or exams before proceeding?	*Explain procedures/exam beforehand*
	Did the staff inform you of the findings from procedures and exams?	*Inform about findings from procedures/exams*
	Did you feel the information given to you during your visit was too little, just about right, or too much?	*Right amount of information*
	Did the staff ask if you have questions?	*Provider asked if any questions*
	Did the staff encourage you to have a support person with you throughout labor and delivery?	*Provider encouraged companion*
	Did you feel comfortable to ask questions during the visit?	*Client comfortable asking questions*
	Summative Index: Did the staff… • Counsel you about danger signs you should look for in yourself such as too much bleeding, fever, or breast pain? • Counsel you about danger signs you should look for in your baby such as refusing to breastfeed, fever, or convulsions (fits)? • Tell you what to do if you or the baby have any problems? • Counsel you on good body hygiene to prevent infections? • Counsel you on breastfeeding? • Counsel you about exclusive breastfeeding (not using any other fluid/food except breastmilk)? • Ask about your reproductive goals? By reproductive goals, we mean did the provider ask about your desire to have children in the future or to use family planning. • Counsel you on when you can have sex with your husband/partner? • Counsel you on when you can bear another pregnancy? • Counsel you on the risks of sexually transmitted infections (STIs), including HIV? • Counsel you on how to prevent sexually transmitted infections (STIs), including HIV? • Tell you when to return for a follow-up visit?	*Index for receipt of post-delivery counseling*
Article III: Every woman has the right to privacy and confidentiality	Do you believe the information you shared about yourself with the health care provider will be kept confidential?	*Client feels provider will keep information confidential*
	Did the staff provide privacy during counseling or exams such as using a private room, screens, curtains, or cloths to cover you?	*Given privacy for exams or counseling*
	When meeting with the health care provider during the visit, do you think other clients could hear what you said?	*Other clients could not hear discussions*

Table 1 Survey questions and variable names included in the respectful maternity care analyses categorized by White Ribbon Alliance Respectful Maternity Care Charter Article—Kigoma Region, Tanzania, April–July 2016 *(Continued)*

White Ribbon Alliance Respectful Maternity Care Charter	Survey Question	Corresponding Variable Name
Article IV: Every woman has the right to be treated with dignity and respect	Did the staff introduce themselves?	*Provider introduced self*
	Did the staff greet you respectfully?	*Greeted respectfully*
	Did any of the staff ever emotionally abuse you during your visit? By emotional abuse, we mean, did they speak or act in an angry or condescending way that made you feel badly about yourself, degraded, embarrassed, or sad?	*Absence of emotional abuse*
	Did the staff interact in a friendly way?	*Interacts in a friendly way*
	Overall, how would you rate the staff's kindness in the way they spoke to you during this visit?	*Kindness*
	Overall, how would you rate the staff's level of encouragement during labor and delivery?	*Encouragement*
	How would you rate the facility's level of cleanliness?	*Level of cleanliness*
	Did the staff advise you on what you could do to make yourself more comfortable when you were in pain?	*Advised of comfort measures*
	Summative Index: What comfort measures did the staff provide to make you more comfortable? • Rubbed back • Offered fluids to drink • Offered food to eat • Assisted in changing position • Helped to walk around • Used encouraging words	*Index for receipt of comfort measures*
Article V: Every woman has the right to equality, freedom from discrimination, and equitable care	None available	None available
Article VI: Every woman has the right to healthcare and to the highest attainable level of health	Did the staff come to attend to you if you called for help?	*Provider came when called*
	Did the staff pay close attention to you throughout labor and delivery?	*Close attention in labor*
	Did the health care staff visit you regularly during the course of labor?	*Visited regularly in labor*
	Was a health care provider with you at the moment of delivery?	*Provider present at delivery*
	Did you feel that your waiting time (when you first arrived at this facility and the time you saw a staff person for a consultation) was reasonable or too long?	*Wait time from arrival to care*
	How long ago was your new baby born? (proxy measure from birth to time from time of exit interview)	*Discharge time 24 h or more after delivery*
	Did the facility provider supplies for your labor and delivery care?	*Facility provided birth supplies*
Article VII: Every woman has the right to liberty, autonomy, self-determination, and freedom from coercion	None available	None available

include the following: race/ethnicity and religion, depending upon context [34–37]; age, with unmarried adolescents [38, 39] and older women of high parity [40, 41] thought to be at particular risk; socioeconomic status (SES), with poor women at perceived higher risk of D&A [42–45]; and medical conditions,

with women with HIV thought to face multiple forms of discrimination [35, 46, 47].

While qualitative studies have identified factors associated with RMC, few studies have quantitatively examined the associations between individual patient characteristics and report of D&A. In Tanzania, women who had attended secondary education or greater, primiparous women, those with experience of low mood in the past year, and those with a personal history of physical abuse or rape were more likely to report experiences of D&A during their delivery; married women were less likely to report D&A [33]. In a follow-up community survey, poor women, women who reported low mood at the time of exit interview, and more educated women were again more likely to report D&A during their delivery, whereas grand multiparas (given birth five or more times) and women with Cesarean sections were less likely to report D&A. Abuya et al., in their exploration of specific forms of D&A during childbirth in Kenya, demonstrated that older women were less likely than younger women to experience non-confidential care, that women of higher parity were more likely to be detained for lack of payment and more likely to have bribes demanded, that married women were less likely to be detained but more likely to be neglected, and that women without a companion were less likely to experience demands for bribes or detention [13].

To our knowledge, published research to date has not modeled relationships between health care provider demographic or practice characteristics and provision of RMC. Qualitative studies, however, including in-depth interviews with providers of maternity care, have generated several hypotheses. Provider training itself is thought to create "distancing" and separation between providers and patients, potentially generating insensitivity toward women in childbirth [39, 48] through lack of attention to patient-provider dynamics, or even through direct rationalization of D&A [49]. Poor provider pay is thought to contribute to lack of RMC provision [17, 50, 51], as is lack of encouragement by facility leadership [17]. Provider demoralization and "moral distress" due to weak health systems, limited supplies, and understaffing have also been well described in relationship to lacking RMC [10, 17, 26, 49].

To date, there is no standardized or widely agreed upon way to define or measure either RMC or D&A. Scales for measurement of RMC have recently been proposed in Ethiopia [52] and in the USA and Canada [53], however, the tools are not yet validated in other contexts. Few studies have attempted to quantitatively identify patient and delivery factors associated with RMC. No identified studies have matched patient and provider interviews or any other form of modeling inclusive of linked patient and provider experience.

This novel study utilizes interviews linked between clients and providers from hospitals, health centers, and dispensaries to describe receipt and delivery of RMC, allowing for description of both patient and provider characteristics and their association with receipt

of RMC. This study also contributes to the science around RMC by constructing measures of RMC based on domains from the WRA RMC Charter.

Methods
Study design and setting
We conducted cross-sectional surveys consisting of facility-based client exit interviews and provider interviews across 61 facilities (6 hospitals, 25 health centers, and 30 dispensaries) in Kigoma Region, Tanzania from April 30 to July 1, 2016.

Kigoma Region covers 45,066 km^2 and is located in the northwest corner of Tanzania, bordering Lake Tanganyika, the Democratic Republic of Congo, and Burundi. Kigoma Region's population in 2012 was 2,127,930 with an annual growth rate of 2.4% and 370,374 households [54]. Approximately 83% of the population live in rural areas where farming is the primary economic activity [54]. Nine out of 10 adults in Kigoma Region have attained a primary school education [54]. Less than two-thirds of births (62.8%) in Kigoma region occur in a health facility [55].

During our study, the Ministry of Health, Community Development, Gender, the Elderly and Children (MoHCD GEC) was implementing a number of efforts to improve maternal health in Tanzania. These efforts included the *National Roadmap Strategic Plan to Accelerate Reduction of Maternal, Newborn and Child Deaths in Tanzania 2008–2015*, the *Big Results Now* (BRN) initiative, and Wazazi Nipendeni ("Parents Love Me"; a safe motherhood multimedia campaign). Additionally, since 2006, the *Project to Reduce Maternal Deaths in Tanzania* has worked in Kigoma Region with the aim of decreasing maternal mortality.

Sampling and data collection
Facility sampling
All hospitals ($n = 6$) and non-refugee camp health centers ($n = 25$) in Kigoma Region were included in the study. A sample of 30 dispensaries (of the approximately 163 dispensaries conducting deliveries in the region) was selected using the following criteria: 1) had an estimated 180 or more births per year; 2) had two or more onsite health providers; 3) was a site for BRN or project partner facility improvements, 4) referred patients to one of the 25 health centers; and 5) to maximize geographic distribution.

Provider sampling
The sampling frame for the provider survey comprised a list of all health care providers in the selected facilities. Providers were recruited if they were

available during the study period and routinely provided labor and delivery care services. Providers were categorized into three cadres: 1) clinicians [Assistant Medical Officers/Clinical Officers/Assistant Clinical Officers], nurses/midwives [Nurse Officers/Assistant Nurse Officers/Registered Nurses/Midwives/Enrolled Nurses], other staff [Medical Attendants/Maternal and Child Health Aides]). Medical Doctors and specialists were excluded from participation due to the small number in the region. A sample of 189 provider interviews was needed to detect a 5% relative mean change in key variables of interest with 90% power and an *alpha* of 0.05.

Client sampling

Convenience sampling was used to enroll women as they exited delivery care services. Clients were eligible if they were 15 to 49 years of age and received delivery care services at the facility. Due to the focus of the project on routine labor and delivery care, clients were excluded if they delivered at home or on the way to the facility, had a cesarean section delivery, or experienced a stillbirth or neonatal death. A sample of 908 client interviews was needed to detect a 15% absolute difference in the variables of interest 90% power and an *alpha* of 0.05 (assuming a 50% reference proportion).

Interview procedures and study tools

Interview guides were developed in English and translated into Swahili. Questionnaires were pre-tested in January 2016. Final questionnaires were translated from English to Swahili and back-translated to English. Informed consent was obtained from each respondent and confirmed with the respondent's thumbprint. All client and provider interviews were administered face-to-face by an interviewer in Swahili. Interviews were conducted at the facility on the day of discharge, most commonly on the same day of delivery or the following day. The *Client Post-Delivery Exit Interview Questionnaire* captured sociodemographic characteristics, perceptions of and satisfaction with services, and pregnancy history and intention. The *Provider Interview Questionnaire* and *Self-administered Knowledge Test* were designed to capture information about provider demographic characteristics, education and training, supervision and mentorship, clinical knowledge, perceptions of the work environment, and current labor and delivery practices.

Development of respectful maternity care measure

An initial 29 items were taken from the survey data to develop the RMC measure; these items were chosen based on domains from the WRA Respectful Maternity Care Charter and previously published research on

RMC [11–14, 19–21, 33, 40]. The RMC items are described in detail in Table 1. Items representing disrespect (rather than respect) were reverse coded prior to inclusion. In initial scale reliability testing, no items were found to be redundant or negatively associated with the scale. Four items with low item-to-scale correlations were dropped (*Discharge time, Facility supplies, Facility cleanliness,* and *Wait time*). The remaining 25-item measure displayed strong internal consistency with Cronbach's alpha of 0.83 and an inter-item correlation of 0.17. In support of criterion validity, Spearman testing found that the RMC measure was positively associated with the variable *Client satisfaction with care* ($rho = 23.8$, p-value < 0.001).

The 25 items were then entered into a Principal Components Analysis (PCA) to establish dimensionality of the scale with the aim of retaining the maximum amount of variance possible. The mean Kaiser-Meyer-Olkin measure of sampling adequacy was 0.81 and all individual item measures were greater than 0.68, indicating strong relationships among scale items [56]. Visualization of the scree plot supported a three-component solution for RMC (Fig. 1); client RMC scores were calculated for each of the first three components.

Items that loaded highest on the first principal component included *Advise on comfort measures, Friendliness, Visit regularly,* and *Pay close attention.* This first component was therefore termed the RMC Dimension 1 (RMC-D1), defined by the domains of Friendliness, Comfort, and Attention. Items that loaded highest on the second principal component included *Consent before procedures/exams, Explain what will happen, Explain procedures/exams beforehand,* and *Post-delivery counseling index.* This second

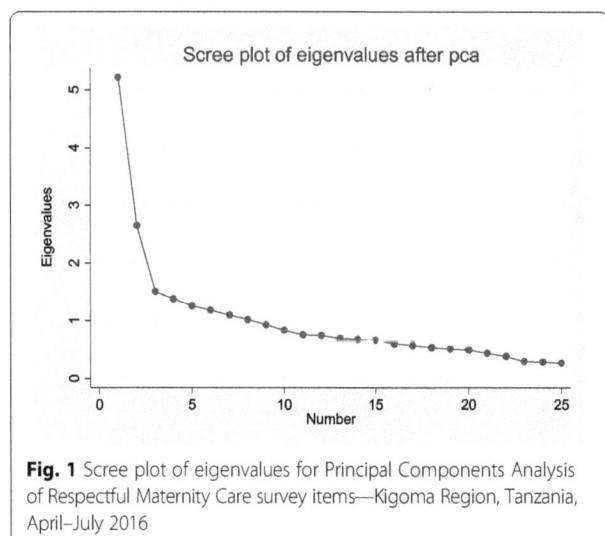

Fig. 1 Scree plot of eigenvalues for Principal Components Analysis of Respectful Maternity Care survey items—Kigoma Region, Tanzania, April–July 2016

component was therefore termed RMC Dimension 2 (RMC-D2), defined by the domains of Information and Consent. Items that loaded highest on the third principal component included *Absence of physical abuse*, *Absence of emotional abuse*, *Encouragement*, and *Kindness*. This component was therefore termed RMC Dimension 3 (RMC-D3), defined by Non-abuse and Kindness.

Outcome variables

The outcome variables of interest included the continuous variables *RMC-D1 score*, *RMC-D2 score*, and *RMC-D3 score* to represent receipt of three dimensions of RMC.

Independent variables

Client-level

The client-level variables of interest included:

- *Client age*: 15 to 19, 20 to 29, 30 to 39, 40 to 49 years of age, age unknown by client;
- *Literacy*: Able to read and write, Unable to both read and write;
- *Highest education attended*: No education, primary, secondary, college or university;
- *Total live births*: Two or fewer, three or more;
- *Marital status*: Not in union, in union;
- *Frequency of attendance at religious services*: Less than once a week, once a week or more often;
- *Companion in labor*: No, yes;
- *Companion at time of delivery*: No, yes;
- *Self-reported delivery complications*[1]: No, yes; and
- *SES*[2]: Low, low middle, middle, high middle, high wealth.

Provider-level

The provider-level variables of interest included:

- *Provider age*: 20 to 29, 30 to 39, 40 to 49, 50 years or older;
- *Sex*: Male, female;
- *Highest education completed*: Primary, secondary, college or university;
- *Cadre*: Clinicians, nurses/midwives, other staff;
- *Years in cadre*: Continuous;
- *Years at the facility*: Continuous;
- *Work hours per week*: Continuous;
- *Number of deliveries attended in last month*: One to 10, 11 to 20, 21 to 30, 31 or more, Don't know;
- *Has on-site supervisor*: No, yes;

- *Job satisfaction*: Very satisfied, a little satisfied, neither satisfied nor dissatisfied, a little dissatisfied, very dissatisfied;
- *Perception paid fairly for job duties*: No, yes;
- *Perception of adequacy of training for job duties*: No, yes;
- *Perception in-service training has helped job performance*: No, yes;
- *Access to Electronic mentoring opportunities*: Access to zero, one, two, or three opportunities related to e-learning, emergency call system, and teleconference;
- *Recent complications summative index*: Has dealt with zero, one, two, three, or four types of complications in the last month related to hemorrhage, eclampsia, obstructed labor, and puerperal sepsis;
- *Delivery ever-training summative index*[3]: Pre- or in-service delivery training in 25 items, continuous;
- *Delivery pre-service summative index*[3]: Pre-service delivery training in 25 items, continuous;
- *Delivery in-service summative index*[3]: In-service delivery training in 25 items, continuous;
- *Recent delivery practice summative index*[3]: Provision of delivery services in 25 items in the last 3 months, continuous; and
- *Clinical knowledge test score*: Percent correct on 64 knowledge questions on the topics of antenatal care, routine delivery, newborn, complications, partograph, and postpartum.

Analytic approach

Client and provider data were matched by asking providers on duty at the time of the delivery and by asking clients which provider most commonly provided their care; only matched client and provider interviews were included in the analysis. Data analyses were conducted using Stata 14.1. Bivariate analyses were conducted to identify client and provider variables associated with the outcome variables of interest; variables with a significant unadjusted relationship ($p < 0.10$) with the dependent variables were included in multivariate modeling. Multilevel, mixed-effects generalized linear models were fitted for the first three RMC PCA scores (*RMC-D1 score*, *RMC-D2 score*, and *RMC-D3 score*) to identify variables with a significant adjusted relationship ($p < 0.05$). Clustering of data by facility was further accounted for through inclusion of a facility identification cluster variable.

Results

From April 30–July 1, 2016, a total of 960 delivery clients and 361 providers (Clinicians $n = 72$, Nurses/

midwives $n = 188$, Other staff $n = 98$) were interviewed. Following exclusion of data from non-matched clients and providers, data from 935 delivery clients and 249 providers (Clinicians $n = 69$, Nurses/midwives $n = 176$, Other staff $n = 85$) were used in the analysis.

Descriptive characteristics

Half of clients were 20 to 29 years of age (50.3%) and received care at a health center (50.6%). The majority of clients included in the study were married (91.0%), attended at least weekly religious services (86.4%), and have attended primary school education (67.3%). Nearly 45% of clients reported having a birth companion with them during labor (44.7%), while only 12% reported having a birth companion with them at the time of delivery. About 13% of clients reported that they experienced delivery complications (12.9%). (Table 2).

With respect to characteristics of RMC, nearly all clients reported that they were greeted respectfully upon admission (96.3%), while less than half reported that the provider introduced themselves (45.6%). Two-thirds of clients reported the provider explained what to expect in labor (63.0%). Regarding procedures and exams, most clients reported that the provider asked for consent (80.4%), explained the procedures and exams ahead of time (70.7%), and gave them the results (87.5%). One-third of clients reported the provider encouraged them to have a companion (32.7%). About three-quarters of clients reported feeling comfortable asking the provider questions (75.4%) and reported believing the information they gave to the provider would remain confidential (77.2%). Nearly all clients reported receiving privacy during exams and counseling (94.2%), although a few reported that other clients could overhear their conversations with the provider (7.9%). On average, clients received 6.7 out of 12 post-delivery counseling elements (Tables 1 and 3).

Most clients reported that the provider was friendly (94.3%), and about three-quarters of clients reported the provider was very kind (76.0%) and very encouraging (79.4%). Nearly nine of 10 clients reported the provider advised them about comfort measures (88.7%); however, receipt of comfort measures from the provider was low at an average of less than two out of six comfort measures (1.3). Clients overwhelmingly reported the provider paid close attention to them during labor (93.5%) and came when they called for them (97.7%). Physical and emotional abuse was reported infrequently by clients at 1.3% and 2.7%, respectively. (Table 3).

Four in 10 providers were 20 to 29 years of age (41.0%), while one-fifth of providers were 50 years or

Table 2 Characteristics of delivery clients included in the respectful maternity care study sample—Kigoma Region, Tanzania, April–July 2016 ($n = 935$)

	Women, n (%)	95% CI
Age in years		
15 to19	163 (17.4)	15.1–20.0
20 to 29	470 (50.3)	47.1–53.5
30 to 39	251 (26.8)	24.1–29.8
40 to 49	38 (4.1)	3.0–5.5
Don't know	13 (1.4)	0.8–2.4
Facility type		
Hospital	254 (27.2)	24.4–30.1
Health center	473 (50.6)	47.4–53.8
Dispensary	208 (22.3)	19.7–25.0
Marital status		
In a union	851 (91.0)	89.0–92.7
Not in a union	84 (9.0)	7.3–11.0
Frequency of attendance at religious services		
Attends at least weekly	808 (86.4)	84.1–88.5
Attends less often than weekly	127 (13.6)	11.5–15.9
Highest education attended		
No education	190 (20.3)	17.9–23.0
Primary	629 (67.3)	64.2–70.2
Secondary	100 (10.7)	8.9–12.8
College or University	16 (1.7)	1.0–2.8
Literacy		
Able to read and write	663 (70.9)	67.9–73.7
Unable to both read and write	264 (28.2)	25.4–31.2
Missing or refused	8 (0.9)	0.4–1.7
Socioeconomic status		
Low wealth	185 (19.8)	17.4–22.5
Low middle wealth	168 (18.0)	15.6–20.6
Middle wealth	186 (19.9)	17.5–22.6
High middle wealth	201 (21.5)	19.0–24.3
High wealth	195 (20.9)	18.4–23.6
Total live births		
Mean (SD)	3.3 (2.3)	3.1–3.4
Companion in labor		
Yes	418 (44.7)	41.5–47.9
No	517 (55.3)	52.1–58.5
Companion at time of delivery		
Yes	112 (12.0)	10.0–14.2
No	823 (88.0)	85.8–90.0
Self-reported delivery complications		
Yes	121 (12.9)	10.9–15.3
No	814 (87.1)	84.7–89.1

NOTE: *CI* Confidence Intervals, *SD* Standard Deviation

Table 3 Receipt of respectful care elements among clients included in the study sample—Kigoma Region, Tanzania, April–July 2016 (n = 935)

	Clients, n (%)	95% CI
Greeted respectfully		
Yes	900 (96.3)	94.8–97.3
No	35 (3.7)	2.7–5.2
Introduced themselves		
Yes	426 (45.6)	42.4–48.8
No	509 (54.4)	51.2–57.6
Explained what to expect		
Yes	589 (63.0)	59.8–66.0
No	346 (37.0)	34.0–40.2
Right amount of information given		
Yes	808 (86.4)	84.1–88.5
No	127 (13.6)	11.5–15.9
Consent before procedures/exams		
Yes	752 (80.4)	77.8–82.9
No	183 (19.6)	17.1–22.2
Explained procedures/exams beforehand		
Yes	661 (70.7)	67.7–73.5
No	274 (29.3)	26.5–32.3
Information given on results of procedures/exams		
Yes	818 (87.5)	85.2–89.5
No	117 (12.5)	10.5–14.8
Encouraged companion		
Yes	306 (32.7)	29.8–35.8
No	629 (67.3)	64.2–70.2
Client felt comfortable asking questions		
Yes	705 (75.4)	72.5–78.1
No	230 (24.6)	21.9–27.5
Client believes information will remain confidential		
Yes	722 (77.2)	74.4–79.8
No	213 (22.8)	20.2–25.6
Received privacy for exams and counseling		
Yes	881 (94.2)	92.5–95.6
No	54 (5.8)	4.4–7.5
Client believes other clients could hear conversations with provider		
Yes	74 (7.9)	6.3–9.8
No	861 (92.1)	90.2–93.7
Post-delivery counseling index, possible range 0 to 12		
Mean (SD)	6.7 (3.4)	6.4–6.9
Providers are friendly		
Yes	882 (94.3)	92.7–95.6
No	53 (5.7)	4.4–7.3

Table 3 Receipt of respectful care elements among clients included in the study sample—Kigoma Region, Tanzania, April–July 2016 (n = 935) *(Continued)*

	Clients, n (%)	95% CI
Perception of kindness		
Very kind	711 (76.0)	73.2–78.7
A little kind, Neither kind nor unkind, a little unkind, very unkind	224 (24.0)	21.3–26.8
Perception of encouragement		
Very encouraging	742 (79.4)	76.6–81.8
A little encouraging, Neither encouraging nor discouraging, a little discouraging, very discouraging	193 (20.6)	18.2–23.4
Provider advised client about comfort measures		
Yes	829 (88.7)	86.5–90.5
No	106 (11.3)	9.5–13.5
Provider Comfort Index, possible range 0 to 6		
Mean (SD)	1.3 (0.9)	1.3–1.4
Provider paid close attention during labor		
Yes	874 (93.5)	91.7–94.0
No	61 (6.5)	5.1–8.3
Provider visited regularly in labor		
Yes	865 (92.5)	90.6–94.0
No	70 (7.5)	6.0–9.4
Provider came when client called for them		
Yes	913 (97.7)	96.4–98.5
No	22 (2.4)	1.6–3.6
Physical abuse		
Yes	12 (1.3)	0.7–2.2
No	923 (98.7)	97.8–99.3
Emotional abuse		
Yes	25 (2.7)	1.8–3.9
No	910 (97.3)	96.1–98.2
Provider present at time of delivery		
Yes	916 (98.0)	96.8–98.7
No	19 (2.0)	1.3–3.2
Respectful maternity care dimension 1 score		
Low (below mean)	337 (36.0)	33.2–39.2
High (at or above mean)	598 (64.0)	60.8–67.0
Respectful maternity care dimension 2 score		
Low (below mean)	430 (46.0)	42.8–49.2
High (at or above mean)	505 (54.0)	50.8–57.2
Respectful maternity care dimension 3 score		
Low (below mean)	428 (45.8)	42.6–49.0
High (at or above mean)	507 (54.2)	51.0–57.4

NOTE: *CI* Confidence Intervals, *SD* Standard Deviation

older (21.7%). The majority of providers included in the study were female (64.7%), college/university educated (66.7%), and in the nurse/midwife cadre (61.0%). On average, providers reported working about 10.3 years in their cadre and 7.5 years at their facility, and reported working an average of 54.8 work hours per week. Two-thirds of providers (63.9%) reported conducting from one to 10 deliveries in the last month. Providers reported receiving in-service training on an average of 8 training elements; almost 9 of 10 providers reported in-service training has helped their job performance. Nearly half of providers reported not having access to electronic mentoring opportunities (48.2%). Less than half of providers stated they were satisfied with their job (44.6%), and less than one-fifth of providers feel they are paid fairly for their job duties (18.5%). On average, providers correctly answered 55.1% of the clinical knowledge questions. (Table 4).

Receipt of respectful maternity care dimension 1 (RMC-D1): *Friendliness, Comfort, and Attention*

Results of bivariate analyses for RMC-D1 – *Friendliness, Comfort, and Attention*, are displayed in Appendix. Based on bivariate analyses for RMC-D1, the following variables were included in the multivariable model: *Client age, Total live births,* and *Self-reported delivery complications; Provider cadre, Ever-training summative index score, Delivery pre-service summative index score, Recent delivery practice summative index score, Number of deliveries attended in last month, Recent complications summative index score, Access to electronic mentoring opportunities, Perception paid fairly for job duties,* and *Perception in-service training has helped job performance.*

In multi-level, multivariate regression analyses, clients aged 30 to 39 years and clients aged 40 to 49 years had significantly higher RMC-D1 scores compared to clients 15 to 19 years (Coefficient [Coef] 0.63, 95% Confidence Intervals [CI] 0.14–1.13; Coef 0.79, 95% CI 0.18–1.39, respectively). Clients who reported that they experienced delivery complications had significantly lower RMC-D1 scores compared to clients who did not report complications (Coef -0.41, 95% CI -0.72-[-0.10]). The client variable of *Total live births* was not found to have a significant adjusted association with *RMC-D1 score.* (Table 5).

Clients of providers who perceived that they were paid fairly for their job duties had significantly higher RMC-D1 scores compared to clients of providers who perceived they are not paid fairly (Coef 0.46, 95% CI 0.04–0.88). Clients of Nurses/midwives had significantly lower RMC-D1 scores compared to clients of clinicians (Coef -0.46, 95% CI -089-[-0.03]). Clients of

providers who reported attending 11 to 20 deliveries in the last month had significantly lower RMC-D1 scores compared to clients of providers who attended 1 to 10 deliveries (Coef -0.35, 95% CI -0.67-[-0.02]). Provider variables not found to have a significant adjusted association with *RMC-D1 score* included the following: *Delivery ever-training summative index, Delivery pre-service summative index, Recent delivery practice summative index, Recent complications summative index, Access to electronic mentoring opportunities,* and *Perception in-service training has helped job performance.* (Table 5).

The intraclass correlation (ICC) defines the proportion of the total variance that can be attributed to the hierarchal grouping by the provider variable. Net of all independent variables included in the final RMC-D1 model, 18% of the total variance (ICC = 0.18) is explained by the provider level.

Receipt of respectful maternity care dimension 2 (RMC-D2): *Information and Consent*

Results of bivariate analyses for RMC-D2 – *Information and Consent*, are displayed in Appendix. Based on bivariate analyses for RMC-D2, the following variables were included in the multivariable model: *Client age, Highest education attended, Total live births, SES, Frequency of attendance at religious services, Companion in labor, Companion at time of delivery; Provider age, Number of deliveries attended in last month, Access to electronic mentoring opportunities, Perception paid fairly for job duties,* and *Work hours per week.*

In multi-level, multivariate regression analyses, clients who had a birth companion in labor had significantly higher RMC-D2 scores compared to clients who did not have a companion in labor (Coef 0.37, 95% CI 0.06–0.68). Clients who reported attending religious services at least weekly had significantly lower RMC-D2 scores compared to clients who reported less than weekly attendance (Coef -0.31, 95% CI -0.06-[-0.02]). Client-level variables found not to have a significant adjusted relationship with *RMC-D2 score* included *Age, Highest education attended, Wealth quintile, Total live births,* and *Companion at time of delivery.* (Table 5).

Clients of providers who perceived they were paid fairly for their job duties had significantly higher RMC-D2 scores compared to clients of providers who perceived they are not paid fairly (Coef 0.37, 95% CI 0.06–0.68). Clients of providers who reported working more hours per week had significantly higher RMC-D2 scores compared to clients of providers who work fewer hours (Coef 0.01, 95% CI 0.00–0.02). Clients of providers aged 30 to 39 and 40 to 49 years had significantly

Table 4 Characteristics of Providers included in the Respectful Maternity Care Study Sample—Kigoma Region, Tanzania, April–July 2016 (*n* = 249)

	Providers, n (%)	95% CI
Age in years		
20 to 29	102 (41.0)	34.8–47.1
30 to 39	37 (14.9)	10.4–19.3
40 to 49	56 (22.5)	17.3–27.7
50 or older	54 (21.7)	16.5–26.8
Sex		
Female	161 (64.7)	58.7–70.6
Male	88 (35.3)	29.4–41.3
Highest education completed		
Primary	12 (4.8)	2.1–7.5
Secondary	71 (28.5)	22.9–34.2
College/university	166 (66.7)	60.8–72.6
Cadre		
Clinician	34 (13.7)	9.4–17.9
Nurse/midwife	152 (61.0)	54.9–67.1
Other staff	63 (25.3)	19.9–30.7
Years in cadre		
Mean (SD)	10.3 (9.4)	9.2–11.5
Years at the facility		
Mean (SD)	7.5 (9.6)	6.3–8.7
Facility type		
Hospital	59 (23.7)	18.4–29.0
Health center	135 (54.2)	48.0–60.4
Dispensary	55 (22.1)	16.9–27.3
Work hours per week		
Mean (SD)	54.8 (14.6)	53.0–56.6
Number of deliveries attended in last month		
1 to 10	159 (63.9)	57.7–69.6
11 to 20	56 (22.5)	17.7–28.1
21 to 30	10 (4.0)	2.2–7.3
More than 30	11 (4.4)	2.5–7.8
Don't know	13 (5.2)	3.0–8.8
Delivery ever-training summative index, possible range 0 to 25		
Mean (SD)	17.7 (5.02)	17.1–18.3
Delivery pre-service summative index, possible range 0 to 25		
Mean (SD)	15.6 (7.1)	14.7–16.4
Delivery in-service summative index, possible range 0 to 25		
Mean (SD)	8.4 (7.0)	7.6–9.3
Recent delivery practice summative index (in last 3 months), possible range 0 to 25		
Mean (SD)	14.9 (4.76)	14.3–15.5

Table 4 Characteristics of Providers included in the Respectful Maternity Care Study Sample—Kigoma Region, Tanzania, April–July 2016 (*n* = 249) *(Continued)*

	Providers, n (%)	95% CI
Perception in-service training has helped job performance		
Yes	221 (88.8)	84.2–92.1
No	28 (11.2)	7.9–15.8
Recent complications summative index (in last 1 month)		
0 of 4 types of complications dealt with - postpartum hemorrhage, eclampsia, obstructed labor, puerperal sepsis (reference)	84 (33.7)	28.1–39.9
1 of 4	70 (28.1)	22.8–34.1
2 of 4	41 (16.5)	12.3–21.6
3 of 4	34 (13.7)	9.9–18.5
4 of 4	20 (8.0)	5.2–12.2
Access to electronic mentoring opportunities		
No access to any of 3 types of electronic mentoring – emergency call system, e-learning, teleconference	120 (48.2)	42.0–54.4
Access to 1 type	62 (24.9)	19.9–30.7
Access to 2 types	38 (15.3)	11.3–20.3
Access to 3 types	29 (11.7)	8.2–16.3
Job satisfaction		
Very satisfied	31 (12.5)	8.9–17.2
A little satisfied	80 (32.1)	26.6–38.2
Neither satisfied nor dissatisfied	31 (12.5)	8.9–17.2
A little dissatisfied	70 (28.1)	22.8–34.1
Very dissatisfied	37 (14.9)	10.9–19.9
Perception paid fairly for job duties		
Yes	46 (18.5)	14.1–23.8
Perception of adequacy of training for job duties		
Yes	169 (67.9)	61.8–73.4
No	80 (32.1)	26.6–38.2
Has an on-site supervisor		
Yes	172 (69.1)	63.0–74.5
No	77 (30.9)	24.5–37.0
Clinical knowledge test score, % correct		
Mean (SD)	55.1 (13.4)	53.4–56.8

NOTE: *CI* Confidence Intervals, *SD* Standard Deviation

lower RMC-D2 scores compared to clients of providers aged 20 to 29 years (Coef -0.34, 95% CI -0.63-[-0.05]; Coef -0.58, 95% CI -0.86-[-0.29]). Provider variables not found to have a significant adjusted association with *RMC-D2 score* included *Number of deliveries attended in last month* and *Access to electronic mentoring opportunities*. Net of all independent variables included in the final RMC-D2 model, nearly one-quarter of the

Table 5 Multilevel Mixed-Effects Generalized Linear Regression Analysis for Receipt of Respectful Care—Kigoma Region, Tanzania, April–July 2016 (Clients n = 935, Providers n = 249)

Fixed Effects - Client Level Variables	Respectful Maternity Care Dimension 1: Friendliness, Comfort, and Attention		Respectful Maternity Care Dimension 2: Information and Consent		Respectful Maternity Care Dimension 3: Non-abuse and Kindness	
	Adjusted Coefficient (95% CI)	P-value	Adjusted Coefficient (95% CI)	P-value	Adjusted Coefficient (95% CI)	P-value
Client age in years						
15 to 19 (reference)						
20 to 29	0.29 (−0.14–0.71)	0.185	−0.20 (−0.45–0.06)	0.131	0.01 (−0.27–0.29)	0.927
30 to 39	0.63 (0.14–1.13)	0.012	−0.17 (−0.52–0.19)	0.361	−0.02 (−0.30–0.27)	0.910
40 to 49	0.79 (0.18–1.39)	0.011	−0.22 (−0.90–0.45)	0.516	−0.20 (−0.67–0.27)	0.393
Don't know	0.51 (−0.09–1.10)	0.094	0.29 (−0.12–0.70)	0.165	−0.85 (−1.87–0.17)	0.103
Highest education attended						
No education (reference)						
Primary	NA		−0.19 (−0.43–0.05)	0.128	NA	
Secondary	NA		0.20 (−0.27–0.68)	0.402	NA	
College or University	NA		−0.24 (−0.78–0.30)	0.385	NA	
Total live births						
0 to 2 (reference)						
3 or more	−0.14 (−0.45–0.17)	0.363	−0.13 (−0.39–0.14)	0.350	NA	
Socioeconomic status						
Low wealth (reference)						
Low middle wealth	NA		−0.12 (−0.47–0.22)	0.486	NA	
Middle wealth	NA		−0.02 (−0.31–0.26)	0.872	NA	
High middle wealth	NA		−0.24 (−0.51–0.04)	0.089	NA	
High wealth	NA		−0.12 (−0.49–0.26)	0.540	NA	
Frequency of attendance at religious services						
Attends less often than weekly (reference)						
Attends at least weekly	NA		−0.31 (−0.60–[−0.02])	0.035	NA	
Marital status						
Not in a union (reference)						
In a union	NA		NA		0.27 (−0.10–0.64)	0.159
Companionship in labor						
No (reference)						
Yes	NA		0.37 (0.06–0.68)	0.020	0.12 (−0.08–0.31)	0.253

Table 5 Multilevel Mixed-Effects Generalized Linear Regression Analysis for Receipt of Respectful Care—Kigoma Region, Tanzania, April–July 2016 (Clients n = 935, Providers n = 249) (Continued)

Fixed Effects - Client Level Variables	Respectful Maternity Care Dimension 1: Friendliness, Comfort, and Attention		Respectful Maternity Care Dimension 2: Information and Consent		Respectful Maternity Care Dimension 3: Non-abuse and Kindness	
	Adjusted Coefficient (95% CI)	P-value	Adjusted Coefficient (95% CI)	P-value	Adjusted Coefficient (95% CI)	P-value
Companionship at time of delivery						
No (reference)						
Yes	NA		0.10 (−0.32–0.52)	0.635	NA	
Self-reported delivery complications						
No (reference)						
Yes	−0.41 (−0.72–[−0.10])	0.010	NA		−0.29 (−0.60–0.02)	0.071
Fixed effects - Provider-level variables						
Provider age in years						
20–29 (reference)						
30–39	NA		−0.34 (−0.63–[−0.05])	0.023	0.14 (−0.06–0.34)	0.178
40–49	NA		−0.58 (−0.86–[−0.29])	0.000	0.03 (−0.20–0.27)	0.777
50+	NA		−0.09 (−0.41–0.23)	0.585	0.34 (0.09–0.58)	0.007
Cadre						
Clinician (reference)						
Nurse/midwife	−0.46 (−0.89–[−0.03])	0.038	NA		−0.02 (−0.27–0.24)	0.881
Other staff	0.33 (−0.27–0.92)	0.287	NA		−0.10 (−0.45–0.25)	0.560
Training and practice						
Delivery ever-training summative index, possible range 0 to 25	0.03 (−0.04–0.09)	0.402	NA		0.01 (−0.01–0.03)	0.356
Delivery pre-service summative index, possible range 0 to 25	0.01 (−0.04–0.06)	0.730	NA		NA	
Delivery in-service summative index, possible range 0 to 25	NA		NA		0.00 (−0.01–0.02)	0.550
Recent delivery practice summative index (in last 3 months), possible range 0 to 25	−0.02 (−0.07–0.02)	0.333	NA		NA	
Number of deliveries attended in last month						
1 to 10						
11 to 20	−0.35 (−0.67–[−0.02])	0.035	−0.30 (−0.61–0.01)	0.059	−0.02 (−0.22–0.19)	0.872
21 to 30	0.03 (−0.82–0.87)	0.947	−0.14 (−0.69–0.40)	0.599	−0.01 (−0.25–0.24)	0.953
More than 30	0.00 (−0.88–0.89)	0.994	0.40 (−0.30–1.11)	0.261	−0.43 (−0.89–0.03)	0.066
Don't know	0.37 (−0.53–1.27)	0.420	−0.07 (−0.61–0.46)	0.792	−0.01 (−0.33–0.32)	0.971

Table 5 Multilevel Mixed-Effects Generalized Linear Regression Analysis for Receipt of Respectful Care—Kigoma Region, Tanzania, April–July 2016 (Clients n = 935, Providers n = 249) (Continued)

Fixed Effects - Client Level Variables	Respectful Maternity Care Dimension 1: Friendliness, Comfort, and Attention		Respectful Maternity Care Dimension 2: Information and Consent		Respectful Maternity Care Dimension 3: Non-abuse and Kindness	
	Adjusted Coefficient (95% CI)	P-value	Adjusted Coefficient (95% CI)	P-value	Adjusted Coefficient (95% CI)	P-value
Types of complications dealt with in last 1 month summative index						
0 of 4 types of complications dealt with - postpartum hemorrhage, eclampsia, obstructed labor, puerperal sepsis (reference)						
1 of 4	0.06 (−0.24–0.37)	0.692	NA		NA	
2 of 4	−0.57 (−1.28–0.15)	0.122	NA		NA	
3 of 4	−0.09 (−0.73–0.56)	0.794	NA		NA	
4 of 4	−0.67 (−1.55–0.22)	0.139	NA		NA	
Access to electronic mentoring opportunities						
Access to 0 of 3 types of electronic mentoring - emergency call system, e-learning, teleconference (reference)						
Access to 1 type	−0.08 (−0.64–0.48)	0.775	0.02 (−0.37–0.40)	0.938	0.10 (−0.10–0.29)	0.334
Access to 2 types	−0.17 (−0.85–0.51)	0.621	−0.05 (−0.48–0.38)	0.827	0.36 (0.07–0.65)	0.014
Access to 3 types	−0.74 (−1.49–0.01)	0.054	0.14 (−0.43–0.71)	0.631	0.25 (−0.08–0.59)	0.134
Work environment						
Perception paid fairly for job duties	0.46 (0.04–0.88)	0.032	0.37 (0.06–0.68)	0.019	NA	
Perception in-service training has helped job performance	−0.31 (−0.74–0.12)	0.156	NA		NA	
Work hours per week	NA		0.01 (0.00–0.02)	0.022	NA	
Random effects						
Provider-level variance (SE)	0.86 (0.29)		0.57 (0.11)		0.04 (0.04)	
Provider-level variance partition coefficient	0.18		0.24		0.03	
Level 1 units	935		935		935	
Level 2 units	249		249		249	
Log likelihood	−2032.0704		−1685.2573		−1492.6216	

NOTE: *CI* Confidence Intervals, *NA* Not Applicable, *SE* Standard Error total variance (ICC = 0.24) is explained by the provider level. (Table 5).

Receipt of respectful maternity care dimension 3 (RMC-D3): *Non-abuse and Kindness*

Results of bivariate analyses for RMC-D3 – *Non-abuse and Kindness*, are displayed in Appendix. Based on bivariate analyses for RMC-D3, the following variables were included in the multivariable model: *Client age, Marital status, Companion in labor, Self-reported delivery complications; Provider age, Cadre, Delivery ever-training summative index score, Delivery in-service summative index score, Number of deliveries attended in the last month*, and *Access to electronic mentoring opportunities*.

In multi-level, multivariate regression analyses, none of the client variables were found to have a significant adjusted association with *RMC-D3 score*. Clients of providers who were aged 50 years or more had significantly higher RMC-D3 scores compared to clients of providers in the 20 to 29 year age group (Coef 0.34, 95% CI 0.09–0.58). Clients of providers who reported access to two types of electronic mentoring had significantly higher RMC-D3 scores compared to clients of providers with no access to electronic mentoring opportunities (Coef 0.37, 95% CI 0.07–0.65). The provider variables of *Age, Cadre, Delivery ever-training summative index score, Delivery in-service summative index score*, and *Number of deliveries attended in the last month* were not found to have a significant adjusted association with *RMC-D3 score*. Net of all independent variables included in the final RMC-D3 model, only 3% of the total variance (ICC = 0.03) is explained by the provider level. (Table 5).

Discussion

As maternal mortality and unskilled birth attendance continue to be high in sub-Saharan Africa, it is essential that the factors that influence health-seeking behavior and their determinants are better understood. In our study, we sought to identify the client and provider factors that predict receipt of three dimensions of RMC among delivery clients in Kigoma, Tanzania. The results provide insights into how dimensions of RMC, including receipt of friendly, comfort, and attention (RMC-D1), information and consent (RMC-D2), and non-abuse and kindness (RMC-D3) during labor and delivery are differentially influenced by characteristics of clients and their providers.

Client factors were significantly associated with the first two dimensions of RMC relating to friendliness,

comfort, and attention (RMC-D1), and information and consent (RMC-D2). In our analyses, client age mattered; clients in their 30's and 40's perceived receiving significantly higher levels of RMC related to friendliness, comfort, and attention compared to clients in their teens. It is possible that health care providers interact and treat teens differently simply because they are younger than the providers are themselves, or it is possible that the providers perceive teens as *too young* to become a mother. Multiple qualitative studies and reviews thereof have pointed to younger women, particularly adolescents, as potential targets of discrimination and potential recipients of less respectful care [10, 11, 14]. Our findings are consistent with the analysis presented by Abuya et al. of D&A during childbirth in Kenya, where younger patients were significantly more likely to receive non-confidential care than older patients [13]. Our findings are in contrast to those by Kruk et al., however, who did not find age associated with receipt D&A in Tanzania [33].

Whether or not the client reported to have had delivery complications also influenced the first dimension of RCM; clients who reported delivery complications had a lower RMC score related to friendliness, comfort, and attention compared to those without perceived complications. There are two potential explanations for this finding: 1) the stress that providers experience during complications and emergencies may make them more likely to exhibit disrespectful behavior; or 2) the experience of complications lowers the client's overall perception of the delivery experience.

Companionship in labor was found to be a positive factor for receipt of RMC related to information and consent; clients with a companion in labor received a higher level of RMC-D2. This finding is not surprising as providers may feel more accountable for providing better information and counseling when someone in addition to the client is present; a companion may also help increase the client's understanding of information. Interestingly, more frequent attendance at religious services was a significant determinant of receipt of a lower level of RMC related to information and consent. It is possible that more religious women may interpret or receive these components differently than their less religious counterparts; alternatively, providers may display a particular bias against giving information to these women. Collectively, these findings provide a better understanding of how client characteristics—or provider perceptions and biases related to those characteristics—may influence provision of respectful care.

Provider factors were also significantly associated with the first two dimensions of RMC, and were the only factors of significance for the third non-abuse and kindness dimension of RMC. Nurses/midwives as compared to clinicians, and providers who attended 11 to 20 deliveries in the last month as compared to providers who attended fewer deliveries, were found to provide lower levels of RMC related to friendliness, comfort, and attention. These findings suggest that the high workload of labor and delivery care—commonly found among nurses/midwives—may lead to less positive interpersonal interactions with clients. Nurse/midwifes may experience prolonged contact with labor and delivery clients, as opposed to the often intermittent contact that clinicians experience, which may reduce a provider's ability to give friendly, comforting, and attentive care day after day. Evidence bolstering this hypothesis comes from psychology research on the depleting effect of decision fatigue on subsequent self-control and active initiative [57]: providers may know that treating clients with respect is important and necessary, but may grow increasingly less able to provide respectful care with the demands of ongoing urgent clinical decision making without respite.

While job satisfaction was not found to be correlated with RMC, providers who perceived they were paid fairly for their work duties as compared to those who did not feel this way provided significantly better RMC related to friendliness, comfort, and attention, and RMC related to information and consent. These findings suggest that the perception of pay equity (versus pay *inequity*) positively influences interpersonal interactions and care provision, and likely reflects an underlying attitude that providers feel appreciated and motivated to do their work. Numerous qualitative studies and reviews thereof have highlighted health worker descriptions of low salaries as a particular stressful aspect of negative work environments resulting in unprofessional behavior [10, 35, 45, 58]. In Tanzania specifically, inadequate compensation for long hours, ineligibility for overtime pay, and lost opportunities to pursue other income-generating activities have been described as contributing to health care providers great dissatisfaction with their working environments [17].

Providers who reported working more as compared with fewer hours per week provided significantly higher levels of RMC related to information and consent. This finding may seem contradictory to the previously discussed finding that nurses/midwives and providers who conduct a higher number of deliveries provide less friendly, comforting, and attentive care. We contend, however, that friendliness/comfort/

attention is a dissimilar construct from information sharing and consent, and therefore, it is not surprising to see disparate patterns of association. It is possible that providers who work more hours take more time to give information during labor and delivery care due to having more work hours, or they may have more opportunity from which to gain expertise communicating with and counseling clients through more frequent experience. Providers in their 30's and 40's provided lower levels of RMC related to information and consent, compared to providers in their 20's. This finding suggests a possible shift in pre-service education whereby client counseling and consent have been emphasized in the education of more recent graduates or perhaps that younger providers simply have more motivation for sharing their knowledge with clients.

With respect to RMC related to non-abuse and kindness, the findings suggest that provider characteristics of age and access to electronic mentoring are protective. Providers aged 50 years and older provided higher levels of RMC care related to non-abuse and kindness than providers in their twenties. A potential explanation for this finding is that older providers, who are more experienced in labor and delivery, may be more patient and therefore less likely to respond negatively. Providers who reported access to two types of electronic mentoring, such as an emergency call line, teleconference, or e-learning, gave significantly better RMC related to non-abuse and kindness compared to clients of providers with no access to electronic mentoring opportunities. It is possible that providers with greater access are more likely to have received RMC training or that access to these types of mentorship opportunities improves provider's underlying attitude toward work and the care of clients.

Strengths and limitations

One strength of our study is the novel way in which we conceptualized and measured RMC. To-date, much of the research and literature around RMC has focused on D&A; we chose to focus on receipt of respectful care as our outcome of interest using the WRA RMC Charter as a conceptual framework. Using PCA to develop our outcomes allowed the identification of three dimensions of RMC in order to identify differences in determinants of RMC by broad dimension. In prior work, disrespect/respect has been operationalized in ways that limit interpretation and implications of findings. First, disrespect has been operationalized as a dichotomous variable where clients having experienced any one or more of a range of disrespectful practices are coded as a "1"

[33]. Results from such an analysis are difficult to interpret because there is no differentiation in degree of disrespect; clients reporting not being greeted respectfully are considered to be equivalent in their experience of RMC with those who reported physical and emotional abuse by providers. Second, respect/disrespect has also been operationalized by running separate regression models for each item of respect/disrespect [13]. This approach results in generation of a large amount of data which may or may not be similar across models, making interpretation of findings and development of recommendations challenging.

A second strength of this study is the use of matched client and provider data. This was a particularly essential strategy given our findings that a larger number provider factors significantly influenced RMC compared to client factors. Identifying provider determinants of RMC allows for the development of recommendations aimed at specific provider characteristics (e.g., new graduates, cadre) or perceptions (e.g., age bias, religious bias) that would not be known otherwise. Another strength of this work is that we operationalized select independent variables in new ways. For example, provider-level *Delivery ever-training index*, *Delivery pre-service index*, and *Recent delivery practice index* variables were operationalized by summing multiple delivery care elements; these variables allowed the analyses to differentiate the importance of both dose and timing of training and practice to provision of RMC.

It is critical to understand the limitations of our work. First, the study was cross-sectional with non-random sampling, eliminating our ability to make causal inferences and generalize findings. Previously collected household-level Reproductive Health Survey (RHS) data in Kigoma from 2016 and a planned 2018 RHS in Kigoma provides a timely opportunity to analyze representative RMC data. Second, our questionnaire did not have items that fit into Article V and Article VII of the WRA RMC Charter, limiting our ability to account for certain known risk factors for receipt of non-respectful care. History of self-reported depression and history of past abuse or rape have both been associated with higher rates of abuse in health care settings in both high-resource [59, 60] and low-resource contexts [33]. Third, while using PCA as a means to create outcome variables has its strengths, it also has its limitations. Interpretation of coefficients is constrained; while we can easily interpret the direction and significance level of relationships, it is more problematic to understand to what extent a change in an independent variable has a *meaningful* change in receipt of RMC. Additionally,

PCA rarely matches conceptual frameworks perfectly, especially for complex constructs such as RMC. Though strong patterns emerged in our PCA, not every item clustered with the most logical component (e.g., *Inform about findings of exam/procedures* loaded highest on the first component, not the second component, as expected).

The site of client interviews at facilities poses an additional important limitation, likely generating an underestimation of true prevalence of D&A and an overestimation of receipt of RMC. Two independent studies of D&A treatment during facility delivery in Tanzania have demonstrated markedly lower reports of D&A from interviewed clients when interviewed at the site of the facility, with significant increases in reporting upon follow up in the community [31, 33]. Another limitation of our data is that some women, particularly those who delivered in hospitals and health centers, may have had more than one care provider. We attempted to control for this issue by matching women with the provider who they reported spending the greatest amount of time with them. Due to budget and time constraints, our questionnaire items used in the development of RMC measures were not developed on the basis of formative work in Kigoma Region. Rather, these items were a compilation of commonly used RMC elements in prior research. Qualitative work ahead of this study may have uncovered local conceptualizations of RMC that would have been important to include in our measure. Finally, the provider-level variables only accounted for 3% of the variance of RMC-D3, and client variables did not have a significant adjusted relationship with this outcome; this suggests that the RMC-D3 model had a poor overall fit. It is important for future work to attempt to explore client and provider characteristics not considered in this study and potential reframing of the non-abuse and kindness dimension.

Programmatic, policy, and research implications

These findings highlight potential areas of focus for programmatic and policy work, as well as future directions to move the RMC research agenda forward. Given our results that Nurses/midwives and providers who conduct a higher number of deliveries provide lower levels of RMC, improving the work environment for labor and delivery providers may improve delivery care. Strategies that aim to reduce workplace stress—including reduction of moral distress and decision fatigue—and improve providers' perceptions of workplace support, self-efficacy in providing quality care, and underlying attitude toward work, may contribute to improved interpersonal interactions between clients and providers. Such approaches might include offering high frequency rotational schedules to give labor and delivery providers short-term respite away from providing maternity care. Strategies that increase access to mentoring and peer-to-peer learning opportunities (with fair access across cadres) may improve workplace support, self-efficacy, and enhance feelings of being a respected and valued member of the team. Pre-service and in-service training on RMC, as well as close mentorship following training, is essential to determine the influence of training on knowledge transfer and behavior change. Additionally, ensuring providers receive equitable pay, on-time, every time may increase provider's sense of worth and underlying attitude towards work.

To move the RMC scientific agenda forward, additional research using matched patient and provider data may improve understanding of the relative importance of patient and provider determinants of RMC. In addition, studies embedded in conceptual models of RMC are needed that aim to standardize and validate measures of RMC. Measures that can be validated across cultural and geographic settings would be particularly valuable so that RMC data can be compared and synthesized across studies. Future analyses would be strengthened through the addition of interaction terms to illuminate the complexities of patient and provider relationships and how these influence respectful care. Given our hypothesis that moral distress and decision fatigue contribute to lack of RMC, future analyses would greatly benefit from inclusion of measures for these constructs. Furthermore, future research may benefit from over-sampling of clinician providers in order to increase the power to detect differences between clinicians and other cadres, and potential differences by gender that were not detected here. Finally, women in low-resource settings may have relatively low expectations of maternity care compared to women in middle- or high-resource settings. Measuring expectations of care and the influence of cultural and gender norms in future research would help advance our understanding of women's experience of RMC and how expectations and context influence measurement and comparison of RMC across settings.

Conclusion

Despite disrespectful maternity care being increasingly recognized as a key deterrent to women seeking facility-based deliveries, there is less consensus about the comparative importance of patient and provider determinants for RMC. Our findings demonstrate that patient and provider factors differentially influence three dimensions of RMC. Future research is needed that aims to standardize RMC measurement through the lens of a conceptual model of RMC and rooted in a human rights perspective. Strategies that promote more equitable pay, offer rotational schedules with short-term respite away from providing maternity care, and increased access to mentoring and peer-to-peer learning platforms may improve RMC and uptake of facility delivery in low-resource settings. An enhanced understanding of the relationships between patient and provider characteristics may improve the provision of quality labor and delivery services and should be considered in the design of maternity care programs, policies, and future research.

Endnotes

[1]Women were asked if they had any complications during labor and delivery. The most common self-reported complications included postpartum hemorrhage, prolonged labor, retained placenta, malpresentation, and lacerations.

[2]The variable for *SES* was developed using principal components analysis (PCA); household assets and characteristics were weighted based on their contribution to the first principal component and summed to create an index score representing five levels of relative household wealth [61].

[3]Providers were asked, "Have you received pre-service training in [...]?"; "Have you received in-service training in [...]?"; and "Have you conducted [...] in the last 3 months?" for the following 25 items: 1) Focused antenatal care; 2) Routine labor and delivery care; 3) Use the partograph; 4) Active management of the third stage of labor; 5) Manual removal of the placenta; 6) Beginning intravenous fluids; 7) Checking for anemia; 8) Administering intramuscular or intravenous magnesium sulfate for the treatment of server pre-eclampsia or eclampsia; 9) Administering intravenous antibiotics; 10) Administering misoprostol or other uterotonic; 11) Bimanual uterine compression (external); 12) Bimanual uterine compression (internal); 13) Suturing an episiotomy; 14) Suturing vaginal lacerations; 15) Suturing cervical lacerations; 16) Vacuum extractor; 17) Forceps; 18) C-section; 19) A blood transfusion; 20) Adult resuscitation; 21) Resuscitating a newborn with bag and mask; 22) Basic Emergency Obstetric and Neonatal Care (BEmONC); 23) Advanced Emergency Obstetric and Neonatal Care; 24) Administering antiretrovirals (ART) for Prevention of Mother-to-Child Transmission (PMTCT); and 25) Rapid diagnostic testing for HIV. Responses were summed to create four indices.

Appendix

Table 6 Bivariate Associations between Client and Provider Characteristics and Receipt of Respectful Maternity Care—Kigoma Region, Tanzania, April–July 2016 (Clients n = 935, Providers n = 249)

	Respectful Maternity Care Dimension 1 – Friendliness, Comfort, and Attention		Respectful Maternity Care Dimension 2 – Information and Consent		Respectful Maternity Care Dimension 3 – Non-abuse and Kindness	
	Unadjusted Coefficient (95% CI)	P-value	Unadjusted Coefficient (95% CI)	P-value	Unadjusted Coefficient (95% CI)	P-value
Client level variables						
Age in years						
15 to 19 (reference)						
20 to 29	0.28 (−0.09–0.66)	0.142	−0.24 (−0.50–0.02)	0.074	0.05 (0.17–0.27)	0.652
30 to 39	0.55 (0.13–0.97)	0.010	−0.27 (−0.56–0.02)	0.072	0.05 (−0.19–0.29)	0.688
40 to 49	0.62 (−0.13–1.37)	0.105	−0.36 (−0.88–0.17)	0.181	−0.11 (−0.54–0.32)	0.616
Don't know	0.22 (−0.99–0.42)	0.727	0.33 (−0.51–1.17)	0.446	−0.83 (−1.52–0.14)	0.019
Highest education attended						
No education (reference)						
Primary	−0.06 (−0.41–0.30)	0.759	−0.31 (−0.56–[−0.07])	0.012	0.00 (−0.20–0.20)	0.997
Secondary	−0.11 (−0.64–0.42)	0.691	0.05 (−0.31–0.42)	0.769	−0.12 (−0.42–0.18)	0.426
College or University	0.44 (−0.66–1.53)	0.434	−0.34 (−1.09–0.40)	0.366	−0.35 (−0.97–0.27)	0.271
Literacy						
Cannot read or write, or can read or write, but not both (reference)						
Can read and write	0.23 (−0.07–0.54)	0.134	−0.15 (−0.37–0.06)	0.158	0.09 (−0.09–0.26)	0.333
Socioeconomic status						
Low wealth (reference)						
Low middle wealth	−0.37 (−0.82–0.07)	0.101	−0.17 (−0.48–0.14)	0.283	−0.06 (−0.31–0.20)	0.653
Middle wealth	−0.28 (−0.72–0.16)	0.212	−0.16 (−0.46–0.15)	0.317	−0.09 (−0.34–0.16)	0.492
High middle wealth	−0.25 (−0.69–0.18)	0.258	−0.34 (−0.64–[−0.04])	0.029	0.09 (−0.16–0.33)	0.485
High wealth	−0.01 (−0.48–0.45)	0.954	−0.17 (−0.49–0.16)	0.312	0.03 (−0.22–0.28)	0.814
Total live births						
0 to 2 (reference)						
3 or more	0.24 (−0.03–0.52)	0.082	−0.16 (−0.35–0.03)	0.097	0.06 (−0.10–0.21)	0.484
Marital status						
Not in a union (reference)						
In a union	0.19 (−0.30–0.67)	0.448	−0.28 (−0.61–0.06)	0.106	0.24 (−0.03–0.52)	0.085

Table 6 Bivariate Associations between Client and Provider Characteristics and Receipt of Respectful Maternity Care—Kigoma Region, Tanzania, April–July 2016 (Clients n = 935, Providers n = 249) (Continued)

	Respectful Maternity Care Dimension 1 – Friendliness, Comfort, and Attention		Respectful Maternity Care Dimension 2 – Information and Consent		Respectful Maternity Care Dimension 3 – Non-abuse and Kindness	
	Unadjusted Coefficient (95% CI)	P-value	Unadjusted Coefficient (95% CI)	P-value	Unadjusted Coefficient (95% CI)	P-value
Frequency of attendance at religious services						
Attends less often than weekly (reference)						
Attends at least weekly	0.28 (−0.12–0.69)	0.165	−0.39 (−0.67–0.12)	0.005	−0.07 (−0.30–0.16)	0.572
Companion in labor						
No (reference)						
Yes	0.15 (−0.17–0.46)	0.360	0.45 (0.23–0.66)	0.000	0.15 (−0.01–0.32)	0.065
Companion at time of delivery						
No (reference)						
Yes	−0.10 (−0.56–0.36)	0.675	0.31 (−0.01–0.63)	0.058	−0.12 (−0.37–0.13)	0.346
Self-reported delivery complications						
No (reference)						
Yes	−0.53 (−0.95–[−0.12])	0.012	−0.11 (−0.41–0.18)	0.439	−0.29 (−0.53–[−0.05])	0.016
Provider-level variables						
Age in years						
20 to 29 (reference)						
30 to 39	−0.05 (−0.62–0.52)	0.868	−0.43 (−0.85–0.02)	0.041	0.17 (−0.07–0.41)	0.175
40 to 49	−0.10 (−0.61–0.40)	0.687	−0.62 (−0.99–[−0.26])	0.001	0.13 (−0.08–0.35)	0.233
50 or older	0.23 (−0.30–0.76)	0.393	−0.07 (−0.46–0.31)	0.700	0.40 (0.17–0.63)	0.001
Sex						
Male (reference)						
Female	−0.31 (−0.72–0.10)	0.142	−0.21 (−0.51–0.10)	0.183	−0.09 (−0.27–0.09)	0.335
Highest education completed						
Primary (reference)						
Secondary	−0.64 (−1.65–0.36)	0.211	0.03 (−0.71–0.77)	0.942	0.31 (−0.15–0.76)	0.185
College/university	−0.49 (−1.46–0.48)	0.326	0.29 (−0.42–1.00)	0.426	0.15 (−0.29–0.59)	0.490
Cadre						
Clinician (reference)						
Nurse/midwife	−0.52 (−1.11–0.08)	0.087	−0.15 (−0.60–0.29)	0.501	−0.24 (−0.51–0.04)	0.091
Other staff	0.36 (−0.31–1.02)	0.290	0.13 (−0.37–0.64)	0.600	−0.29 (−0.60–0.02)	0.064
Years in cadre	0.01 (−0.01–0.03)	0.360	−0.01 (−0.02–0.01)	0.245	0.01 (−0.00–0.02)	0.119

Table 6 Bivariate Associations between Client and Provider Characteristics and Receipt of Respectful Maternity Care—Kigoma Region, Tanzania, April–July 2016 (Clients n = 935, Providers n = 249) (Continued)

	Respectful Maternity Care Dimension 1 – Friendliness, Comfort, and Attention		Respectful Maternity Care Dimension 2 – Information and Consent		Respectful Maternity Care Dimension 3 – Non-abuse and Kindness	
	Unadjusted Coefficient (95% CI)	P-value	Unadjusted Coefficient (95% CI)	P-value	Unadjusted Coefficient (95% CI)	P-value
Years at the facility	0.01 (−0.01–0.03)	0.200	−0.00 (−0.02–0.01)	0.824	0.01 (−0.00–0.02)	0.105
Work hours per week	0.01 (−0.00–0.02)	0.140	0.02 (0.01–0.03)	0.000	−0.00 (−0.01–0.00)	0.114
Delivery ever-training summative index, possible range 0 to 25	−0.04 (−0.08–[−0.01])	0.025	−0.00 (−0.03–0.03)	0.998	0.01 (−0.00–0.03)	0.097
Delivery pre-service summative index, possible range 0 to 25	−0.03 (−0.06–0.00)	0.034	0.00 (−0.02–0.02)	0.650	0.00 (−0.01–0.01)	0.624
Delivery in-service summative index, possible range 0 to 25	−0.01 (−0.04–0.01)	0.352	−0.01 (−0.03–0.01)	0.302	0.01 (0.00–0.02)	0.046
Recent delivery practice summative index, (in last 3 months), possible range 0 to 25	−0.07 (−0.11–[−0.03])	0.000	0.00 (−0.03–0.03)	0.831	0.01 (−0.00–0.03)	0.124
Number of deliveries attended in last month						
1 to 10 (reference)						
11 to 20	−0.65 (−1.11–[−0.20])	0.005	−0.26 (−0.61–0.08)	0.129	0.03 (−0.17–0.23)	0.794
21 to 30	−0.34 (−1.26–0.57)	0.462	−0.06 (−0.75–0.63)	0.861	−0.05 (−0.45–0.35)	0.821
More than 30	−0.82 (−1.71–0.08)	0.074	0.60 (−0.07–1.27)	0.080	−0.37 (−0.76–0.03)	0.066
Don't know	−0.10 (−0.93–0.73)	0.814	−0.20 (−0.82–0.43)	0.535	0.06 (−0.31–0.42)	0.766
Recent complications summative index (in Last 1 Month)						
0 of 4 types of complications dealt with: postpartum hemorrhage, eclampsia, obstructed labor, puerperal sepsis (reference)						
1 of 4	−0.21 (−0.71–0.28)	0.402	−0.06 (−0.44–0.32)	0.750	0.02 (−0.21–0.25)	0.874
2 of 4	−0.89 (−1.44–[−0.35])	0.001	−0.32 (−0.74–0.10)	0.134	−0.17 (−0.41–0.08)	0.186
3 of 4	−0.68 (−1.28–[−0.09])	0.025	−0.18 (−0.64–0.28)	0.438	−0.02 (−0.29–0.25)	0.858
4 of 4	−1.06 (−1.75–[−0.36])	0.003	−0.39 (−0.92–0.15)	0.159	0.18 (−0.13–0.48)	0.260
Access to electronic mentoring opportunities						
Access to 0 of 3 types of electronic mentoring: emergency call system, e-learning, teleconference (reference)						
Access to 1 type	−0.10 (−0.57–0.36)	0.664	−0.00 (−0.35–0.35)	0.994	0.13 (−0.07–0.34)	0.198
Access to 2 types	−0.35 (−0.92–0.22)	0.227	−0.03 (−0.45–0.40)	0.903	0.37 (0.12–0.62)	0.004
Access to 3 types	−0.92 (−1.53–−0.30)	0.003	0.43 (−0.03–0.89)	0.068	0.22 (−0.05–0.49)	0.111

Table 6 Bivariate Associations between Client and Provider Characteristics and Receipt of Respectful Maternity Care—Kigoma Region, Tanzania, April–July 2016 (Clients n = 935, Providers n = 249) (Continued)

	Respectful Maternity Care Dimension 1 – Friendliness, Comfort, and Attention		Respectful Maternity Care Dimension 2 – Information and Consent		Respectful Maternity Care Dimension 3 – Non-abuse and Kindness	
	Unadjusted Coefficient (95% CI)	P-value	Unadjusted Coefficient (95% CI)	P-value	Unadjusted Coefficient (95% CI)	P-value
Perception in-service training has helped job performance						
No (reference)						
Yes	−0.69 (−1.32−[−0.06])	0.033	−0.34 (−0.81−0.13)	0.157	0.13 (−0.16−0.42)	0.384
Job satisfaction						
Very dissatisfied (reference)						
A little dissatisfied	−0.07 (−0.68−0.54)	0.820	−0.03 (−0.49−0.42)	0.895	−0.05 (−0.32−0.22)	0.707
Neither satisfied nor dissatisfied	−0.16 (−0.93−0.61)	0.682	−0.40 (−0.97−0.17)	0.165	0.02 (−0.33−0.37)	0.916
A little satisfied	−0.45 (−1.06−0.15)	0.142	−0.22 (−0.67−0.23)	0.334	0.06 (−0.21−0.32)	0.680
Very satisfied	−0.09 (−0.83−0.65)	0.814	0.10 (−0.45−0.65)	0.730	0.15 (−0.18−0.48)	0.379
Perception paid fairly for job duties						
No (reference)						
Yes	0.57 (0.07−1.07)	0.027	0.46 (0.08−0.83)	0.016	−0.06 (−0.29−0.16)	0.584
Perception of adequacy of training for job duties						
No (reference)						
Yes	−0.02 (−0.44−0.40)	0.925	−0.16 (−0.47−0.15)	0.310	0.02 (−0.16−0.21)	0.810
Has an on-site supervisor						
No (reference)						
Yes	0.07 (−0.35−0.49)	0.732	−0.17 (−0.48−0.14)	0.292	−0.05 (−0.24−0.14)	0.599
Clinical knowledge test score	−0.63 (−2.06−0.81)	0.392	−0.31 (−1.38−0.76)	0.568	0.41 (−0.23−1.05)	0.211

NOTE: CI Confidence Intervals

Abbreviations

BRN: Big results now; CDC: Centers for disease control and prevention; CI: Confidence intervals; Coef: Coefficient; D&A: Disrespect and abuse; ICC: Intraclass correlation; MOHCDGEC: Ministry of health, community development, gender, the elderly, and children; NBS: National bureau of statistics; PCA: Principal components analysis; RHS: Reproductive health survey; RMC: Respectful maternity care; RMC-D1: Respectful maternity care-dimension 1; RMC-D2: Respectful maternity care-dimension 2; RMC-D3: Respectful maternity care-dimension 3; SD: Standard deviation; SE: Standard error; USAID: United States agency for international development; WHO: World Health Organization; WRA: White ribbon alliance

Acknowledgements

We are grateful to the postpartum women and health providers who gave of their time to participate in the survey. The authors would also like to acknowledge the support of our in-country partner, AMCA Inter Consult, and CDC colleagues Erin Bernstein, Susanna Binzen, Fernando Carlosama, Jonetta Mpofu, Alicia Ruiz, Michelle Schmitz, and intern from Emory University Rollins School of Public Health, Hannah Nguyen.

Funding

This study was funded by Bloomberg Philanthropies and the Fondation H & B Agerup.

Authors' contributions

MD was responsible for the study design, undertook the fieldwork and data collection, analysis, and helped interpret findings and write the manuscript. ET was responsible for the literature search and helped interpret findings and write the manuscript. LK participated in data analysis and helped interpret findings and write the manuscript. AAM helped with data collection and interpret findings. FS helped with the study design, interpret findings, and write the manuscript. GM, SAD, PC, and NM helped interpret findings. All authors read and approved the final manuscript submitted for publication.
The findings and conclusions in this report are those of the authors and do not necessarily represent the official position of the US Centers for Disease Control and Prevention.

Competing interests

All authors declare that they have no competing interests.

Author details

[1]Centers for Disease Control and Prevention, Division of Reproductive Health, Atlanta, Georgia. [2]Bloomberg Philanthropies Tanzania, Kigoma, Tanzania. [3]AMCA Inter Consult, Dar es Salaam, Tanzania. [4]Thamini Uhai, Kigoma, Tanzania. [5]Kigoma Region Ministry of Health, Kigoma, Tanzania. [6]Ministry of Health Community Development Gender Elderly and Children, Dar es Salaam, Tanzania.

References

1. WHO, UNICEF, UNFPA, The World Bank and United Nations Population Division. Trends in maternal mortality: 1990 to 2015. Generva; 2015. Access at: http://apps.who.int/iris/bitstream/10665/194254/1/9789241565141_eng.pdf?ua=1.
2. Adegoke AA, van den Broek N. Skilled birth attendance—lessons learnt. BJOG. 2009;116(Suppl 1):33–40.
3. Harvey SA, Ayabacab P, Bucaguc M, Djibrinad S, Edsona WN, Gbangbadee S, et al. Skill birth attendant competence: an initial assessment in four countries, and implications for the safe motherhood movement. Int J Gynecol Obstet. 2004;87:203–10.
4. Koblinksy MACO, Heichelheim J. Organizing delivery care: what works for safe motherhood? Bull World Health Organ. 1999;77:399–404.
5. Ronsmans C, Graham WJ. Maternal mortality: who, when, where, and why. Lancet. 2006;368(9542):1189–200.
6. World Health Organization. Beyond the numbers: reviewing maternal deaths and complications to make pregnancy safer. Geneva: Department of Reproductive Health and Research, World Health Organization; 2004.
7. De Brouwere V, Tonglet R, Van Lerberghe W. Strategies for reducing maternal mortality in developing countries: what can we learn from the history of the industrialized west? Tropical Med Int Health. 1998;3:771–82.
8. Ministry of Health, Community Development, Gender, Elderly and Children (MoHCDGEC) [Tanzania Mainland], Ministry of Health (MoH) [Zanzibar], National Bureau of Statistics (NBS), Office of the Chief Government Statistician (OCGS), and ICF. Tanzania demographic and health survey and malaria indicator survey (TDHS-MIS) 2015–16. Dar es Salaam: MoHCDGEC, MoH, NBS, OCGS, and ICF; 2016.
9. Kujawski S, Mbaruku G, Freedman LP, Ramsey K, Moyo W, Kruk ME. Association between disrespect and abuse during childbirth and women's confidence in health facilities in Tanzania. Matern Child Health J. 2015;19(10):2243–50.
10. Bohren M, Vogel JP, Hunter EC, Lutsiv O, Makh SK, Souza JP, Aguiar C, Saraiva CF, Diniz AL, Tuncalp O, Javadi D, Oladapo OT, Khosla R, Hindin MJ, Gulmezoglu AM. The mistreatment of women during childbirth in health facilities globally: a mixed-methods systematic review. PLoS Med. 2015;12(6):e10001847.
11. Bowser D, Hill K. Exploring evidence for disrespect and abuse in facility based childbirth: a report of a landscape analysis. USAID-TRAction Project, Harvard School of Public Health and University Research Co., 2010. Access at: https://cdn2.sph.harvard.edu/wp-content/uploads/sites/32/2014/05/Exploring-Evidence-RMC_Bowser_rep_2010.pdf.
12. Asefa A, Bekele D. Status of respectful and non-abusive care during facility-based childbirth in a hospital and health centers in Addis Ababa. Ethiop Reprod Health. 2015;12:33.
13. Abuya T, Warren CE, Miller N, Njuki R, Ndwiga C, et al. Exploring the prevalence of disrespect and abuse during childbirth in Kenya. PLoS One. 2015;10(4):e0123606.
14. Warren CE, Njue R, Ndwiga C, Abuya T. Manifestations and drivers of mistreatment of women during childbirth in Kenya: implications for measurement and developing interventions. BMC Preg Childbirth. 2017;17:102.
15. Gabrysch S, Campbell OM. Still too far to walk: literature review of the determinants of delivery service use. BMC Preg Childbirth. 2009;9:34.
16. Gebrehiwot T, Coicolea I, Edin K, San SM. Making pragmatic choices: women's experiences of delivery care in northern Ethiopia. BMC Preg Childbirth. 2012;12:1113.
17. Mselle LET, Moland KM, Mvungi A, Evjen-Olsen B, Kohi TW. Why give birth in a health facility? Users' and providers' accounts of poor quality of birth care in Tanzania. BMC Health Ser Res. 2013;13:174.
18. Kruk ME, Paczkowsi M, Mbaruku G, de Pinho H, Galea S. Women's preferences for place of delivery in rural Tanzania: a population-based discrete choice experiment. Am J Public Health. 2009;99(9):1666–72.
19. Bohren MA, Ec H, Munthe-Kaas HM, Souza JP, Vogel JP, Gulmezoglu AM. Facilitators and barriers to facility-based delivery in low- and middle-income countries: a qualitative evidence synthesis. Reprod Health. 2014;11(1):71.
20. Shiferaw S, Spigt M, Godefrooij M, Melkamu Y, Tekie M. Why do women prefer home births in Ethiopia? BMC Preg Childbirth. 2013;13:5.
21. Rosen HE, Lynam PF, Carr C, Reis V, Ricca J, Bazant ES, Bartlett LA. Direct observation of respectful maternity care in five countries: a cross-sectional study of health facilities in east and southern Africa. BMC Preg Childbirth. 2015;15:306.
22. Okafor II, Ugwu EO, Obi SN. Disrespect and abuse during facility-based childbirth in a low-income country. Int J Gynaecol Obstet. 2015;128(2):110–3.
23. Misago C, Kendall C, Freitas P, Haneda K, Silveira D, Onuki D, Mori T, Sadamori T, Umenai T. From 'culture of dehumanization of childbirth' to 'childbirth as a transformative expereince': changes in five municipalities in north-East Brazil. Int J Gynaecol Obstet. 2001;75(Suppl 1):S67–72.
24. Lukasse M, Laanpere M, Karro H, Kristjansdottir H, Schrolla AM, Van Parys AS, Wangel AM, Schei B. Bidens study, group, pregnancy intendedness and the association with physical, sexual and emotional abuse – a European mulit-country cross-sectional study. BMC Pregnancy Childbirth. 2015;15:120.
25. Silal S, Penn-Kekana L, Barnighausen T, Schneider H, Harris B, Birth S, McIntyre D. Exploring inequalities in access to and use of maternal health services in South Africa. BMC Health Serv Res. 2012;12:120.

26. Ishola F, Owolabi O, Filippi V. Disrespect and abuse of women during childbirth in Nigeria: a systematic review. PLoS One. 12(3):e0174084.

27. D'Ambruoso L, Abbey M, Hussein J. Please understand when I cry out in pain: women's accounts of maternity services during labor and delivery in Ghana. BMC Public Health. 2005;5:140.

28. Avorti GS, Beke A, Abekah NG. Predictors of satisfaction with child birth services in public hospitals in Ghana. Int J Health Care Qual Assur. 2011;24(3):223–37.

29. Freedman LRK, Abuy T, Bellows B, Ndwiga C, Warren CE, Kujawski S, Moyo W, Kruk ME, Mbaruku G. Defining disrespect and abuse of women in childbirth: a research, policy and rights agenda. Bull World Health Organ. 2014;92(12):915–7.

30. FCI. Care-seeking during pregnancy, delivery and the postpartum period: a study in Homa Bay and Migori districts, Kenya; FCI 2005. New York: The Skill Care Initiative Technical Brief: Compassionate Maternity Care: Provider Communication and Counselling Skills; 2005.

31. Sando D, Ratcliffe H, McDonald K, Spiegelman D, Lyatuu G, Mwanyika-Sando M, Emil F, Wegner MN, Chalamilla G, Langer A. The prevalence of disrespect and abuse during facility-based childbirth in urban Tanzania. BMC Preg Childbirth. 2016;16:236.

32. White Ribbon Alliance. Respectful maternity care: the universal rights of childbearing women. Washington, D.C.: 2011. Access at: http://www.healthpolicyproject.com/pubs/46_FinalRespectfulCareCharter.pdf.

33. Kruk ME, Kujawski S, Mbaruku G, Ramsey K, Moyo W, Freedman LP. Disrespectful and abusive treatment during facility delivery in Tanzania: a facility and community survey. Health Policy Plan. 2014:1–8.

34. Janevic T, Sripad P, Bradly E, Dimitrievska V. "There's no kind of respect here" a qualitative study of racism and access to maternal health care among Romani women in the Balkans. Int J Equity Health. 2011;10:53.

35. Human Rights Watch. "Stop making excuses": accountability for maternal health care in South Africa. New York: Human Rights Watch; 2011.

36. Hulton LA, Matthews Z, Stones RW. Applying a framework for assessing the quality of maternal health services in urban India. Soc Sci Med. 2007;64:2083–95.

37. Jomeen J, Redshaw M. Black and minority ethnic women's experiences of contemporary maternity care in England. J Reprod Infant Psychol. 2011;29:e9.

38. Atuyambe L, Mirembe F, Johansson A, Kirumira EK, Faxelid E. Experiences of pregnant adolescents—voices from Wakiso district, Uganda. Afr Health Sci. 2005;5:304–9.

39. Jewkes R, Abrahams N, Mvo Z. Why do nurses abuse patients? Reflections from south African obstetric services. Soc Sci Med. 1998;47:1781–95.

40. McMahon SA, George AS, Chebet JJ, Mosha IH, Mpembeni RN, Winch PJ. Experiences of and responses to disrespectful maternity care and abuse during childbirth; a qualitative study with women and men in Morogoro region, Tanzania. BMC Preg Childbirth. 2014;14:268.

41. Ng'anjo PS, Fylkesnes K, Ruano AL, Moland KM. 'Born before arrival': user and provider perspectives on health facility childbirths in Kapiri Mposhi district, Zamiba. BMC Preg Childbirth. 2014;14:323.

42. Moyer CA, Adongo PB, Aborigo RA, Hodgson A, Engmann CM. 'They treat you like you are not a human being': maltreatment during labour and delivery in rural northern Ghana. Midwifery. 2014;30:262–8.

43. Ith P, Dawson A, Homer CSE. Women's perspective of maternity care in Cambodia. Women Birth. 2013;26:71–5.

44. Oyerinde K, Harding Y, Amara P, Garbrah-Aidoo N, Kanu R, Oulare M. A qualitative evaluation of the choice of traditional birth attendants for maternity care in 2008 Sierra Leone: implications for universal skilled attendance at delivery. Maternal Child Health. 2013;17:862–8.

45. Rahmani Z, Brekke M. Antenatal and obstetric care in Afghanistan—a qualitative study among health care receivers and health care providers. BMC Health Ser Res. 2013;13:166.

46. Turan JM, Miller S, Bukusi EA, Sande J, Cohen CR. HIV/AIDS and maternity care in Kenya: how fears of stigma and discrimination affect uptake and provision of labor and delivery services. AIDS Care. 2008;20:938–45.

47. Sando D, Kendall T, Lyatuu G, Ratcliffe H, McDonald K, Mwanyika-Sando M, et al. Disrespect and abuse during childbirth in Tanzania: are women living with HIV more vulnerable? JAIDS. 2014;67(Suppl 4):S228–34.

48. Uzochukwu BS, Onwujekwe OE, Akpala CO. Community satisfaction with the quality of maternal and child health services in southest Nigeria. East Afr Med J. 2004;81(6):293–9.

49. Rominski SD, Lori J, Nakua E, Dzomeku V, Moyer CA. When the baby remains there for a long time, it is going to die so you have to hit her small for the baby to come out: justification of disrespectful and abusive care during childbirth among midwifery students in Ghana. Health Policy Plan. 2017;32:215–24.

50. Onah HE, Ikeako LC, Iloabachie GC. Factors associated with the use of maternity services in Enugu, southeastern Nigeria. Soc Sci Med. 2006;63(7):1870–8.

51. Knight HE, Self A, Kennedy SH. Why are women dying when they reach hospital on time? A systematic review of the 'third delay'. PLoS One. 2013;8(5):e63846.

52. Sherefaw ED, Mengesha TZ, Wase SB. Development of a tool to measure women's perception of respectful maternity care in public health facilities. BMC Preg Childbirth. 2016;16:67.

53. Vedam S, Stoll K, Rubashkin N, Martin K, Miller-Vedam Z, Hayes-Klein H, Jolicoeur G, the CCinBC Steering Committee. The mothers on respect (MOR) index: measuring quality, safety, and human rights in childbirth. SSM Population Health. 2017;3:201–10.

54. National Bureau of Statistics & Office of Chief Government Statistician. The United Republic of Tanzania, Kigoma region: basic demographic and socio-economic profile: Population and Housing Census; 2012. p. 2016. http://www.nbs.go.tz/nbs/takwimu/census2012/2012_CENSUSVol3DATAsheet.pdf.

55. Centers for Disease Control and Prevention. Kigoma reproductive health survey: Kigoma region, Tanzania. Atlanta: Centers for Disease Control and Prevention; 2016. p. 2017.

56. MacCallum RC, Widaman KF, Zhang S, Hong S. Sample size in factor analysis. Psychol Methods. 1999;4(1):84–99.

57. Vohs KD, Baumeister RF, Schmeichel BJ, Twenge JM, Nelson NM, Tice DM. Making choices impairs subsequent self-control: a limited-resource account of decision making, self-regulation, and active initiative. J Pers Soc Pschycol. 2008;94(5):883–98.

58. Ganle J, Parker M, Fitzpatrick R, Otupiri E. A qualitative study of health system barriers to accessibility and utilization of maternal and newborn healthcare services in Ghana after user-fee abolition. BMC Pregnancy Childbirth. 2014;14:425.

59. Swahnberg K, Wijma B, Wingren G, Hilden M, Schei B. Women's perceived experiences of abuse in the health care system: their relationship to childhood abuse. BJOG. 2004;111:1429–36.

60. Swahnberg K, Schei B, Hilden M, Halmesmäki E, Sidenius K, Steingrimsdottir T, Wijma B. Patients' experiences of abuse in health care: a Nordic study on prevalence and associated factors in gynecological patients. Acta Obstet Gynecol Scand. 2007;86:349–56.

61. Filmer D, Pritchett LH. Estimating wealth effects without expenditure data—or tears: an application to educational enrollments in states of India. Demography. 2001;38(1):115–32.

14

Qualitative evaluation of the Saleema campaign to eliminate female genital mutilation and cutting in Sudan

Andrea C. Johnson[1], W. Douglas Evans[1*], Nicole Barrett[1], Howida Badri[2], Tamador Abdalla[2] and Cody Donahue[2]

Abstract

Background: Female genital mutilation and cutting (FGM/C, herein FGM) is a widespread and harmful practice. The Government developed a national campaign in Sudan, called Saleema, to change social norms discouraging FGM. Saleema translates to being "whole", healthy in body and mind, unharmed, intact, pristine, and untouched, in a God-given condition. An interim evaluation was conducted using focus groups among Sudanese adults. The primary aim was to explore perceptions of the Saleema poster exemplars and to assess if the desired themes were being communicated. Secondary aims were to understand more about participants' information sources, values, and suggestions for the campaign broadly.

Methods: The Saleema campaign evaluation included four focus groups from each of the 18 states in Sudan (72 total). Participants were presented with three poster stimuli from the Saleema campaign and asked about the content and their reactions. Themes were coded inductively by concepts that arose through content in the transcripts. Codes were also reviewed in conjunction with themes from the broader Saleema evaluation framework.

Results: Participants reported the most common source of information or admiration was from local leaders who are responsive to a community, media-based outlets, and discussions among community members. Participants held high value for education, community solidarity, and/or religious devotion. Participants had positive opinions of Saleema and responded positively to the branding elements in the posters and the campaign as a whole. The most common suggestion was continued awareness. Advocacy, training, and posters were suggested to highlight the harms of FGM through leaders or in community settings. Individuals suggested that these activities target older women and individuals in rural villages. There was also a burgeoning theme of targeting youth for support of the campaign.

Discussion: The results of this focus group analysis demonstrate support for future Saleema campaign efforts promoting awareness and community engagement. The campaign could capitalize on partnerships with young people and those who are respected in the community (e.g., religious leaders) or continue promoting common values aligning with the support of education and community solidarity. Continuing campaign efforts have promise to decrease the harms of FGM in Sudan.

Keywords: Female genital mutilation and cutting, Social marketing, Branding, Social norms, Focus groups, Qualitative research

* Correspondence: wdevans@gwu.edu
[1]Milken Institute School of Public Health, The George Washington University, 950 New Hampshire Avenue, NW, Washington, DC 20052, USA
Full list of author information is available at the end of the article

Plain English summary

Female genital mutilation and cutting (FGM/C, herein FGM) is a widespread and harmful practice. The Government developed a national campaign in Sudan, called Saleema, to change social norms discouraging FGM. Saleema translates to being "whole", healthy in body and mind, unharmed, intact, pristine, and untouched, in a God-given condition. The Saleema campaign evaluation included four focus groups within 18 states in Sudan (72 total). Participants were presented with three poster stimuli from the Saleema campaign and asked about the content and their reactions. The primary aim was to explore perceptions of the Saleema poster exemplars and to assess if the desired themes were being communicated. Secondary aims were to understand more about participants' information sources, values, and suggestions for the campaign broadly. Participants had positive opinions of Saleema and responded positively to the branding elements in the posters and the campaign as a whole. The most common suggestion was continued awareness. Advocacy, training, and posters were suggested to highlight the harms of FGM through leaders or in community settings. Individuals suggested that these activities target older women and individuals in rural villages. There was also a burgeoning theme of targeting youth for support of the campaign. The results of this focus group analysis demonstrate support for future Saleema campaign efforts promoting awareness and community engagement. The campaign could capitalize on partnerships with young people and those who are respected in the community (e.g., religious leaders) or continue promoting common values aligning with the support of education and community solidarity. Continuing campaign efforts have promise to decrease the harms of FGM in Sudan.

Background

The World Health Organization (WHO) and other global health and development organizations, including the Department for International Development (DFID) and US Agency for International Development (USAID), note female genital mutilation and cutting (FGM/C, herein FGM) is a widespread and harmful practice [1]. There are 4 main types of FGM, ranging in severity from Type I to IV [2]. FGM prevalence is highest in 27 countries in Africa and the Middle East [2, 3]. In Sudan, FGM is highly prevalent among all age groups of girls and women, with a national prevalence rate of 87% [4].

There is a steady, though modest, decline among the younger age cohorts (age 25 and below) and 52% of women believe the practice should stop [4]. The social practice of FGM has deep cultural and historical roots and has connotations with religious practice. When a social norm such as FGM is in place, families and individuals engage in the practice because they believe that it is

expected of them and is prevalent. Without these perceptions, the social norm would be weakened and practice would become less widespread and may eventually cease to exist. Changing social norms is thus a key step in behavior change [5].

Health communication and branding is a common intervention modality to change social norms. The study team developed a national campaign in Sudan, called Saleema, to change social norms discouraging FGM. Saleema translates to being "whole" (e.g., physically, emotionally). The campaign uses health branding theory (HBT) [6]. In part, HBT holds that creating positive mental associations with the alternative to unhealthy or anti-social behavior promotes behavior change [6–8]. There is evidence that creating positive brand identifications, or brand equity, mediates the effects of interventions on behavior change [9]. After formative testing, campaign messaging and activities targeted the entire population including all age groups using an expansive branding strategy. The campaign primarily focused on messages of community cohesion, strength, and change to reject FGM norms. The campaign held local events in each state and used a variety of channels, such as the radio, television, and billboards to show posters communicating the various messages.

Within the longitudinal, mixed methods campaign evaluation, the authors conducted a qualitative analysis using focus groups among Sudanese adults. The primary aim was to explore perceptions of the Saleema poster exemplars and to assess if the desired themes were being communicated as well as if there was any identification with the Saleema brand. Secondary aims were to understand more about participants' information sources, values, and suggestions for the campaign broadly.

Methods

Setting and materials

The Saleema campaign evaluation plan is a longitudinal mixed methods design. For the first round of the qualitative component, the evaluation included four nationally representative focus groups from each of the 18 states in Sudan using a pre-defined sampling framework. Following a cluster randomized sample plan, the study team randomly sampled two administrative units within each state to collect a sample [10]. The focus groups for this study were sampled using a Primary Sampling Unit (PSU) and randomly sampled from households in the same PSU. As a result, each state included focus groups in two geographically separate localities. Within each locality, there was a focus group composed of Sudanese adult males and females. Focus group moderators completed training and followed a focus group guide designed by the study team and UNICEF partners.

Participants were presented with three graphical poster stimuli from the Saleema campaign used in print advertisements and asked about the content and their reactions. The three posters represented common themes designed for the Saleema campaign and included bright red and green colors to represent those who supported the campaign. The Saleema campaign was branded with positive, gain-frame messaging, with themes focusing on changing norms and preventing FGM by way of choice and community cohesion. The first poster, "I am not afraid of change" represented changing norms within a community, showcasing a lack of fear in progress away from FGM. In particular, it seeks inclusivity of family members and community irrespective of age and sex. The second poster, "Because I am strong in my decision", represents a young woman taking a stand against FGM and stating her desire to remain uncircumcised. Lastly, the third poster "Saleema" includes a circumcised woman holding her infant daughter. The mother is happy because she is choosing to not circumcise her daughter, thereby changing the trend of FGM in her family for the next generation.

The focus group guide also inquired about information sources and values. Importantly, questions also asked about support of and suggestions for the campaign. Focus group questions were designed using a conceptual framework drawn from common health behavior theories. Specifically, this included Health Branding Theory (e.g., brand equity) and Social Marketing principles (e.g., product, price, place, promotion) [6, 11]. This structure sought to assist in organizing suggestions around message content, channels for delivery, target populations, and methods of promotion for greater receptivity.

Analysis and validation

All focus groups were recorded, transcribed, and translated by a team from Ahfad University from Arabic to English. This step was completed by a UNICEF staff member in Sudan. Transcript coding was conducted in an iterative fashion by a primary coder (ACJ) who was independent of the study design and data collection. Analysis was broadly organized by question in the focus group guide (e.g., information sources and values, campaign engagement, poster reactions, campaign suggestions). The focus group transcripts were coded first using axial coding where codes were provided "in vivo" labels, or words participants used [12]. As new transcripts were reviewed, the codes were iteratively grouped together into categories and themes. As a result, the themes were coded inductively using Grounded Theory by concepts that arose through content in the transcripts [13, 14]. Themes are presented descriptively using the codes with highest frequency. Finally, codes were

deductively aligned back to the themes based on the concepts applied from the broader Saleema evaluation framework (e.g., Social Marketing principles). Codes were not mutually exclusive and were assigned to multiple codes if the text represented multiple concepts. A final codebook was developed by the primary coder.

The codebook was validated using a second coder (NB) on 10% of the transcripts. The second coder was also not involved with the study design or data collection. The coding comparison showed high agreement between the two coders through an average kappa of 0.80, generated using NVIVO 11.4 software. Coding discrepancies were discussed and resolved as needed by the Principal Investigator (WDE). This type of qualitative analysis technique has been utilized in various disciplines [13, 14]. Themes and exemplars italicized quotes are presented in the results. The number of coding instances, not necessarily the number of individuals, is listed next to the code only to illustrate the estimated magnitude of each theme [15].

Results

The present qualitative evaluation included four focus groups within $N = 18$ states in Sudan. Each state included focus groups in two geographically separate localities. There were a total of 71 focus groups across all states, with roughly 5-10 individuals per group. This excluded one female group in Blue Nile for which recorded data was incomplete and consequently not included in the analysis. A tracking summary for each state is presented in Table 1. The coding results below represent high-level themes with specific codes outlined below. For each code, the results first are presented numerically in parentheses (source, reference). The source shows the magnitude of the number of sources, or number of states with the code. Then the reference is the frequency the code was endorsed across states. Quotes were not outlined by gender and locality to protect participant identities due to small sample sizes within each group.

Information sources and values

Participants discussed individuals and sources where they typically acquire information. The most common source of information or admiration was through leaders in the community ($n = 16$, $n = 53$), particularly religious ($n = 17$, $n = 83$) or local administrators ($n = 18$, $n = 123$). Other individuals were those in positions of authority, including family members ($n = 14$, $n = 65$) or clinicians ($n = 13$, $n = 29$). Individuals noted, "*The elderly people, the one who leads the prayers, the mayor of the neighborhood, not necessarily someone who came from outside, but anyone whose speech is accepted*" (Blue Nile) and "*Mayors and neighborhood wise men and wise women*

Table 1 Focus Groups by State

Sudan State	Male Focus Group	Female Focus Group	Focus Group Total
Blue Nile	2	1	3
Central Darfur	2	2	4
East Darfur	2	2	4
Gadarif	2	2	4
Gezira	2	2	4
Kassala	2	2	4
Khartoum	2	2	4
North Darfur	2	2	4
North Kordofan	2	2	4
Northern State	2	2	4
Red Sea	2	2	4
River Nile	2	2	4
Sennar	2	2	4
South Darfur	2	2	4
South Kordofan	2	2	4
West Darfur	2	2	4
West Kordofan	2	2	4
White Nile	2	2	4
TOTAL	36	35	71

because women listen to them, and imams all people listen to them." (West Darfur).

The most common source of information or admiration via entertainment was through music ($n = 11$, $n = 33$). Frequent information channels used were the internet (e.g., Facebook, WhatsApp, Google), ($n = 17$, $n = 88$), telephones ($n = 14$, $n = 95$), TV ($n = 18$, $n = 94$) and radio (n = 17, n = 88), word of mouth ($n = 13$, $n = 62$), and print materials ($n = 15$, $n = 40$). One individual in West Darfur mentioned, "*Back in the days, you chat with you friends and find information, but now information comes through the internet and everyone who find new information comes and tells the others.*" However, there was some discussion of the radio or community events being more common for rural and disadvantaged areas. "*Some people their phones are not smart, so they get their information from radio and TV*" (Sennar) and "*Coffee sessions, the events in the village where the information are disseminated*" (Gadarif).

Participants were most inclined to mention they admire individuals who are responsive to their community ($n = 12$, $n = 67$) and/or have power ($n = 10$, $n = 36$). Other similar attributes included respect ($n = 14$, $n = 43$) or admiring those with talent ($n = 9$, $n = 20$). One participant in West Darfur described these trends by saying, "*A famous personality in the community especially the simple community. He is a local administration man, and*

he has contributions and served the community a lot. He is also a man of religion and his word is listen to, and is local man who can solve many problems with his wisdom.*" Additionally, "*He [A regional leader] has been able to achieve security, peace and stability in the region. He has been able to assert his authority in the state despite the ongoing conflict between tribes*" (East Darfur).

Common values centered on education ($n = 17$, $n = 96$), comfort or stability ($n = 13$, $n = 42$), community solidarity ($n = 16$, $n = 91$), and religious devotion (n = 13, $n = 66$). There was a theme in Central Darfur of associating family and community health as interchangeable, "*[The community is] Important because the society where people live and its stability means the stability of the families and individuals. The community is the large family.*" Similarly, another individual described, "*Education: because without education you cannot help create a health and sound community, cannot choose good friends, cannot get a good job*" (North Darfur).

Saleema campaign brand equity and engagement

There was strong communal receptivity of and identification with the Saleema message of not circumcising women ($n = 16$, $n = 107$). One participant in the Gezira outlined this by saying, "*The village took a decision to abandon it. We are now thinking of Saleema. Now about seventy percent of the people have stopped the circumcision.*" Yet, even with many identifying with the campaign's message of not circumcising women, there were some individuals who felt comfortable discussing their support of circumcision ($n = 12$, $n = 33$). One mother in South Darfur mentioned,

"*The idea and habit of circumcision has appeared in our society, but I will circumcise my daughter due to social stigma, because circumcision reduces sexual desire, and if the boys knew that the girl is uncircumcised they will [be] looking for her and practice adultery with her, so I will circumcised my daughter.*"

Common sources of campaign awareness came by way of media (e.g., advertising, radio) ($n = 17$, $n = 79$), word of mouth (e.g., family or community) ($n = 13$, $n = 41$), and local Saleema events ($n = 6$, $n = 30$). For instance, one individual in North Darfur stated, "*I saw a national jazz singer in a poster, wearing Saleema's standard, I was intrigued, so I looked it out in the internet, and discovered that he and the rest of the people in the poster were Saleema's ambassadors. Then I attended the workshop and learned more.*" Almost half of the states had individuals who mentioned they would like to be engaged with the campaign and promote the Saleema message ($n = 7$, $n = 11$). In particular, one participant from Gezira mentioned, "*As youth, any service you want it from us, we are ready to do it for you. We do not have any problem to offer you the help you need. We will stand together with you, for promoting the campaign, such as by advertising, and anything required from us, we will not hesitate to help together with the People's Committee."*

Saleema campaign poster content and reactions

As outlined above, common themes designed for the posters related to individuals with bright colored clothes emitting happiness through their choice to keep women Saleema and not circumcised. The branding was intended to embody change and cohesion toward anti-FGM attitudes and norms through fictitious leaders in a typical community. The themes arising out of the focus groups are presented numerically in Table 2 with exemplar quotes in Table 3. There were other themes which arose from coding but were lower in frequency and not shown.

Not being circumcised was a prominent theme across all three posters. It was mentioned most frequently across states in poster 2 ($n = 13$, $n = 48$). Happiness was the most common theme across the posters. This theme was most discussed in poster 1 ($n = 11$, $n = 35$) and poster 2 ($n = 12$, $n = 34$). The code representing community cohesion, or "merging communities" was shown only in poster 1. However, there also seemed to be confusion ($n = 10$, $n = 29$) about what type of ceremony was occurring (e.g., circumcision ceremony or a wedding). Regarding the codes of strength and choice, poster 2 was the only one eliciting such responses. Lastly, the concept of change was most common in poster 3 ($n = 7$, $n = 33$), yet there was some confusion about the messaging across states where some thought the mother was "sad" ($n = 8$, n = 10).

More broadly, some mentioned the posters were "beautiful" and that they wanted to be like the people in them. This was shown most prominently in poster 2 ($n = 8$, $n = 18$). One individual in North Kordofan stated, *"I felt that my family should be as healthy, happy and beautiful as they are."* There was also some discussions of the Saleema colors, where many had a clear interpretation that the bright colors represented being Saleema ($n = 11$, $n = 48$). One individual in North Kordofan stated, *"Those dressed in colors are*

uncircumcised and those in black are circumcised." There were only a few locations which interpreted the black as those who do not agree with Saleema (versus being circumcised). For instance, an individual in the Red Sea said, *"The ones in blacks were either didn't hear about Saleema or they are afraid"* and conversely in East Darfur, *"The people who are wearing the campaign's logo are convinced of the campaign's theme."*

Campaign suggestions

Across states, participants most commonly suggested awareness to prevent FGM ($n = 13$, $n = 76$). We aligned this suggestion within social marketing principles (product, price, place, promotion) ad hoc to assist in organizing the suggestions from participants. Specifically, with regard to the mode in which messaging should be communicated (product), the most common theme came in the form of advocacy ($n = 15$, $n = 72$). As stated in Gezira, *"It is important to keep this project going on and you can choose four young women and four young men from this locality to be the focal points, with whom you can continue the communications, they raise our concerns and you give them ideas to convey, and to provide them with the posters to distribute."* Additionally, trainings ($n = 15$, $n = 55$), and posters ($n = 13$, $n = 37$) were themes that arose as well. In Central Darfur one individual outlined, *"Education is the foundation and it is necessary to raise our daughters in a good way. It is important to raise them to be decent, Saleema, educated and understanding, in order to lead the society and help their people."*

Participants said that messaging should highlight the harms of FGM or compare people who were circumcised versus not (n = 13, $n = 35$) (price). In Sennar, *"We explain to people all the consequences after circumcision like acute inflammation, accumulation of menstruation, difficulties in giving a baby and so, and we expose all this in the society."* Participants commonly desire to hear more from doctors ($n = 7$, n = 22) and religious groups ($n = 14$, $n = 37$) on the topic as well as institute trainings or education in schools

Table 2 Poster Content Coding Summary

Code	Poster 1 States (count)	Codes (count)	Poster 2 States (count)	Codes (count)	Poster 3 States (count)	Codes (count)
Not circumcised	10	36	13	48	9	24
Happy	11	35	12	34	11	18
Merging Communities	9	17	0	0	0	0
Strong	0	0	12	39	0	0
Choice	0	0	13	39	0	0
Change	2	3	0	0	7	33

Table 3 Poster Coding Exemplar Quotes

Code	Exemplar Quote
Not circumcised	*Wearing Saleema's logo, and they ae convinced to stop circumcision and that the entire community should remain whole (Poster 1, West Darfur).*
	A mother holding her child, and she hopes her daughter to grow healthy and be Saleema (Poster 2, South Darfur)
Happy	*People are happy the father, mother and children because they are healthy and the father is happy with his children because they are sound. I felt that my family should be as healthy, happy and beautiful as they are (Poster 1, North Kordofan).*
	The girl is happy. Those in black are not healthy. I like her because she is Saleema and proud of that. I wish that all girls are like her (Poster 2, North Kordofan).
	The mother is happy because her daughter is SALEEMA (Poster 3, Northern State).
Merging Communities	*It means to me that it matters to everyone, and people join efforts men, women and children for it (Poster 1, South Darfur).*
Strong	*The shape of women who wears the tone of Saleema establishes the message and means that the woman is strong and has a determination and can deliver her message (Poster 2, Central Darfur).*
Choice	*A happy life, of course, because she is a strong woman in her decisions, convinced by her decisions, because she has taken the right decision (Poster 2, Gezira).*
Change	*The woman in black is not Saleema but if she is convinced by the idea, she will leave her girl in hand Saleema and in this way the coming generation will be Saleema (Poster 3, Sennar).*

($n = 11$, $n = 33$), the media ($n = 14$, $n = 72$), or communal settings ($n = 15$, $n = 66$) (place). In West Kordofan, "*Broadcasted programs, as most of the people in these areas depend on only on radio. They don't have TV set due to lack of electricity*" and East Darfur,

"*After the thorough discussions and the information that we have heard for the first time, we have become totally convinced. If anything, this indicates that the community is in need of workshops, symposiums and discussion groups, which stand for the yield good results in terms of our safety and the safety for our daughters in the future.*"

With regard to whom should be the target of message, the focus groups commonly mentioned men to marry ($n = 6$, $n = 11$), midwives ($n = 10$, $n = 28$), older women ($n = 10$, $n = 28$), and people in rural villages ($n = 10$, $n = 34$) (promotion). In the Central Darfur, "*Women are the main cause of the spread and persistence of circumcision. The grandmothers as well insist on the circumcision of their daughters. In their view, the uncircumcised is a disgrace and shame. She will be discarded and stigmatized by words... If the women were sensitized and become active in the campaign, certainly the campaign will be successful.*" In

North Kordofan, "*Changing people opinions depends to the area if in countryside the most influenced were the teachers, sheikh of the village, imam of the mosque those can raise the awareness in a simple way to explain its harms and negatives.*" Additionally, though not common in all states, youth were specifically mentioned ($n = 3$, $n = 6$) as targets as well. In Gezira, "*Your messages are very good. Just you need to have a special unit for the youth. The messages targeting them should be direct and clear.*" And East Darfur, "*We have already reached old age and what we have learnt is more than what is yet be learnt. It is the youth's turn to act now.*"

Discussion

The primary purpose of the current evaluation was to assess qualitative responses to the Saleema campaign. The campaign as a whole reflects an integrated strategy, employing all 4 Ps of social marketing, including place-based strategies through community-events, participatory activities in the form of public declarations to abandon FGM, mass media and digital media messages, and public advocacy. The current study was limited in scope. Results are based on qualitative focus groups assessed Sudanese perceptions of the information sources, values, and reactions to three Saleema campaign posters that were chosen to be representative of the primary campaign messages. The most common source of information or admiration was local leaders who are responsive to their community, media-based outlets, and discussions among community members. Special consideration of dissemination outlets when targeting rural areas was discussed as well provided their lack of access to technology and available resources. Participants held high value for education, community solidarity, and/or religious devotion. These findings were consistent across a majority of the states.

With respect to the primary aim of this study, we found that participants had positive opinions of Saleema and the concepts that it conveyed. Participants responded positively to the Saleema brand and branding elements in the posters and the campaign as a whole. In particular, individuals were most receptive to the bright colors and positive messaging. It seems there could be increased clarity surrounding specific activities as well as the connotations of those individuals wearing black in the posters. In addition, there was still a sizeable group across states that was vocal about their support of FGM due to social stigma. It could be useful to consider addressing specific stigma-related topics directly in future iterations of the campaign messaging.

Overall, participants had a positive response to the posters. There were some mixed responses to each individual poster, but poster 2 was most successful in eliciting interpretations aligning with the intended message design. Many understood Saleema inferred a happy life. Poster 1 was most successful in representing merging of communities. There could be more clarity about the activity in Additional file 1: poster 1 specifically to enhance effectiveness. Additional file 2: Poster 2 was most effective in eliciting interpretations of strength and choice. Additional file 3: Poster 3 was best at conveying change of FGM norms. Combined, the posters capture the full spectrum of the campaign. Though there seemed to be high brand equity, as noted previously responses indicated there were still a substantial group supporting FGM. Therefore, there is still room to expand the campaign and decrease social norms encouraging FGM.

Focus group questions also asked about suggestions for the campaign. The most common suggestion was in the form of continued awareness. The results outlined suggestions in line with Social Marketing principles (product, price, place, promotion). Advocacy, training, and posters were suggested to highlight the harms of FGM through leaders or in community settings. Individuals suggested that these activities target older women and individuals in rural villages. However, a burgeoning theme of targeting youth for support of the campaign came through as well.

The results should be interpreted in the light of its limitations. This study presents qualitative results only and may be subject to selection bias. However, the sampling strategy utilized mitigated this issue to an extent. Of course with such a sensitive topic there could also be bias with the results for those that felt comfortable to discuss FGM in front of others or more confident in their interpretation of the posters. There is one focus group missing and results are cross-sectional. Consequently, they do not represent perceptions over time. There are also potential drawbacks to the focus groups being coded with individuals not living in Sudan. Yet, the transcripts were translated by individuals who are bilingual in Sudan. Coding questions that arose about specific wording and culture were discussed and resolved prior to summarizing the results. Lastly, generalizability of the results outside of Sudan or other localities is limited. Evaluations of the Saleema campaign at other time points as well as work on FGM in other countries and populations can refine the interpretation.

Conclusions

The results of this focus group analysis demonstrate support for future Saleema campaign efforts promoting awareness and community engagement. In particular, there was a rising theme of community involvement by engaging youth. The campaign could capitalize on partnerships with young people and those who are respected in the community (e.g., religious leaders) or continue promoting common values aligning with the support of education and community solidarity. Efforts could also engage those willing to get involved as well as continue to utilize or adapt to those channels depending on the locality. Continuing campaign efforts have promise to decrease the harms of FGM in Sudan. Moving forward, this information should also be triangulated with quantitative results to assess campaign effectiveness in relation to attitudes and social norms.

Abbreviations
DFID: Department for International Development; FGM/C: Female Genital Mutilation and Cutting; UNICEF: United Nations International Children's Emergency Fund; USAID: US Agency for International Development; WHO: World Health Organization

Acknowledgements
The study authors would like to acknowledge all the individuals who engaged as study participants and provided their feedback.

Funding
Funding for this project was provided by UNICEF Communication For Development (C4D) program, Sudan office. The funding assisted with the developed of the study design and collection but not analysis, interpretation of data, or in writing the manuscript.

Authors' contributions
WDE designed the study and trained the focus group moderators. HB collected the focus group data and transcribed the transcripts from Arabic to English. TA and CD reviewed and provided input on the study design. ACJ and NB analyzed and interpreted the data. WDE was the principal investigator and oversaw data collection and analysis. All authors read and approved the final manuscript.

Authors' information
ACJ is a PhD student at The George Washington University.
WDE is a Professor at The George Washington University.
NB is a Senior Research Associated at The George Washington University.
HB is with UNICEF Sudan.
TA is with UNICEF Sudan.
CD is with UNICEF.

Competing interests
The authors declare that they have no competing interests.

Qualitative evaluation of the Saleema campaign to eliminate female genital mutilation and cutting...

167

Author details
[1]Milken Institute School of Public Health, The George Washington University, 950 New Hampshire Avenue, NW, Washington, DC 20052, USA. [2]UNICEF, Kassala, Sudan.

References
1. World Health Organization, Department of Gender, Women and Health. Health complications of female genital mutilation including sequelae in childbirth: a systematic review. 2000.
2. UNICEF. Female genital mutilation/cutting: a statistical overview and exploration of the dynamics of change. 2013.
3. Elmusharaf S, Elhadi N, Almroth L. Reliability of self reported form of female genital mutilation and WHO classification: cross sectional study. BMJ. 2006; 333(7559):124.
4. Central Bureau of Statistics (CBS), UNICEF Sudan. Multiple indicator cluster survey 2014 of Sudan, final report. 2016;Khartoum, Sudan: UNICEF and Central Bureau of Statistics (CBS), February 2016.
5. Cialdini RB. Descriptive social norms as underappreciated sources of social control. Psychometrika. 2007;72:236.
6. Evans WD, Hastings G. Public health branding: applying marketing for social change. London, United Kingdom: Oxford University Press; 2008.
7. Evans WD. Social marketing research for global public health: methods and technologies. New York: Oxford University Press; 2016. ISBN 9780199757398.
8. Berg RC, Denison EM. A realist synthesis of controlled studies to determine the effectiveness of interventions to prevent genital cutting of girls. Paediatr Int Child Health. 2013;33(4):322–33. https://doi.org/10.1179/2046905513Y.0000000086.
9. Evans WD, Blitstein J, Vallone D, Post S, Nielsen W. Systematic review of health branding: growth of a promising practice. Transl Behav Med. 2015; 5(1):24–36. https://doi.org/10.1007/s13142-014-0272-1.
10. Evans WD. Quasi-Experimental and Heavy-Up Experiments in Social Marketing. Chapter 8 In Social Marketing for Global Public Health: Methods and Technologies. New York: Oxford University Press; 2016.
11. Kotler P, Roberto EL, Roberto N. Social marketing: Strategies for changing public behavior. Free Press; 1989. ISBN-13: 978-0029184615.
12. Saldana J. The coding manual for qualitative researchers. Thousand Oaks, CA: Sage; 2013.
13. Creswell JW. Qualitative inquiry and research design: choosing among five approaches. 3rd ed. Thousand Oaks, CA: SAGE Publications, Inc; 2013. ISBN-13: 978-1412995306.
14. Patton MQ. Qualitative research & evaluation methods: integrating theory and practice. 4th ed. Thousand Oaks, CA: SAGE Publications, Inc; 2015. ISBN-13: 978-1412972123.
15. Tong A, Sainsbury P, Craig J. Consolidated criteria for reporting qualitative research (COREQ): a 32-item checklist for interviews and focus groups. Int J Qual Health Care. 2007;19(6):349–57.

15

Why ethnicity and gender matters for fertility intention among married young people: a baseline evaluation from a gender transformative intervention in rural India

Tina Khanna[*] ⓘ, Murari Chandra, Ajay Singh and Sunil Mehra

Abstract

Background: Social inequities in early child bearing persist among young married people, especially among tribal populations in India. Rural women belonging to tribal groups and those coming from poor households are more likely to give birth before age 18. This paper explores the connection between ethnicity, gender and early fertility intention among young married people in rural India.

Methods: The data is drawn from a cross sectional baseline evaluation of an intervention programme in rural India. A sample of 273 married young people was taken. Respondents were selected using systematic random sampling. Logistic Regression was used to assess the effect of being a tribal on early fertility intention and also to determine if covariates associated with early fertility intention differed by tribal status. Qualitative data was analysed using deductive content analysis approach.

Results: Bivariate and logistic regression results indicated that young married people from tribal communities had higher odds of planning a child within one year of marriage than non-tribals (OR = 1.47, p-value-0.079). Findings further suggest that early fertility intention among tribals is driven by gender factors and higher education and among non-tribals, higher education and awareness on contraception are key predictors. Among tribals, the odds of planning a child within one year of marriage was strongly associated with inequitable gender norms (OR = 1.94, p-value-0.002). Higher education showed significant positive association with non-tribals (OR = 0.19, p-value-0.014) and positive association with tribals (OR = 0.56, p-value-0.416). Qualitative investigation confirms that fertility desires of young married people are strongly influenced by gender norms especially among tribal populations.

Conclusion: Early child bearing was underpinned by complex ethnic factors and gender norms. Preference for early child bearing was seen most among tribal communities. Gender attitudes were a cause of concern especially among tribal groups. These results suggest that efforts to improve early child birth will require changing gender norms related to fertility among tribals as well as social equity issues including higher education among non-tribals and tribals.

Keywords: Tribal, Fertility, Young men and women, Gender, Education, India

[*] Correspondence: tina@mamtahmc.org
MAMTA Health Institute for Mother and Child, B-5, Greater Kailash Enclave-II, New Delhi 110048, India

Plain English Summary

Despite increase in age of marriage and declining fertility, social inequities in early child bearing exist among young married women and men, especially among tribal populations in India. This study sought to understand ethnic variation in early fertility preference among young people in rural India. This study utilizes mixed method approach to assess the effect of being tribal on early fertility intention and also whether determinants associated with early fertility intention differed among tribals and non-tribals. The data was collected through a survey of young married women (ages 14–18) and men (ages 15–21) and also through qualitative interviews with young married women and men, community health workers and parents. Results showed that preference for early child bearing is significantly associated with tribal communities who had early marriages and low contraceptive use. This is attributable to inequitable gender norms associated with early child bearing among tribals. Also, the role of higher education in influencing fertility intention among non-tribal and tribal cannot be neglected. The analysis underscores the need to address gender inequitable attitude among tribals and to amplify efforts to promote higher education among tribals and non-tribals for delaying early child birth.

Background

In India, rates of early childbearing are persistently high, especially among ethnic and caste minorities and women from socio-economic disadvantaged backgrounds. Analysis of the National Family and Health Survey (NFHS-3) data indicates that rural women - those belonging to Scheduled Tribes (ST), and those coming from poor households were more likely to have had a birth before age 18 [1]. Fertility rates are higher for rural women in STs in comparison to Scheduled Caste (SCs), Other Backward Classes (OBCs), and general category [2]. Couples in tribal communities report some of the lowest rates of contraceptive use in India [2, 3].

Despite India's recent economic growth, health and human development indicators of STs or *Adivasi* lag behind the national averages [4, 5]. Among the social groups in India, tribes are the most socio-economically deprived groups with low literacy and poor economic conditions and low access to health services [4–6]. The latest NFHS-4 (2015–2016) data also highlighted that reproductive health services are least accessed by women from ST groups. Tribal women also had lower rates of antenatal care visits and institutional births among all social groups [7].

Although there is extensive literature on various aspects of population, fertility, and family planning, it is noteworthy that only a limited number of empirical studies have attempted to explain tribal reproductive health (especially among young people) systematically in India [8–10]. A recent study of adolescent fertility in Africa highlights that first birth among young people is most common among the poorest and least educated, and progress in reducing rates within this group has not been made over the last few decades [11]. It further highlighted that it is valuable to examine fertility behaviour of different cultural groups to target programmes at the people most at risk, in order to reduce young people's fertility [11].

A few micro-level studies in India demonstrate that being from a tribal community positively influenced the probability of early child bearing. Panel data from Andhra Pradesh [12] demonstrates that young married women from the tribal groups were 10.5% more likely to give birth by the time they were 19 years old than women from other castes [12]. Some studies in India highlighted that early age at marriage, son preference, lower education, and low access to services are some of the reasons for low contraceptive use among tribals [13]. Gender norms are an important aspect of early fertility desires, which are largely overlooked in interventions, especially for marginalised sections. Gender relations among Indian tribes have historically been more balanced and equitable; however there is an increasing trend of gender bias in tribal culture emerging due to the assimilation and modernising process [14]. In consonance with the recent declines of tribal female-male ratio (FMR) there is growing evidence to showcase the disadvantages that tribal females have been undergoing due to expansion of developmental activities and integration. A recent study suggests that the sharp drop in tribal FMR is due to assimilation into the patriarchal norms of higher castes through ongoing processes of sanskritisation and detribalisation -all contributing to an emerging culture of discrimination against women among tribal people [15, 16]. Therefore, the present paper tries to understand reproductive behaviour among young married people of tribal communities in India and explore the inter-connection between ethnicity and gender with early fertility intention, an important factor that has not been well established or investigated systematically.

The specific objectives of the paper are: (a) To explore fertility intention among tribal and non-tribal young married people (b) To assess the effect of being a member of tribal community on early fertility intention among young married people. (c) To assess gender and social determinants of early fertility intention among tribal and non-tribal young married people in rural India.

Method

Study design

This study involved analysis of cross-sectional baseline (using quantitative and qualitative methods) data from young married people[1] in a family planning evaluation study in rural India. This paper is based on the analyses of young married people living in marital home aged 14 to 21 (Total = 273, tribal = 108, non-tribal = 165). The survey was conducted in two states of India – Madhya Pradesh (MP) and Rajasthan (two districts each) where early marriage (55–60%) and total fertility rate in rural areas fertility was higher (3.3- MP and 3.6- Rajasthan) than national estimates (National Family Health Survey, 2007–08). A three-stage sampling design was implemented in selecting six blocks across study districts and further from each blocks, 10 villages were selected using Probability Proportion to Size. Systematic random sampling was used to randomly select the respondents from completed household list of selected villages.

Data

The quantitative data was collected through a structured questionnaire by trained male and female field investigators, taking an average time of 40 min. Male investigators interviewed young married men, and young married women were interviewed by female investigators. Survey data assessed determinants of fertility intention among these people by tribal and non-tribal groups. The survey tool contained questions on socio-demographic information (including age, sex, ethnic group, education, age at marriage) and also on fertility intention, decision making, gender attitudes, use of contraceptives etc. The instrument was verbally translated into Hindi and was field-tested to ensure language and cultural contexts.

Qualitative methods

A total of 40 in-depth interviews (IDIs) were conducted among young married men and women (10 each) and parents (10 each - father and mother). We also conducted key informant interviews (KIIs) (8) with health care providers. Under the National Rural Health Mission, the government of India has employed Accredited Social Health Activist (ASHA) and Anganwadi workers (AWW) who act as community health workers. They provide counselling to married couples for use of family planning methods and also support community to access public health services. ASHA and AWW were purposively selected for KIIs since they are first point of contact with young married people in village for health care counselling and services including family planning.

We included perspectives of both young men and women and parents of young men and women to better understand emergence of early fertility norms within their particular social environments. For IDIs it took approximately 60 min and around 40 min for KIIs. The qualitative instruments contained questions relating to cultural norms and practices around early marriage and fertility, knowledge, access and use of family planning

methods, gender barriers, etc. Purposive sampling was followed to select participants for IDIs and KIIs. We selected married young girls (aged 14–18) and married young boys (15–21) who were married in last 1 year without any children/not currently pregnant (married young women and wife of married young men) from tribal and non-tribal communities. For the health care providers, we recruited community health workers who had more than two years of working experience in the community. The senior research team (qualitative) in collaboration with field team with extensive experience conducted interviews.

Ethics, consent and permissions

All study participants provided consent and/or assent to participate in the study. Verbal informed consent of parents, health care providers, young men and women was sought prior to the survey. Respondents aged below 18 provided assent, while verbal informed consent was sought from their parents. The questionnaires did not request the name or other identifying variables, to ensure anonymity of data for research purpose only. Participants did not receive any material compensation. Ethical permission was obtained from the Institutional Review Board (IRB) of MAMTA- Health Institute for Mother and Child (India) prior to data collection. Since young men and women aged 14–17 years are the most vulnerable populations in research, hence the study minimised all possible risks to the participants during the survey. Every effort was made to ensure protection and confidentiality and to reduce any potential adverse consequence to the participants.

Measurement

Outcome variable: The response (dependent) variable was chosen to investigate early child bearing plan among married young people. This was categorised into two levels: intention to have child within one year of marriage and after one year. Hence, the dependent variable was coded dichotomously within one year (coded as 1) and after one year (coded as 0).

Explanatory variables

Selected socio-demographic factors that may affect early child plan at young ages were controlled in an adjusted model. These variables were: gender of respondent, age at marriage, age at *gauna*, caste, education and economic status and gender attitudes. Since the data consists of young married men and women, hence fertility choices by genders was taken in an adjusted model. *Gauna* is a traditional custom in rural India (performed in marriage that occurs at very young age) where a married couple consummate their marriage and cohabit together. Education level was grouped as till primary level (0–5 years), secondary (6–10 years); and senior secondary and higher (11 years and above). Economic status was measured by household having Below Poverty Line (BPL) card or Antyodhaya card (extreme poor) provided by Government of India. Social-ethnic group was grouped/categorized as tribal (STs) and non-tribals (OBCs and SCs). Awareness of modern contraceptive method such as condoms, IUD, pills and injectable was computed. Anganwadi centers (AWC) is the nearest and the most feasible place that provides basic health care in Indian villages including contraceptive counseling and supply and reproductive health education hence awareness about AWC was coded as 1 and 0 otherwise. Exposure to mass media (measured as mobile/internet and books/magazine) was also computed.

Gender attitude of young married people was measured through Gender Equitable Men Scale (GEMS) on 10 statements related to early child bearing, contraceptive use, family planning, autonomy, reproductive rights, etc. The statements were a mix of attitudes that were gender equal and non-equal. For each statement, the response options were 'agree', 'partially agree' and 'do not agree'. All the statements were made unidirectional before assigning the scores to a gender discriminatory statement. A score of 0 was given to the most negative statement and a score of 2 was assigned to the most positive statement. Factor analysis was done using Principle Component Analysis (PCA) and factor loading was performed to identify the most important variables with highest variability explained (Eigenvalues) in particular factor (index) created with higher reliability value ($\alpha = 0.81$). Hence the predicted scores on the scale were distributed in three equal fragments assigning as low, moderate and high gender equitable attitudes. Of these, the two very relevant statements were chosen after bivariate tests were used in an adjusted model. This methodology of creating a GEM scale has been used and validated in previous research in India as well as other countries [17, 18].

Statistical analysis
Bivariate analysis and Chi square assessed associations between tribal status and selected socio-demographic variables, early fertility intention, contraceptive use and gender norms. Adjusted Logistic Regression was used to assess effect of tribal status on early fertility intention. Intention to conceive after one year was taken as a reference category. Further, separate models were developed to determine if covariates associated with early fertility intention differed by tribal status.

Qualitative analysis
For the qualitative data analysis, all the interviews were recorded, transcribed and subsequently translated into English. Professional translators well versed with English and Hindi translated the Hindi transcript into English. The first author (Indian speaking English and Hindi) cross checked all English translated transcripts with hindi transcripts (also checked with the audio files whenever necessary) to ensure quality of translation. Hindi transcripts were read several times to get acquainted with raw data and checked at random by the first author. The translated text was coded inductively, and ambiguities in meaning were resolved by consulting project staff. Data were organised using Atlas-ti software following a content analysis approach. Themes emerging during review of the transcripts were sorted and grouped according to key categories.

Results
Socio-economic characteristics, education and exposure
Participants ($n = 273$) were 39.5% tribal and 60.5% non-tribal. The mean age for tribal and non-tribal young people were 18.7 and 18.6 The socio-demographic characteristics varied among tribal and non-tribal groups. The majority of young married tribal people (77.8%) belonged to either poor or extremely poor families. Compared to non-tribal groups, young people from the tribal community received less education. More than 40% of the young tribal people had either no education or only primary education compared to nearly one-fourth of young non-tribal people. Only about 17% of the young tribal people reached education levels above class 10th as against one third of young non-tribal people (33.3%). The exposure to media through mobile/internet and books/magazine was also very low among tribal as compared to non-tribal people. Young tribal people (55.6%) had less access to mobile and internet than their non-tribal counterparts (61.8%).

Early marriage, fertility preference and contraceptive use: Bivariate analysis
Tribal status of young people was significantly associated ($p < 0.001$) with younger age at marriage; and younger age at cohabitation with spouse (Gauna). Around half of tribal young women (46.6%) were married before age 16 in comparison to non-tribal (27.1%). Also, the majority of young tribal men (63.5%) were married before age 18 as compared to nontribal (46.4%). Importantly, 23.3% of young tribal women and majority of young tribal men (42.8%) start cohabiting as married couples before age 16 and 18 years respectively in comparison to non-tribal young women (12.9%) and non-tribal young men (24.6%) as reflected in Table 1.

Data on fertility preference indicate a significant association between tribal status and intentions for early child bearing. Within the study sample, 27.4% of young married tribal people expressed the desire for having a child within one year of marriage compared to 18.7% of

Table 1 Socio demographic and family planning characteristics among tribals and non-tribals

	Tribal (n = 108)	Non-tribal (n = 165)	p-value
Mean age*	18.7 *.54	18.6 *.53	
Socio-Economic characteristics			
Below Poverty Line and extreme poor	77.8	52.1	0.001
Education			0.002
None	15.7	9.1	
Primary (1-5th standard)	25.9	13.3	
Up to Secondary (6-10th Standard)	41.7	44.2	
Higher secondary & above (10th Standard and above)	16.7	33.3	
Exposure to media			
Mobile/ Internet	55.6	61.8	0.303
Books/magazines	5.6	21.8	0.001
Marriage			
Young women married below 16 years	46.6	27.1	0.001
Young men married below 18 years	63.5	46.4	0.001
Age at *gauna* (young women) below 16 years	23.3	12.9	0.001
Age at *gauna* (young men) below 18 years	42.8	24.6	0.001
Family planning characteristics			
Plan to have child within one year of marriage	27.4	18.7	0.088
Awareness of modern contraception methods: condom	46.3	55.4	0.152
Awareness of modern contraception Methods: Pills	82.4	93.9	0.002
Awareness about place to get contraceptives near village (AWC)	27.8	45.4	0.003
Currently using any method	15.7	24.2	0.091
Methods of use (modern method)	14.8	23.0	0.096
Reasons for not using contraception			0.053
Lack of knowledge of modern contraceptive methods	24.7	14.1	
Planning to conceive	55.3	53.9	

*Standard deviation

their non-tribal counterparts. A difference was also observed on awareness of modern contraceptive methods (condoms and pills) between tribal and non-tribals. Also, less percentage of young married people who belonged to tribal families (27.8%) were aware of AWC as the place

within or near the village where one could get modern contraceptives in comparison to non-tribals (45.4%). Likewise, the current contraceptive (modern method) use among tribals (15.7%) was less than among non-tribals (24.2%).

Gender Attitudes towards early child bearing among tribal and non-tribal young married people

Tribal and non-tribal young married people were asked whether they agree, partially agree or disagree with specific gender statements related to early child bearing which provides deeper insight into the effect of gender-related attitudinal differences among tribal and non-tribal young people, on fertility intention. Gender attitudes of young married people and especially in tribal groups were biased against women when it comes to planning for the first child. As reflected in Table 2, a vast majority of young married tribal people (68.5%) agreed to the statement that '*it is husbands who can decide when to have a first child*' in comparison to 50.3% of non-tribal young people. There was a difference in the attitudes of young people, especially among tribal groups towards the pressure of early child bearing for young women, with tribals displaying more rigid and biased attitudes. Half of young tribal people agreed that '*women should conceive within one year of marriage to avoid shame*' in comparison to only 31.5% non tribals. Also more than half of young tribal people were in agreement with the statement '*Early child bearing makes women valuable in family and society,*' than their non-tribal counterparts (37%).

Further, a Gender Equitable Men Scale (from the individual statements) was developed (as explained in methodology section) whereby individual scores of members were placed in one of three categories (low, moderate and high) reflecting their level of support for gender equity. The GEMS scale (Fig. 1) shows that a majority of young tribal people fall into low and moderate gender equity category, meaning that they hold attitudes that were less or moderately supportive of gender equity towards early child bearing ($p < 0.001$). As seen in Fig. 1, young non-tribal people were more gender equitable than their tribal counterparts.

Multivariate Analysis: Logistic regression (adjusted Model) for combined and separate ethnic groups

The logistic regression analyses showed that tribal status was a significant predictor for intention to have early child birth while adjusting with other confounders (Table 3). Young people from tribal communities had 47% higher odds to plan a child within one year of marriage than their non-tribal counterparts (OR-1.47, $p < 0.079$). In the combined model, gender measures (norms) and education were other significant predictors. Young married people with restrictive gender attitudes had higher odds to plan a child within

Table 2 Gender attitudes on early child bearing (percent who agreed to selected statements) among tribals and non-tribals young married people

Statements	Tribal %	Non-tribal %	P-value (Chi-square)
If a couple doesn't have a child then it's a woman's fault	27.8	18.2	0.061
It's a woman's responsibility to avoid getting pregnant	59.3	51.5	0.209
Women should conceive within one year of marriage to avoid shame	50.0	31.5	0.002
It is husbands who can decide when to have first child	68.5	50.3	0.003
The real man is the one who has child within one year of marriage	23.2	16.9	0.207
Early child bearing makes women valuable in family and society	51.9	37.0	0.015

one year of marriage. For example, young married people who agreed with the statement 'The real man is the one who has a child within one year of marriage' had 78% higher odds of planning a child within one year of marriage than those who disagreed with the statement (OR = 1.78, $p < 0.004$), given that the other predictors in the model held constant. Also, overall, the young married women had higher odds to plan a child within one year of marriage as compared to men (OR-1.55, $p < 0.067$). Young married people with higher level of education (senior secondary and higher), had lower odds to go for early child bearing (both tribals and non-tribals in the combined model) than those who had low level of education (OR-0.39, $p < 0.025$).

Further, separate models were developed to determine if covariates associated with early fertility intention differed by tribal status. Among tribal groups, early fertility intention was significantly associated with gender factors unlike their non-tribal counterparts. Young people from tribal group who agreed with the statement 'The real man is the one who has a child within one year of marriage' had 94% higher odds of early child bearing than those who disagreed with the statement (OR-1.94, $p < 0.002$). Within the tribal group, women had 82% higher odds of planning a child within one year of

marriage as compared to their male counterparts (OR-1.82, $p < 0.020$).

Early fertility intention was positively associated with increase in education among both tribal and non-tribal groups. Table 3 reflects that with increase in level of education the odds of planning a child early after marriage decreased irrespective of ethnic groups. Among non-tribals higher education had positive and significant association (OR-0.19, $p < 0.014$) with early fertility intention, however among tribals it showed only positive association (OR-0.56, $p < 0.416$). Among non-tribals, young married people who were not aware of contraceptive methods had 71% higher odds of planning a child within one year of marriage (OR-1.71, $p < 0.026$). Thus among non-tribals, early fertility intention was significantly associated with education and awareness about contraception and not with gender factors.

Qualitative findings

The qualitative investigation found that the desire for young people to bear children early was influenced by social and gender norms, especially among tribal populations.

Social and family related factors

The pressure to fulfill the social demand to conceive early to prove their worth soon after marriage was found among young women, and this was particularly high for tribal women who were married early and had less education. Parents from both tribal and non-tribal communities shared that it is a common trend for a married couple to have a first child early, and therefore no birth control measures were taken. They were taken only after the second child for spacing. However, in the context of tribals, parents and families were more averse towards imparting family planning to newly married couples and feared using family planning methods. These respondents (parents) also had less education (primary education) and less exposure. They shared that talking about sexual relations, family planning issues is neither needed nor acceptable in the community. It is considered a cultural taboo and some parents even feared and

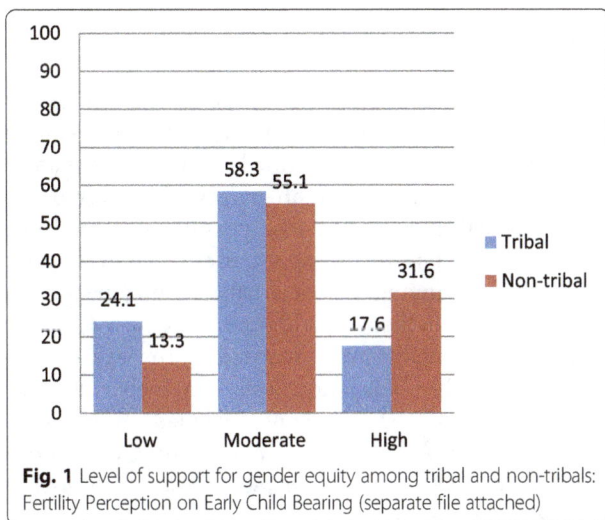

Fig. 1 Level of support for gender equity among tribal and non-tribals: Fertility Perception on Early Child Bearing (separate file attached)

Table 3 Odds Ratio (OR) of Fertility Intention within one year by selected predictors for combined and separate ethnic groups

	Model 1: Combined ethnic groups	Model 2: Tribal	Model 3: Non-tribal
	OR	OR	OR
Gender			
Boy	1	1	
Girl	1.55*	1.82**	1.63
Caste			
Non-tribal	1	1	
Tribal	1.47*		
Education level			
Up to primary (0-5th standard)	1	1	1
Secondary (6-10th Standard)	0.88	0.80	0.93
Senior secondary & higher (10th standard and above)	0.39**	0.56	0.19**
Duration of cohabitation after marriage (years)	1.00	1.20	0.95
Awareness about contraception methods:			
Yes	1	1	1
No	1.52**	1.46	1.71**
Gender statements			
The real man is the one who has a child within one year of marriage			
Disagree	1	1	1
Agree	1.78***	1.94***	1.33
Early child bearing makes women valuable in family and society			
Disagree	1	1	1
Agree	1.08	0.37	1.42
Constant	0.015	0.0666	0.031
Adjusted R^2	0.115	0.2101	0.181

Note: Response outcome for early fertility preference 0(ref) = after 1 year, 1 = within 1 year, results are controlled for other predictors such as current age, BPL status, family support @reference category. *$p < 0.1$, ** $p < 0.05$, ***$p < 0.01$

questioned the relevance of providing this knowledge. As shared by an elder woman from the tribal community:

"No one talks about these things in a village. It is considered a wrong and sinful practice. You should not give this information otherwise newly married will know about ways to delay pregnancy and they will delay their first child. You should give this information to those who have at least one child."

Young married tribal women shared that there is strong family pressure on them to conceive early especially for the first child. They explained that they have limited decision-making powers in family planning; these decisions are mostly taken by the husband. As shared emphatically by a married tribal girl (19):

I: What will you do if you don't want to have a child now?

R: I/my husband will have to use birth control methods.

I: Will you face any difficulty in using contraceptives?

R: My in-laws can stop me; they will say we want to have a grandchild now.

I: What will you do? What support would you need?

R: I would definitely need my husband's support to refuse to have a child now. If my husband wants it, then I will have to conceive and deliver a child, and if he doesn't then I will not conceive.

Young men were also influenced by social norms about early fertility and perceived attitudes of people in their social networks. Young married men also stated that there are negative repercussions that a woman has to bear if she doesn't conceive within two years of marriage, including facing negative remarks and abandonment. This was shared by both tribal and non-tribal men. The young tribal men who were married early (at 16–17 years) and had less education, were found more bound by traditional community norms for early child bearing.

"It is expected to have a child within one year of marriage. If she doesn't conceive within 1-2 years then such a woman is taunted, taken to doctors and may be abandoned."

Married boy (19 years), Scheduled Tribe.

Among tribal populations, around two-thirds of interviewed young married tribal men and women (n = 6) lacked correct knowledge about pregnancy. Few of them thought that pregnancy can never occur in one sexual contact and it is possible after multiple contacts. The knowledge about use of contraception was also less among married tribal young people as less than half of them were aware of it (n = 4). Most of these respondents were married at the age of 15–16 years and had education less than higher secondary. As shared by a young married tribal man (18 years): *"No I have not used a condom, and I also don't know how to use it. In fact, I will never use; it looks horrible to me."*

Factors related to service provision/health care providers

The qualitative interviews with health care workers highlighted their apprehension to provide family planning knowledge and services to young married men and women and their limited outreach to tribal communities. Many village health care providers expressed disapproval at using contraceptive methods to delay the first pregnancy and spoke of community challenges and the non-acceptability of it.

"The first child should be born after two years - we can counsel the couple on this but we can't go against society. Even if the couple is educated and aware, they will be forced to have the first child soon. They can delay the second child not the first."

Community health worker (Female, 34 years).

Community health workers also expressed that young married men and women from tribal communities lacked awareness and access to health care services. They explained that they were not able to reach them as they lived on the periphery of the village, far from the health centre.

Tribal communities live far from the main village, and the health centre. We are less in contact with them and they also don't come to the centre.

Community health worker (Female, 28 years).

Discussion

The findings from bi-variate analysis and adjusted logistic regression also reinforced from qualitative analysis indicate that preference for early child bearing is significantly associated with tribals in comparison to non-tribal. The current findings indicate that young married people from tribal community have higher odds of planning a child early within one year of marriage. These findings have also been recognised in earlier studies that have found more cases of early marriage and child bearing among tribal populations than other socio-ethnic groups [1, 2, 12]. Studies on tribal population in south and west India have also found low contraceptive use, misconceptions and lack of access to various contraceptive methods to be the causes of early child bearing [2, 14, 19]. The tribal populations have less education, which further makes them vulnerable to low contraceptive use and high unmet need than other social groups [12, 19]. The bi-variate association between tribal status and gender inequitable attitudes was also significant. Overall, tribals had greater gender inequitable and patriarchal attitudes on early child-bearing as compared with their non-tribal counterparts.

This study contributes to a growing body of studies on reproductive behaviour and is one of the few studies using the GEM scale to understand gender-equitable attitudes of tribals and non-tribals. Existing studies have reflected gender equitable attitude for equitable reproductive decision-making and increased contraceptive use [20, 21]. However, such linkages are explored less among tribal populations. While historically gender relations among tribals have been more egalitarian as compared to other social groups, anti-female patterns of discrimination are now increasing among some tribal communities as their lives become integrated into mainstream culture and social practices, generally through the conversion to Hinduism [11, 15]. These studies have pointed out the growing trend of gender deficit of females and gender bias among tribal communities [11, 15].

Further, findings also indicate that tribals who were more likely to plan child early was attributable to inequitable gender norms associated with early child bearing. This reflects that not only do gender attitudes influence the perception of young married people among tribals for early child bearing but they also impact the planning of a child within one year of marriage. The present findings have reaffrmed this connection on a firmer footing. This is particularly noteworthy in light of the current findings. Gender attitudes of young married people were a cause of concern especially among tribal groups and therefore support the need for involvement of both men and women for addressing traditional gender inequitable norms for reproductive behavior. This finding also corroborates with a recent study conducted among tribal populations in rural India on reproductive behavior, where tribals were less likely to practice spacing contraceptive use (SCU) than their non-tribal counterparts. The lower SCU among tribal was driven by gender inequalities and social vulnerabilities (higher son preference, higher fertility preference and low education) [19].

The finding also confirms that the pressures for early child bearing among tribals fall more on young married women than men. Young married women had higher odds of planning a child within one year in comparison to their male counterparts. Qualitative findings congruently found that young married women were more influenced by negative prejudices around delayed childbearing and obliged to have at least one child before seeking family planning services. This was also found in previous studies in India [22]. The role of higher education in influencing fertility intention among non tribal and tribal cannot be neglected, although it was positively associated with tribal status however not significant. The results reflect that higher education (above class 10th) matters in determining fertility behavior among young married people in both non-tribal and tribal groups. Qualitative accounts further demonstrated that young married people from tribal communities had less access to health services and modern contraceptives. There was also poor outreach of reproductive services by community health workers to tribal communities. A review also highlights that tribal people face geographical isolation and limited interactions and exposure, along with poor access to healthcare in India [8].

Limitations of the study

The current findings should be viewed in context of certain limitations, which are important to state. The sample taken for the analysis was small ($n = 273$) and from the larger data on young men and women thus, the findings currently described may not hold true across other geographic and socioeconomic contexts and hence there can be limited generalisations. Further, the use of selective cross-sectional data limits our ability to make causal inferences at macro level. Therefore, further research will be required to extend and validate this analysis by including larger representative sample across different contexts.

Conclusion

This paper reaffirms that efforts need to be directed towards the tribal populations the most. These findings call for pursuing gender transformative strategies for promoting gender equitable attitudes for reproductive decision making especially among tribals. The focus of health and population interventions should not only be to target young married tribals, but also to improve their gender attitudes for the purpose of delaying early childbirth. Efforts should also be intensified for providing access to higher education among tribals and non-tribals as it can significantly influence fertility intention. There is also a need to reduce disparities in access to family planning health services that exist between tribals and other social groups, strengthening outreach for family planning programmes. The findings are relevant to design and tailor appropriate family planning interventions for young married people to meet their current and future fertility desire needs.

Endnotes

[1]Adolescence is defined by WHO as between 10 and 19 years, while youth refers to 15–24 years. Young people refer to the 10–24-year-old age group. For the purpose of this paper, we have used the term young people throughout to refer to 14–21 years of boys and girls in the study population.

Abbreviations

AWC: Anganwadi Center; BPL: Below Poverty Line; FMR: Female-male ratio; GEMS: Gender Equitable Men's Scale; IDIs: In-depth interviews; KIIs: Key informant interviews; NHFS: National Family and Health Survey; OBC: Other Backward Classes; OR: Odds Ratio; SC: Scheduled Caste; SCU: Spacing Contraceptive Use; ST: Scheduled Tribes

Acknowledgements

First and foremost, the authors thank all the study participants and field staff. The authors would like to thank Dr. Rachana Patel for assisting with the analysis. The authors would also like to thank Mr. Praveer Goyal for coordinating the study in the field, Ms. Shilpa Jain, Mr. Mohammed Ahmed and Mr. Shubham Rai for ensuring quality checks during the data collection and assisting in field management.

Funding

The baseline study was conducted from the intervention project funded by American Jewish World Services (AJWS).

Authors' contributions

TK, MC, and SM conceived the study. TK and MC were involved in tool development and data acquisition. TK undertook the analysis and wrote the manuscript. AS and MC contributed to the interpretation of the findings providing inputs for the background, analysis and conclusion section. SM provided overall guidance and review of manuscript draft. All authors read and approved the final manuscript.

Ethics approval and consent to participate

All study participants provided informed consent and/or assent to participate in the study. Verbal informed consent was taken from parents, health care providers and young married men and women prior to the study. Respondents aged below 18 provided assent, while verbal informed consent was sought from their parents.

Ethical permission was obtained from the Institutional Review Board of MAMTA- Health Institute for Mother and Child for conducting research. The following members of the institutional ethics committee approved the study:
1. Dr. Ravi Verma, Chairperson, Ethics Committee, Regional Director (Expert in Gender and Research studies), International Centre for Research on Women (ICRW), Asia Regional Office, Delhi, India.
2. Dr. Sushanta Banerjee, (Expert in Social and behavioral sciences Senior) Advisor, IPAS, New Delhi, India.
3. Dr. U.V. Somayajulu: Expert in Biostatistics Statistics. CEO and Executive Director, SIGMA Research and Consulting Pvt. Ltd., New Delhi, India.
4. Dr. AK Sharma: (Expert in social and behavioral sciences) Professor of Sociology, Department of Humanities and Social Sciences, Indian Institute of Technology, Kanpur. India.
5. Dr. Anita Acharya, Associate Professor, Lady Harding Medical College, Delhi, India.
6. Ms. Sauda Begam, Community Member and Frontline Worker, India.
7. Dr. Sunil Mehra, (Medical Expert on RMNCH+A) Executive Director, MAMTA Health Institute for Mother and Child.

Competing interests

The authors declare that they have no competing interests.

References

1. Daniel EE, Masilamani R, Rahman M. The effect of community-based reproductive health communication interventions on contraceptive use among young married couples in Bihar, India. Int Fam Plan Perspect. 2008; 34(4):189–97.
2. National Family Health Survey (NFHS-3), 2005–06. India, vol. I. Mumbai: IIPS: International Institute for Population Sciences (IIPS) and Macro International; 2007.

3. Prusty RK. Use of contraceptives and unmet need for family planning among tribal women in India and selected hilly states. Journal of Health. Population and Nutrition (JHPN). 2014;32:342–55.

4. Sarkar S, Mishra S, Dayal H, Nathan D. Development and deprivation of Scheduled Tribes. Econ Polit Wkly. 2006;18:4824–7.

5. Subramanian SV, Davey Smith G, Subramanyam M. Indigenous health and socioeconomic status in India. PLoS Med. 2006;3:1794–804.

6. Agarwal S. Health and nutritional disadvantage among tribal women and children of Orissa, India: a situational analysis. Journal of Community Health and medicine. 2013; 317-339. file:///C:/Users/newuser/AppData/Local/Packages/Microsoft.MicrosoftEdge_8wekyb3d8bbwe/TempState/Downloads/2.Heallthandnutritionaldisadvantage%20(2).pdf.

7. National Fact Sheet BF. NFHS-4 (National Family Health Survey-4). International Institute for Population Studies. 2016.

8. Mohindra KS, Labonté R. A systematic review of population health interventions and Scheduled Tribes in India. BMC Public Health. 2010;10:438.

9. Maharatna A. Fertility, mortality and gender bias among tribal population: an Indian perspective. Soc Sci Med. 2000;50:1333–51.

10. Maharatna A. Tribal fertility in India: Socio-cultural influences on demographic behaviour. Econ Polit Wkly. 2000;19:3037–47.

11. Neal SE, Chandra-Mouli V, Chou D. Young people first births in East Africa: disaggregating characteristics, trends and determinants. Reprod Health. 2015;12(1):13.

12. Singh A, Revollo PE. Teenage Marriage, Fertility, and Well-being: Panel Evidence from India. 2016.

13. Susuman SA. Son preference and contraceptive practice among tribal groups in rural south India. Studies of Tribes and Tribals. 2006;4:31–40.

14. Maharatna A. How Can 'Beautiful 'Be' Backward'? Tribes of India in a Long-term Demographic Perspective. Econ Polit Wkly. 2011;22:42–52.

15. Xaxa V. Women and Gender in the Study of Tribes in India. Indian Journal of Gender Studies. 2004;11:345–67.

16. Bramley D, Hebert P, Tuzzio L, Chassin M. Disparities in indigenous health: a cross-country comparison between New Zealand and the United States. Am J Public Health. 2005;95(5):844–50.

17. Barker G, Contreras M, Heilman B, Singh A, Verma R, Nascimento M. Evolving Men: Initial Results from the International Men and Gender Equality Survey (IMAGES). In. Washington, DC and Rio de Janeiro: International Center for Research on Women (ICRW) and Instituto Promundo; 2011. p. 47.

18. Verma RK, Pulerwitz J, Mahendra VS, Khandekar S, Singh AK, Das SS, Nura A, Barkar G. "Promoting Gender Equity as a Strategy to Reduce HIV Risk and Gender-Based Violence among Young Men in India". In Horizons Final Report. Washington, DC: Population Council; 2008.

19. Battala M, et al. Association between tribal status and spacing contraceptive use in rural Maharashtra, India. Sexual & Reproductive Healthcare. 2016:78–80.

20. Mishra A, Nanda P, Speizer IS, Calhoun LM, Zimmerman A, Bhardwaj R. Men's attitudes on gender equality and their contraceptive use in Uttar Pradesh India. Reprod Health. 2014;4; 11(1):41.

21. Khan ME, Patel BC. Male Involvement in Family Planning: A Knowledge Attitude Behaviour and Practice Survey of Agra District. New Delhi: Population Council, June 1997. https://pdfs.semanticscholar.org/95b5/c9516040efc472f6dde5f777abccc5a40fe6.pdf. Accessed 2 Feb 2017.

22. Mathur S, Greene M, Malhotra A. Too Young to Wed: The Lives, Rights, and Health of Young Married Girls. International Centre for Research on Women. 2003; Accessed 10 Feb 2017.

16

A randomized controlled trial of an intervention delivered by mobile phone app instant messaging to increase the acceptability of effective contraception among young people in Tajikistan

Ona McCarthy[1*], Irrfan Ahamed[1], Firuza Kulaeva[2], Ravshan Tokhirov[2], Salokhiddin Saibov[2], Marieka Vandewiele[3], Sarah Standaert[3], Baptiste Leurent[4], Phil Edwards[1], Melissa Palmer[1] and Caroline Free[1]

Abstract

Background: Unintended pregnancy is associated with poorer health outcomes for women and their families. In Tajikistan, around 26% of married 15–24 year old women have an unmet need for contraception. There is some evidence that interventions delivered by mobile phone can affect contraceptive-related behaviour and knowledge. We developed an intervention delivered by mobile phone app instant messaging to improve acceptability of effective contraceptive methods among young people in Tajikistan.

Methods: This was a randomized controlled trial among Tajik people aged 16–24. Participants allocated to the intervention arm had access to an app plus intervention messages. Participants allocated to the control arm had access to the app plus control messages. The primary outcome was acceptability of at least one method of effective contraception at 4 months. Secondary outcomes were use of effective contraception at 4 months and during the study, acceptability of individual methods, service uptake, unintended pregnancy and induced abortion. Process outcomes were knowledge, perceived norms, personal agency and intention. Outcomes were analysed using logistic and linear regression. We conducted a pre-specified subgroup analysis and a post-hoc analysis of change in acceptability from baseline to follow-up.

Results: Five hundred and seventy-three participants were enrolled. Intervention content was included on the app, causing contamination. Four hundred and seventy-two (82%) completed follow-up for the primary outcome. There was no evidence of a difference in acceptability of effective contraception between the groups (66% in the intervention arm vs 64% in the control arm, adjusted OR 1.21, 95% CI .80–1.83, $p = 0.36$). There were no differences in the secondary or process outcomes between groups. There was some evidence that the effect of the intervention was greater among women compared to men (interaction test $p = 0.03$). There was an increase in acceptability of effective contraception from baseline to follow-up (2% to 65%, $p < 0.001$).

(Continued on next page)

* Correspondence: ona.mccarthy@lshtm.ac.uk
[1]Department of Population Health, Faculty of Epidemiology and Population Health, London School of Hygiene & Tropical Medicine, Keppel Street, London WC1E 7HT, UK
Full list of author information is available at the end of the article

(Continued from previous page)

Conclusions: The whole intervention delivered by instant messaging provided no additional benefit over a portion of the intervention delivered by app pages. The important increase in contraceptive acceptability from baseline to follow-up suggests that the intervention content included on the app may influence attitudes. Further research is needed to establish the effect of the intervention on attitudes towards and use of effective contraception among married/sexually active young people.

Keywords: Randomized controlled trial, Tajikistan, Contraception, Smart phone, Reproductive health, Young adults

Plain English summary

Unintended pregnancy is associated with poor health and social outcomes for women and their families. Despite wide availability of contraception, many women globally face barriers in realizing their fertility desires. A woman has an unmet need for modern contraception if she wants to avoid a pregnancy but currently uses no method or a traditional method. In Tajikistan, unmet need for contraception is approximately 26% among married 15–24 year olds. Oppositional attitudes towards contraception (both their own and others') is a common reason women provide for not using contraception.

We developed an intervention delivered by mobile phone to increase the acceptability of effective contraception among young people in Tajikistan. The intervention was developed with young people using an established approach grounded in behavioural science. We conducted a randomized controlled trial to evaluate the effect of the intervention on acceptability of effective contraception. Participants allocated to the intervention group had access to an app plus the intervention messages. Participants allocated to the control group had access to the app plus control messages. The app contained a proportion of the intervention messages that targeted knowledge of and attitudes towards effective contraception. This was different from what was planned in the trial protocol.

The intervention instant messages did not have an added benefit over the app with regards to any of the outcomes. When data from both groups were analysed together, there was a large increase in acceptability of effective contraception from baseline to follow-up (2% at baseline to 65% at follow-up). While we cannot attribute this increase unequivocally to the intervention content, it suggests that providing accurate information and targeting beliefs that influence contraceptive use may be sufficient in changing attitudes towards these methods among young people in Tajikistan. Further research is needed to reliably establish the effect of the intervention on attitudes towards and use of effective contraceptive methods among married/sexually active young people.

Background

Unintended pregnancy persists as a global health problem, with people in lower income countries experiencing them at a higher rate [1]. Unintended pregnancy is associated with a multitude of negative health and economic outcomes for women and their families [2–11]. It is estimated that modern contraceptive use currently prevents 307 million unintended pregnancies each year in developing regions [12]. Satisfying unmet need for modern contraception in these regions would reduce unintended pregnancies by 74% [12]. A woman has an unmet need for modern contraception if she wants to avoid a pregnancy but currently uses no method or a traditional method [13].

Despite a number of governmental policy initiatives and strategies aimed at improving reproductive health in Tajikistan, young people in the country face challenges in gaining accurate information about contraception and in accessing services [14, 15]. The 2012 Tajikistan Demographic and Health Survey is the most reliable resource for family planning data in the country at present [16]. The survey estimates that Tajik women have an average of half a child more than their desired number, implying that if unintended pregnancies were avoided, the total fertility rate would be 3.3 births per woman rather than the actual 3.8 [16]. The effective contraceptive methods available in Tajikistan are oral contraceptive pills (OCs), intrauterine devices (IUDs), injectables and implants ('effective methods are methods with a less than 10% typical use failure rate at 12 months [17–19]). Though these methods are available, around 26% of married 15–24 year old women have an unmet need for contraception [16]. Unmet need is the highest between the ages of 20 to 29 [20]. The main reason women with an unmet need provide for not using contraception are oppositional attitudes towards contraception, both their own and others' [20]. The next common reasons relate to low perceived pregnancy risk and negative attitudes about the methods, such as fear of side-effects [20].

Over the past few decades, the dramatic global increase in mobile phone ownership has engendered enthusiasm amongst researchers and health care providers regarding the use of mobile phones for health care delivery [21–32]. Trials have provided some evidence that interventions delivered by mobile phone can improve contraceptive-related behaviours [33–36] and knowledge [37–39], however others have failed to find an effect [40–43]. The London School of Hygiene and Tropical Medicine (LSHTM) and the Tajik Family Planning Association (TFPA), a Member Association of the International Planned Parenthood Federation (IPPF) collaborated to develop and evaluate an intervention delivered by mobile phone to improve attitudes towards the effective contraceptive methods among young people in Tajikistan.

To evaluate the intervention, we conducted a randomized controlled trial from November 2016 to July 2017. This paper reports the results of the trial. To the best of our knowledge, this is the first trial to evaluate a contraceptive behavioural intervention delivered by mobile phone in Tajikistan. The results contribute to an understanding about how to help young people in Tajikistan avoid unintended pregnancies.

Methods

The methods reported in this section were first published in the trial protocol [44] and the statistical analysis plan [45].

Study design and participants

This was a parallel group, individually randomized superiority trial with a 1:1 allocation ratio. The aim of this trial was to assess the effect of the intervention on the acceptability of effective contraceptive methods among young people in Tajikistan. Participants were eligible to take part in the trial if they were between the ages of 16 and 24, owned a personal Android mobile phone, lived in Tajikistan, could provide informed consent and could read Tajik or Russian. Participants must also have been willing to download a mobile phone app and receive instant messages about contraception through the app. Participants provided informed consent though the secure online trial database and randomization system. All participants received usual care (the normal care that a young person would receive if they attended a sexual and reproductive health service in Tajikistan) and were free to seek any other support.

Intervention and control

The intervention was developed with young Tajik people in 2015–2016 guided by an established approach grounded in behavioural science [46]. It consisted of short mobile phone instant messages delivered through TFPA's 'healthy lifestyles' app over 4 months. It was informed by the Integrated Behavioural Model (IBM) [47] and contained 10 behaviour change methods (BCM)

(belief selection, facilitation, anticipated regret, guided practice, verbal persuasion, tailoring, cultural similarity, arguments, shifting perspective and goal setting) [48], adapted for delivery by mobile phone. The messages provided information about contraception, targeted beliefs identified in the development phase that influence contraceptive use and aimed to support young people in believing that they can influence their reproductive health.

The messages are tailored according to marital status and gender, resulting in four sets of messages (female-married, female-not married, male-married and male-not married). The majority of the messages in the four sets are the same, with minor tailoring so that the messages are relevant to these groups. (Marital status was used as a proxy for sexual activity because the target group and TFPA considered it inappropriate to ask directly about sexual activity.) Further details about the intervention are presented in the trial protocol [44] and in a forthcoming intervention development publication.

Contamination

Participants allocated to the intervention arm had access to the app plus the intervention instant messages. Participants allocated to the control arm had access to the app plus control instant messages about trial participation. Contrary to what was planned in the trial protocol [44], the app contained intervention content. The app was intended to contain only basic information about contraception and no behaviour change methods. This contamination occurred due to a misunderstanding between the partners collaborating in the research.

The app contraception pages included just under a third of the intervention content. Specifically, 57% of the female-married intervention messages that provide accurate information about the effective contraceptive methods and 36% of the messages that use the BCM 'belief selection' were included on the app. Forty-four percent of the female-married intervention content included on the app used the same words as the intervention messages (56% did not use the same words but was very similar and conveyed the same meaning). The intervention content included on the app aimed to help individuals: name the effective methods, describe how the effective methods work, list services that provide effective contraception, list the risks and benefits of the effective methods, describe how methods are used, express positive attitudes towards the effective methods and differentiate between real potential side-effects and misconceptions about the methods.

Allocation and intervention delivery

After providing informed consent, participants completed the baseline questionnaire through the database and randomization system. The allocation sequence was generated by the remote computer-based randomization software. Randomization occurred immediately after baseline data was submitted. All participants downloaded the app immediately after they submitted their baseline data. The delivery of the intervention (and control) instant messages began on the same day if participants downloaded the app before 13:00 and the following day if they downloaded it after 13:00.

Protecting against bias

Due to the nature of the intervention, participants would have been aware of the allocation soon after they started receiving the messages. Local research staff collecting outcome data were masked to allocation unless the participant revealed it to them. Researchers that analysed the data were masked to treatment allocation.

Outcomes

Primary outcome

The primary outcome was the proportion of participants reporting that at least one method of effective contraception was acceptable at 4 months post randomization. The primary outcome measure was constructed based on guidelines for measuring IBM constructs [47, 49, 50] and tested for face validity with the target group. The acceptability of each method was measured by the following stems: Using the [method] ...causes infertility, ...causes unwanted side effects, ...is easy, ...is a good way to prevent pregnancy and I would recommend the [method] to a friend. The IUD and implant include an additional stem: The [method] insertion would not be a problem. The response options for each scale were strongly disagree, disagree, not sure, agree, strongly agree and I do not know what the [method] is. A method was acceptable if participants reported 'agree' or 'strongly agree' for all scales except for '...causes infertility' and '...causes unwanted side effects' stems, for which 'disagree' or 'strongly disagree' indicated acceptability.

Secondary outcomes

Secondary outcomes were: use (or partner's use) of effective contraception; acceptability of individual methods; use (or partner's use) of effective contraception at any time during the 4 months; service uptake; unintended pregnancy and induced abortion.

Process outcomes The process outcomes were: knowledge of effective contraception; perceived norms in relation to using and communicating with partners about contraception; personal agency in using (women only) and communicating with partners about contraception; intention to use effective contraception (women only) and intervention dose received. Details about the

scales used to measure knowledge, perceived norm, personal agency and intention are reported in the trial protocol [44].

Data collection

Data was collected at baseline and at 4 months post-randomization using questionnaires. At baseline, we collected personal and demographic data and acceptability of at least one method of effective contraception (using the same scales as the primary outcome measure). All baseline data was entered onto the trial database system by the participant on their mobile phone. At 4 month follow-up, we collected all outcomes and the following data: if participants report using an effective method, where they obtained it; current pregnancy intention; whether they knew someone else that took part in the study and if so, if they read each other's messages; if they stopped the messages; if they experienced physical violence since being in the study and if anything good or bad happened as a result of receiving the messages. An instant message that included a link to the database to complete the follow-up questionnaire was sent to all participants through the app 4 months after downloading the app. If participants did not complete the follow-up questionnaire themselves, local research staff contacted them by telephone to collect their data.

Sample size

The trial was powered to detect a 15% increase in acceptability of effective contraception in the intervention group compared with the control group. Four hundred and fifty-four participants allowed for 90% power to detect a 15% absolute increase in acceptability, assuming 50% acceptability in the control group (i.e. 50% in the control vs 65% in the intervention, an odds ratio of 1.86). Allowing for 20% loss to follow-up, we aimed to randomize 570 people.

Statistical analysis

The trial protocol was accepted for publication on 21 July 2017 [44] and the statistical analysis plan was publicly released on 16 August 2017 [45]. The analysis was conducted using Stata 15. Analyses were according to randomized arm and only participants with complete outcome data were included in the principal analysis. All statistical tests were two-sided and considered significant at the 5% level. Unmasking occurred on 29 August 2017, after the analyses outlined within the analysis plan were complete.

Loss to follow-up and missing data

We used a chi-squared test to investigate whether loss to follow-up differed by arm. We used logistic regression to compare baseline characteristics of participants that completed follow-up against participants that did not. We investigated whether predictors of loss to follow-up differed by arm by testing for an interaction.

Principal analysis

Analysis of the primary outcome

We compared the proportion that reported that at least one method was acceptable in each group using logistic regression. We report the crude and adjusted odds ratio (OR) along with the 95% confidence interval (CI) and *p*-value. We adjusted the primary analysis regression for the following pre-specified baseline covariates: pregnancy intention (wants to avoid/other); gender (female/male); age (16–19/20–24); highest education level completed (university/other) and acceptability of effective contraception (at least one method acceptable/ no methods acceptable) [44, 45].

Analysis of the secondary outcomes

The analysis of the secondary outcomes was similar to the analysis of the primary outcome. We estimated the difference between the groups using logistic regression and report odds ratios with 95% CIs and *p*-values. Regressions were adjusted for the baseline covariates pregnancy intention, gender, age, education level and acceptability (of at least one method or with acceptability of individual methods, of the corresponding method).

Analysis of the process outcomes

The process outcomes perceived norms, personal agency and intention were comprised of ordinal scales. Each scale was analysed individually using ordered logistic regression to estimate proportional ORs. For knowledge, each correct answer received one point. The points were summed and an overall score was produced. We used linear regression to test for a difference in mean scores between the arms. To assess the 'dose' of the intervention that the intervention participants received, we analysed the number of messages that participants reported to have read (all, most, some, none) and whether they stopped the messages.

Additional analyses

Sensitivity analyses

We conducted two sensitivity analyses regarding the missing data. In the first, we considered that participants lost to follow-up did not find at least one method acceptable. In the second, we adjusted for the main baseline predictors of missingness. Both sensitivity analyses were adjusted for the baseline covariates pregnancy intention, gender, age, education level and acceptability.

Subgroup analysis

We conducted an exploratory subgroup analysis for the primary outcome to determine if the intervention effect varied by baseline characteristics. The pre-specified subgroups were gender (female/male); age (split at the median); marital status (married/not married); number of children (0/1+); ethnicity (Tajik/other); occupation (in education/other); highest education level completed (university/other) and pregnancy intention (wants to avoid/other). Within the subgroups, we assessed heterogeneity of treatment effect with a test for interaction [51–55]. We estimated ORs along with 95% CIs for each subgroup.

Contamination

To assess the potential for contamination, we report the proportion of control group participants that reported that they read another participant's messages and the proportion of intervention participants that reported that their messages were read by another participant.

Change from baseline

In addition to the analyses specified in the statistical analysis plan, we tested for a change in the primary outcome from baseline to follow-up, using McNemar's χ^2 test for paired data. This post hoc non-randomized analysis was conducted to explore the increase in acceptability overall, as the app included intervention content (see Discussion).

Results

Recruitment, randomization, exclusions

Between 16 November 2016 and 1 March 2017, there were 580 randomizations. During the analysis, we discovered that five participants enrolled and were randomized twice. For the three participants that were allocated to the same arm on both randomizations, we kept them in the analysis using the baseline data from their first record. For the two participants that were allocated to different arms, we excluded them from the analysis. This resulted in 573 participants included in the trial (see Discussion).

Two hundred and seventy-five participants were allocated to the intervention arm and 298 participants were allocated to the control arm (Fig. 1). No participants withdrew from the trial after allocation.

Baseline characteristics

Baseline characteristics of trial participants are reported in Table 1. Mean age was 20 years, and 53% were male. Ninety-four percent were not married (259/573), and only 2% (13/573) found at least one method of effective

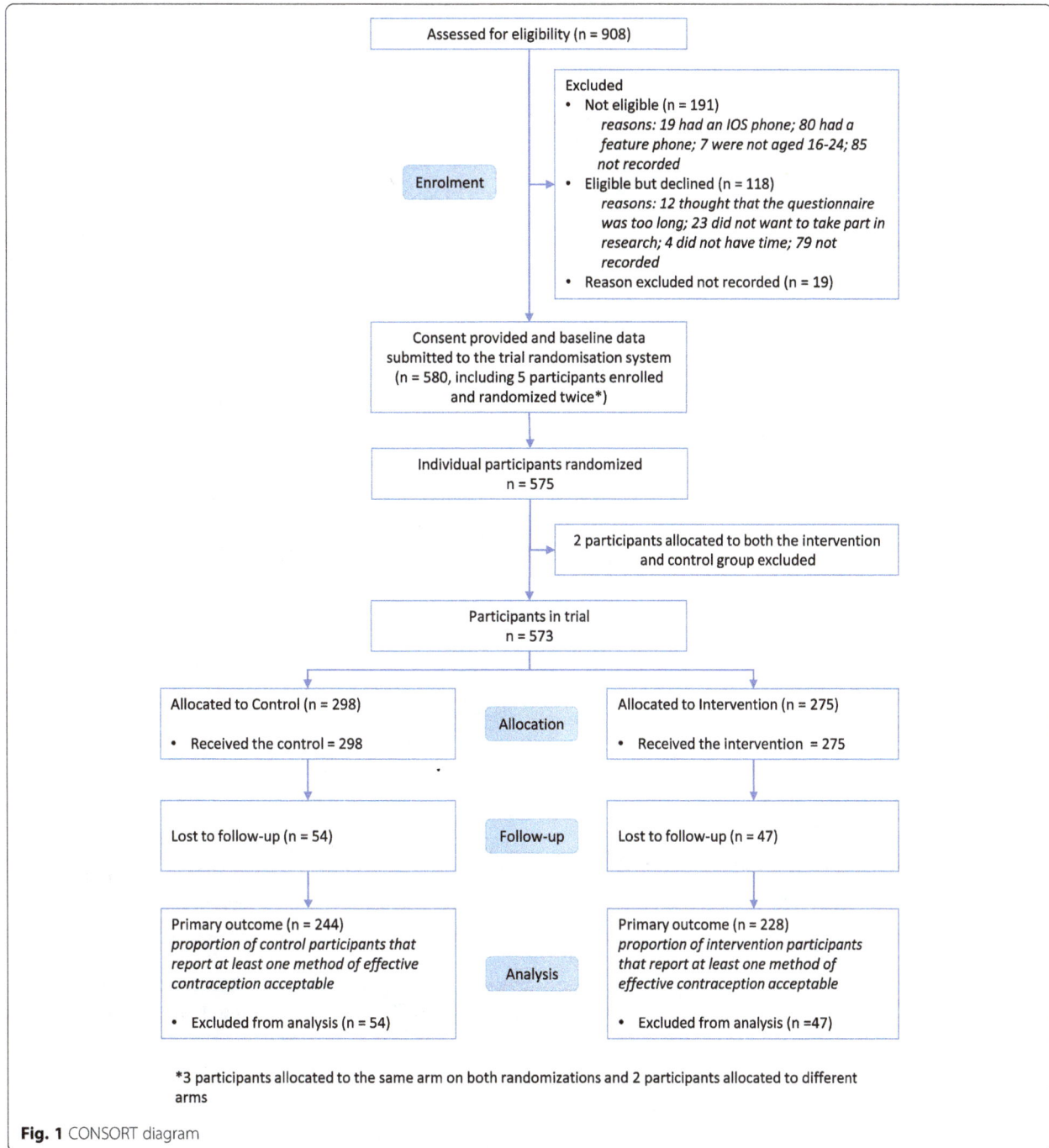

Fig. 1 CONSORT diagram

contraception acceptable. Characteristics were similar between the two groups.

Loss to follow-up

Four hundred and seventy-six participants total (83%) contributed follow-up data. Four hundred and seventy-two participants (82%) completed the trial follow-up for the primary outcome (intervention, $n = 228$; control, $n = 244$) (Fig. 1). Retention did not differ between the arms (83% in the intervention vs 82% in the control, $p = 0.75$). The main predictors of retention were male gender (OR 1.78, $p = 0.01$), Tajik ethnicity (OR 2.22, $p - 0.03$) and having completed a level of education lower than university at enrolment (OR 1.79, $p = 0.02$). The effect of these predictors did not differ by arm (interaction test p-values: gender, $p = 0.72$; ethnicity, $p = 0.41$; education level, $p = 0.98$). Detailed characteristics of follow-up completers and non-completers are reported in Additional file 1.

Table 1 Baseline characteristics

		Control N = 298, % (n)	Intervention N = 275, % (n)	All participants N = 573, % (n)
Age	mean [sd]	20.00 [2.41]	19.93 [2.24]	19.98 [2.33]
	16–19	53.02 (158)	56.73 (156)	54.80 (314)
	20–24	46.98 (140)	43.27(119)	45.20(259)
Gender	female	45.97(137)	47.27 (130)	46.60 (267)
	male	54.03 (161)	52.73 (145)	53.40 (306)
Marital status	married	6.71 (20)	5.82 (16)	6.28 (36)
	not-married	93.29 (278)	94.18 (259)	93.72 (537)
Number of children	0	95.64 (285)	97.09 (267)	96.34 (552)
	1	2.01 (6)	2.18 (6)	2.09 (12)
	2 or more	2.35 (7)	0.73 (2)	1.57 (9)
Ethnicity	Tajik	92.62 (276)	93.82 (258)	93.19 (534)
	Russian	2.35 (7)	0.36 (1)	1.40 (8)
	Uzbek	5.03 (15)	5.45 (15)	5.24 (30)
	other	0 (0)	0.36 (1)	0.17 (1)
Occupation	school	17.79 (53)	17.09 (47)	17.45 (100)
	university	68.46 (204)	70.55 (194)	69.46 (398)
	working	10.74 (32)	10.55 (29)	10.65 (61)
	training	0.67 (2)	0 (0)	0.35 (2)
	parent	0.34 (1)	0 (0)	0.17 (1)
	not working	1.68 (5)	1.82 (5)	1.75 (10)
	university & working	0.34 (1)	0 (0)	0.17 (1)
Highest level of education completed	primary	12.75 (38)	13.09 (36)	12.91 (74)
	secondary	66.11 (197)	59.64 (164)	63.00 (361)
	university	19.46 (58)	25.82 (71)	22.51 (129)
	other	1.68 (5)	1.45 (4)	1.57 (9)
Current pregnancy intention ('Do you want a pregnancy now?')	yes	3.02 (9)	4.00 (11)	3.49 (20)
	no	12.42 (37)	5.82 (16)	9.25 (53)
	unsure	1.01 (3)	0.73 (2)	0.87 (5)
	not married[a]	83.56 (249)	89.45 (246)	86.39 (495)
Baseline method	none	31.88 (95)	29.45 (81)	30.72 (176)
	male condom	2.01 (6)	1.09 (3)	1.57 (9)
	IUD[b]	0.67 (2)	0 (0)	0.35 (2)
	not married[a]	65.10 (194)	69.09 (190)	67.02 (384)
	LAM[c]	0 (0)	0.36 (1)	0.17 (1)
	other	0.34 (1)	0 (0)	0.17 (1)
At least one effective method is acceptable	yes	2.68 (8)	1.82 (5)	2.27 (13)
	no	97.32 (290)	98.18 (270)	97.73 (560)
Pill acceptability	yes	1.34 (4)	0.73 (2)	1.05 (6)
	no	98.66 (294)	99.27 (273)	98.95 (567)
IUD acceptability	yes	1.34 (4)	0 (0)	0.70 (4)

Table 1 Baseline characteristics (Continued)

		Control N = 298, % (n)	Intervention N = 275, % (n)	All participants N = 573, % (n)
	no	98.66 (294)	100 (275)	99.30 (569)
Injection acceptability	yes	0.67 (2)	1.45 (4)	1.05 (6)
	no	99.33 (296)	98.55 (271)	98.95 (567)
Implant acceptability	yes	0.34 (1)	0.73 (2)	0.52 (3)
	no	99.66 (297)	99.27 (273)	99.48 (570)

[a]The response 'not married' was used as a proxy for not being sexually active
[b]IUD Intrauterine device
[c]LAM Lactational amenorrhea method

Primary outcome

In the intervention arm, 66% (151/228) reported that at least one method of contraception was acceptable compared to 64% (156/244) in the control arm (Table 2). There was no evidence of a difference in acceptability between the groups (crude OR 1.11, 95% CI .76–1.62, $p = 0.60$; adjusted OR 1.21, 95% CI .80–1.83, $p = 0.36$).

Secondary outcomes

There were no significant differences in any of the secondary outcomes between the groups (Table 3).

Process outcomes

There were no significant differences in any of the process outcomes between the groups (Table 4).

Potential for contamination

Three percent (8/243) of control participants said that they read the messages of someone else in the study. Nine percent (21/227) of intervention participants said that someone else in the study read their messages.

Participants' report of physical violence during the study

Overall, 0.85% (4/470) reported that they experienced physical violence since being in the study (0.41% in the control and 1.32% in the intervention, $p = 0.57$).

Sensitivity analyses

The effect of the intervention on the primary outcome observed in the principal analysis did not change when we considered participants lost to follow-up did not find

Table 2 Primary outcome

	Control N = 244, % (n)	Intervention N = 228, % (n)	OR (95% CI)	p-value
At least one effective method is acceptable[a]	63.93 (156)	66.23 (151)	1.21 (.80–1.83)	0.36

[a]adjusted for pregnancy intention, gender, age, education level and acceptability at baseline

Table 3 Secondary outcomes

	Control % (n/N)	Intervention % (n/N)	OR (95% CI)	p-value
Use of effective contraception[a]	3.66 (9/246)	1.30 (3/230)	.35 (.06–1.42)	0.18
Pill acceptability[b]	56.56 (138/244)	60.53 (138)	1.32 (.88–2.00)	0.18
IUD acceptability[b]	52.87 (129/244)	51.32 (117/228)	1.00 (.67–1.50)	0.98
Injection acceptability[b]	54.51 (133/244)	55.26 (126/228)	1.14 (.76–1.70)	0.52
Implant acceptability[b]	48.77 (119/244)	48.68 (111/228)	1.08 (.73–1.59)	0.71
Effective contraceptive use during the 4 months[a]	2.88 (7/243)	1.76 (4/227)	.61 (.13–2.42)	0.62
Service uptake[c] (attended a service one or more times)	10.29 (25/243)	7.93 (18/227)	.76 (.39–1.46)	0.41
Unintended pregnancy[c]	0 (0)	0 (0)	–	–
Induced abortion[c]	0 (0)	0 (0)	–	–

[a]based on unadjusted exact logistic regression, due to small numbers
[b]adjusted for pregnancy intention, gender, age, education level and the corresponding method acceptability at baseline
[c]adjusted for pregnancy intention, gender, age, education level and acceptability at baseline

at least one method acceptable (OR 1.20, 95% CI .84–1.73, $p = 0.31$) or when we adjusted the model for the predictors of missingness (OR 1.21, 95% CI .80–1.85, $p = 0.35$).

Subgroup analysis
There was some evidence that the effect of the intervention was greater among women compared to men (interaction test $p = 0.03$). (Fig. 2).

Change from baseline analysis
Among the 472 participants who completed follow-up 2% ($n = 10$) thought that at least one method was acceptable at baseline, which increased to 65% at follow-up ($n = 307$, $p < 0.001$) (Fig. 3). Acceptability for the individual methods increased from 1% at baseline to 49%–58% at follow-up ($p < 0.001$).

Discussion
Main results
Contrary to what was planned in the trial protocol, the app contained intervention content. Both intervention and control participants received intervention content targeting knowledge and attitudes towards effective contraception, including the BCM 'belief selection'. The trial therefore evaluated the effect of the whole intervention with all ten BCMs (belief selection, facilitation, anticipated regret, guided practice, verbal persuasion, tailoring, cultural similarity, arguments, shifting perspective and goal setting) delivered by instant messaging, compared to a proportion of the intervention delivered on the app pages with the BCM belief selection.

The trial found no evidence of a difference in acceptability of at least one effective contraceptive method between the intervention and control groups. There was also no evidence of a difference in any of the secondary and process outcomes between the groups (use of effective contraception, service uptake, knowledge,

perceived norms, personal agency and intention to use effective contraception). This indicates that the intervention content delivered by the intervention messages only (includes nine additional BCMs targeting attitudes and personal agency) did not have an additional benefit over the app regarding these outcomes. The subgroup analysis suggests that the intervention delivered by instant messaging could be more effective among women compared to men. When data from both groups were analysed together, there was a large statistically significant increase in acceptability from baseline to follow-up.

Comparisons with other research
Trials that have evaluated interventions delivered by mobile phone to improve contraceptive-related outcomes have had mixed results [33–43]. We are conducting trials in Bolivia and Palestine that are evaluating the effect of interventions similar to the Tajik intervention on acceptability and use of effective contraception [56, 57]. The results of the three trials together should contribute to a better understanding of the effect of the intervention evaluated in this Tajik trial.

Our trial shows no additional benefit on the outcomes from the nine BCMs deliver by instant messaging. No previous research reports the effectiveness of these BCMs aimed at improving contraceptive-related outcomes delivered by mobile phone [58].

Ongoing trials of interventions delivered by mobile phone to improve reproductive health are measuring participants' experience of violence during their participation in the trial [56, 57, 59]. In this Tajik trial, we found no association between the intervention and experience of violence. While this is reassuring, both groups had access to the app so we are unable to assess the effect of the app on partner violence.

Table 4 Process outcomes

		Control % (n/N)	Intervention % (n/N)	proportional OR* (95% CI), p-value
Knowledge of effective contraception		Mean = 4.00 [sd = 2.04]	Mean = 4.08 [sd = 2.02]	.08** (−.29–.44), 0.69
My friends would use the pill, IUD, injection or implant if they wanted to prevent pregnancy	strongly disagree	3.70 (9/243)	1.33 (3/226)	1.40 (.97–2.01), 0.07
	disagree	4.53 (11/243)	5.31 (12/226)	
	not sure	17.28 (42/243)	16.37 (37/226)	
	agree	64.61 (157/243)	59.29 (134/226)	
	strongly agree	9.88 (24/243)	17.70 (40/226)	
My friends would talk to their husband/wife about contraception if they wanted to prevent a pregnancy	strongly disagree	1.23 (3/243)	1.33 (3/226)	1.09 (.76–1.57), 0.64
	disagree	5.35 (13/243)	6.64 (15/226)	
	not sure	16.05 (39/243)	15.93 (36/226)	
	agree	65.02 (158/243)	59.29 (134/226)	
	strongly agree	12.35 (30/243)	16.81 (38/226)	
If you wanted to use the pill, IUD, injection or implant, how easy would it be for you to use it? (women only)	very difficult	7.62 (8/105)	5.83 (6/103)	1.43 (.87–2.34), 0.16
	difficult	17.14 (18/105)	9.71 (10/103)	
	not sure	27.62 (29/105)	29.13 (30/103)	
	easy	38.10 (40/105)	43.69 (45/103)	
	very easy	9.52 (10/105)	11.65 (12/103)	
If you wanted to talk to your husband/wife about contraception, how easy would it be for you to talk to him/her?	very difficult	3.70 (9/243)	3/10 (7/226)	1.22 (.86–1.73), 0.26
	difficult	6.17 (15/243)	7.52 (17/226)	
	not sure	14.81 (36/243)	14.16 (32/226)	
	easy	60.49 (147/243)	53.10 (120/226)	
	very easy	14.81 (36/243)	22.12 (50/226)	
If you wanted to use the pill, IUD, injection or implant, how certain are you that you could use it? (women only)	very certain I could not	2.86 (3/105)	5.83 (6/103)	.99 (.60–1.63), 0.96
	certain I could not	6.67 (7/105)	7.77 (8/103)	
	not sure	38.10 (40/105)	32.04 (33/103)	
	certain I could	40.00 (42/105)	41.75 (43/103)	
	very certain I could	12.38 (13/105)	12.62 (13/103)	
If you wanted to talk to your husband/wife about contraception, how certain are you that you could talk to him/her?	very certain I could not	1.23 (3/243)	2.65 (6/226)	1.10 (.78–1.53), 0.60
	certain I could not	13.17 (32/243)	12.39 (28/226)	
	not sure	16.46 (40/243)	16.81 (38/226)	
	certain I could	50.62 (123/243)	44.25 (100/226)	
	very certain I could	18.52 (45/243)	23.89 (54/226)	
I intend to use the pill, IUD, injection or implant	strongly disagree	4.76 (5/105)	2.91 (3/103)	1.37 (.84–2.25), 0.21
	disagree	10.48 (11/105)	12.62 (13/103)	
	not sure	31.43 (33/105)	25.24 (26/103)	
	agree	39.05 (41/105)	34.95 (36/103)	
	strongly agree	14.29 (15/105)	24.27 (25/103)	
Number of messages read	all		32.16 (73/227)	
	most		43.61 (99/227)	
	some		18.50 (42/227)	
	none		5.73 (13/227)	
Proportion of intervention participants that stopped the intervention			29.07 (66/227)	

*estimated from ordered logistic regression
**mean difference

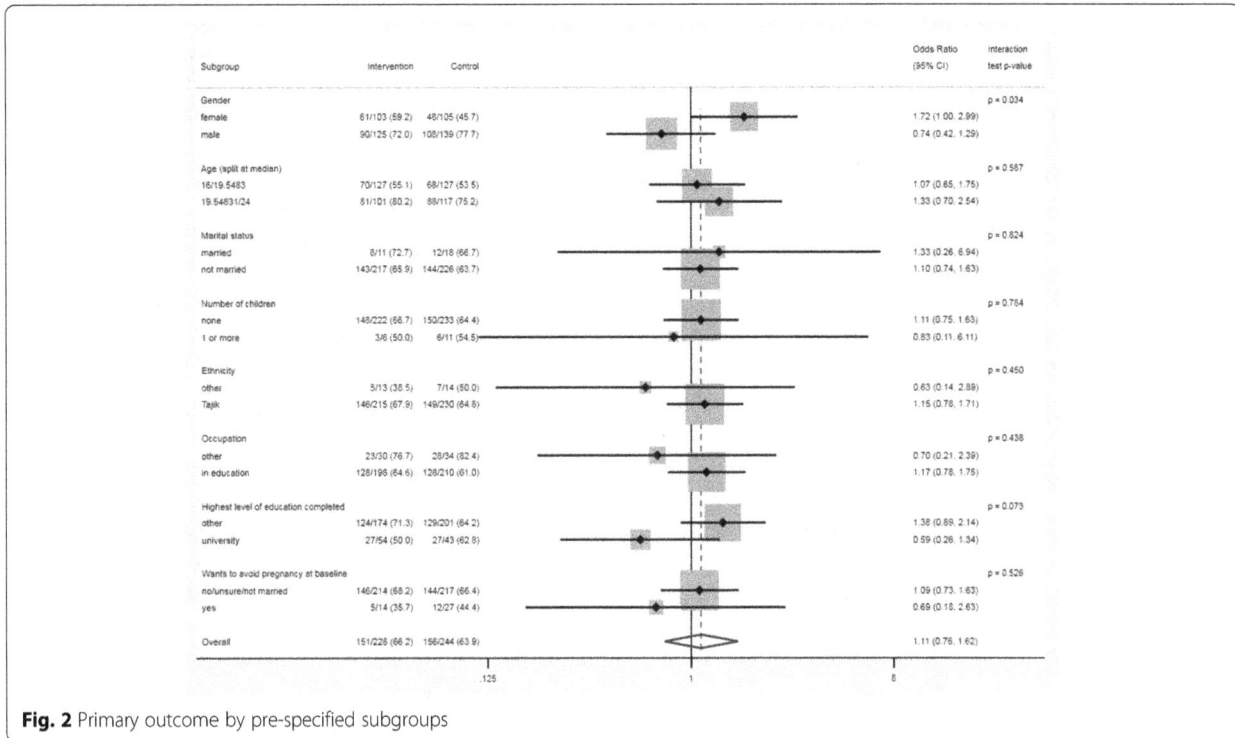

Fig. 2 Primary outcome by pre-specified subgroups

Strengths and limitations

The trial conduct has a number of strengths. We recruited our target number of participants and were able to collect follow-up data for an acceptable proportion of them, given that the sample size allowed for 20% loss. We developed and tested a remote trial database and randomization system, which successfully generated and concealed the allocation sequence and achieved well-balanced groups. An important limitation is that the app included intervention content, as discussed above. This constitutes a protocol deviation and the trial was therefore not able to answer the primary question it aimed to answer. Because the self-reported acceptability scales were collected by telephone by the research staff, participants may have been more likely to report positive attitudes than they were at baseline where

they completed the questionnaire by themselves on their phones. Regarding the large increase in acceptability from baseline to follow-up, we cannot rule out the possibility that at least a portion of this increase was due to participation in the trial as opposed to the intervention itself; participants were aware that the trial involved changing attitudes towards contraception. Five participants enrolled and were randomized twice.

There were inconsistencies in participants' self-reporting of marital status. The proportion that responded 'not married' to the current pregnancy intention (495/573, 86%) and the baseline method question (384/573, 67%) is lower than the proportion that responded 'not married' when asked directly about their marital status (537/573, 94%). We cannot say why

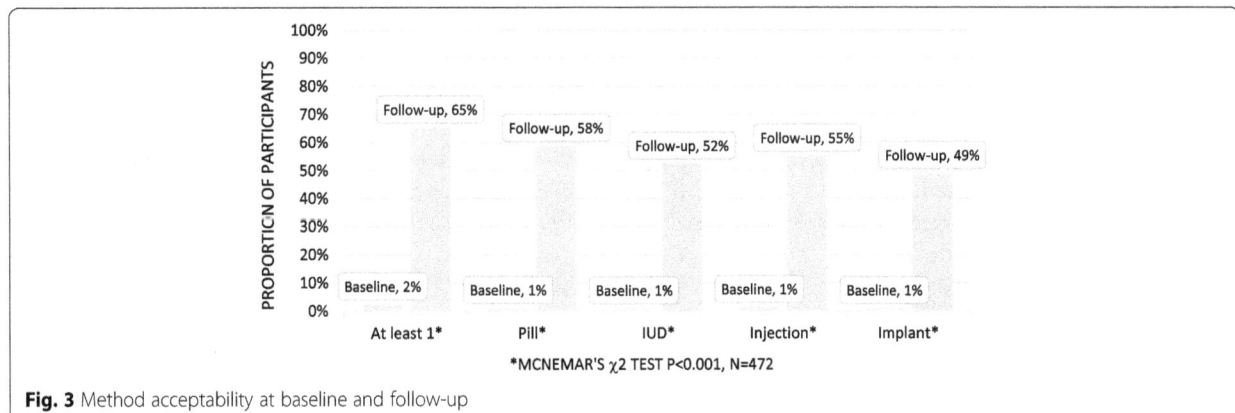

Fig. 3 Method acceptability at baseline and follow-up

these inconsistencies occurred. However, we can specu-late that some participants who responded 'not married' to the marital status question were sexually active and responded to the other two questions with responses other than 'not married'.

Thirty six percent of people assessed for eligibility (328/908) were excluded from the study. The reason for ineligibility was not recorded for 85 people, which could limit the generalizability of the trial findings. While the recording of this information was not complete, of those that are known, the majority appear to have been excluded because they either did not have an Android phone ($n = 99$). If those who do not own a smartphone are less likely to find at least one method of effective contracep-tion acceptable, this could affect the generalisability of the results. Smartphone ownership is rapidly in-creasing however, and ownership could be an option for a greater proportion of young people across different socioeconomic communities in the near future.

Implications of the findings

The finding that the intervention instant messages did not have an additional benefit over the app along with the large increase in acceptability from baseline to follow-up suggests that participants read the app contra-ception pages. It may be that in a context such as Tajikistan, where young people have limited access to information and support about reproductive health, they are willing to read static app pages about this topic. In comparison, a trial in the United Kingdom found that young people did not engage heavily with a sexual and reproductive health website [60, 61]. In contexts such as the United Kingdom where information and support are more accessible, interventions delivered on app pages and websites may be utilized less frequently than in contexts such as Tajikistan.

Because the intervention content included on the app aimed to improve knowledge of and attitudes towards effective contraception, it is not surprising that there was no evidence of a difference between the groups regarding these outcomes. Though the large increase in acceptability from baseline to follow-up cannot be unequivocally attributed to the intervention content, an increase this large suggests that the intervention content included on the app at least was partially effective in improving attitudes to-wards the effective methods. Because the intervention is well-specified, we were able to identify the components of the intervention that may have been effective in producing this change (accurate informa-tion and targeting beliefs using the BCM belief selection) [46, 48].

Despite the contamination that occurred, interven-tion participants received content that control partici-pants did not. The secondary outcomes use and service uptake and the process outcomes personal agency and intention are related to the content that only intervention participants received. There are a number of potential explanations for why we did not observe a difference between the groups in these outcomes. The first is that the BCMs targeting these outcomes did not work. This could have been because the conditions under which the methods have been shown to be effective were not fully satisfied [46, 48]. In addition, because a large proportion of meaning comes from visual cues in face-to-face interaction [46], some of the meaning of the BCMs may have been lost when delivered by mobile phone. For ex-ample, the BCM 'guided practice' requires skill dem-onstration, enactment and individual feedback. While the intervention messages demonstrated and provided instruc-tion, we were not able to observe the participant enacting the behavior or to provide individual feedback. This may have resulted in a loss of effectiveness of the BCM. Another explanation is that intervention could be more effective on these secondary and process outcomes with people where the behaviour is salient, such as with those who are mar-ried/sexually active or soon to be. In this trial however, only 6% (36/573) were married/sexually active, which was too small to explore this possibility. Alternatively, the app alone may have been effective in influencing these secondary and process outcomes; in the Tajik context, providing accurate information from a credible source and targeting the pre-identified beliefs may be sufficient. Finally, these secondary and process outcomes could have be so strongly influenced by environmental conditions (e.g. stigma regarding sexual activity before marriage and pressure to bear children) that they are not amenable to change by a mobile phone inter-vention only.

While caution is necessary in interpreting the results of the subgroup analysis, it suggests that the whole inter-vention delivered by instant messaging could be more effective among women compared to men. The trials in Bolivia and Palestine involve women only so the results should provide additional evidence of the intervention's effectiveness in women.

We are currently conducting qualitative interviews with trial participants to explore their experiences in receiving the intervention and app content. If partici-pants were positive about receiving the intervention messages, this could support the delivery of the messages with the download of the app. The fact that the intervention is already developed and therefore inex-pensive to deliver, plus the fact that it does not appear to cause harm, also supports the delivery of the messages with the download of the app.

Conclusions

This trial demonstrated that the whole intervention delivered by app instant messaging provided no additional benefit over a portion of the intervention delivered by the app pages. An analysis of participants randomized to the control and intervention groups together showed a large significant increase in acceptability from baseline to follow-up. Further research is needed to establish the effect of the intervention on attitudes towards and use of effective contraceptive methods among married/sexually active young people.

Abbreviations
BCM: Behaviour change method; CI: Confidence interval; IPPF: International Planned Parenthood Federation; LSHTM: London School of Hygiene & Tropical Medicine; OR: Odds ratio; TFPA: Tajik Family Planning Association

Acknowledgements
We would like to thank the young people in Tajikistan who participated in both the intervention development phase and the trial. We would also like to thank Matlyuba Salikhova, Safarbek Saidov, Ramziyor Saydaliev and Khusrav Bobobekov who promoted the study and assisted with collection of the follow-up data. We are extremely grateful for their hard work and volunteering their time. Finally, we would like to thank the International Planned Parenthood Federation for funding the trial and Alison McKinley, the Senior Research and Evaluation Officer for the Innovation Programme, for her support throughout the project.

Funding
The trial was supported by the International Planned Parenthood Federation Innovation Programme. IPPF had some influence over the study design (MV and SS) but were not involved in the data collection or analysis.

Authors' contributions
OLM designed and managed the trial, conducted the analysis and wrote the manuscript. FK coordinated and conducted the trial recruitment and follow-up and contributed to planning discussions regarding the trial. RT facilitated trial implementation, contributed to planning discussions regarding the trial and took overall local responsibility for the project. SSa facilitated trial implementation and contributed to planning discussions regarding the trial. MV and SSt contributed to planning discussions regarding the trial. IA developed the trial database and randomization system. BL provided advice regarding the statistical analysis and reviewed the Stata analysis code. PE provided oversight regarding the statistical analysis. MP reviewed the primary outcome Stata analysis code. CF provided guidance regarding the trial design and took overall academic responsibility for the project. All authors revised the work, approved the version to be published and agree to be accountable for all aspects of the work.

Competing interests
The authors declare that they have no competing interests.

Author details
[1]Department of Population Health, Faculty of Epidemiology and Population Health, London School of Hygiene & Tropical Medicine, Keppel Street, London WC1E 7HT, UK. [2]Tajik Family Planning Association, 10 Rudaki Avenue, TC 'Sadbarg', 7th floor, Dushanbe, Tajikistan. [3]International Planned Parenthood Federation European Network, Rue Royale 146, 1000 Brussels, Belgium. [4]Department of Medical Statistics, Faculty of Epidemiology and Population Health, London School of Hygiene & Tropical Medicine, Keppel Street, London WC1E 7HT, UK.

References
1. Sedgh G, Singh S, Hussain R. Intended and unintended pregnancies worldwide in 2012 and recent trends. Stud Fam Plan. 2014;45(3):301–14.
2. Tsui AO, McDonald-Mosley R, Burke AE. Family planning and the burden of unintended pregnancies. Epidemiol Rev. 2010;32:152–74.
3. Logan C, Holcombe E, Manlove J, Ryan S. The consequences of unintended childbearing: a white paper. Washington, DC: Child Trends; 2007.
4. Khajehpour M, Simbar M, Jannesari S, Ramezani-Tehrani F, Majd HA. Health status of women with intended and unintended pregnancies. Public Health. 2013;127(1):58–64.
5. Gipson JD, Koenig MA, Hindin MJ. The effects of unintended pregnancy on infant, child, and parental health: a review of the literature. Stud Fam Plan. 2008;39(1):18–38.
6. Nakku JEM, Nakasi G, Mirembe F. Postpartum major depression at six weeks in primary health care: prevalence and associated factors. Afr Health Sci. 2006;6(4):207–14.
7. Cheng D, Schwarz EB, Douglas E, Horon I. Unintended pregnancy and associated maternal preconception, prenatal and postpartum behaviors. Contraception. 2009;79(3):194–8.
8. Marston C, Cleland J. Do unintended pregnancies carried to term lead to adverse outcomes for mother and child? An assessment in five developing countries. Popul Stud. 2003;57(1):77–93.
9. Shah PS, Balkhair T, Ohlsson A, Beyene J, Scott F, Frick C. Intention to become pregnant and low birth weight and preterm birth: a systematic review. Matern Child Health J. 2011;15(2):205–16.
10. Mohllajee AP, Curtis KM, Morrow B, Marchbanks PA. Pregnancy intention and its relationship to birth and maternal outcomes. Obstet Gynecol. 2007; 109(3):678–86.
11. Brown SS, Eisenberg L, editors. The Best Intentions: Unintended Pregnancy and the Well-Being of Children and Families. Washington D.C.: National Academies Press; 1995.
12. Darroch JE, Audam S, Biddlecom A, Kopplin G, Riley T, Singh S, et al. Adding it up: the costs and benefits of investing in sexual and reproductive health 2017 (Investing in contraception and maternal and newborn health fact sheet): Guttmacher Institute; 2017.
13. Singh S, Darroch J, Ashford L. Adding it up: the costs and benefits of investing in sexual and reproductive health 2014. New York: Guttmacher Institute; 2014.
14. UNFPA Tajikistan country Programme 2010–2015 evaluation report. United Nations Population Fund; 2014.
15. Country programme document for Tajikistan. United Nations Population Fund; 2015.
16. Tajikistan Demographic and Health Survey 2012. Dushanbe, Tajikistan, and Calverton, Maryland, USA: SA, MOH, and ICF International.: Statistical Agency under the President of the Republic of Tajikistan (SA), Ministry of Health [Tajikistan], and ICF International., 2013.
17. Cleland J, Ali MM. Reproductive consequences of contraceptive failure in 19 developing countries. Obstet Gynecol. 2004;104(2):314–20.
18. Trussell J. Contraceptive efficacy. In: Hatcher R, Trussell J, Nelson A, Cates W, Kowal D, Policar M, editors. Contraceptive technology: twentieth revised edition. 20th ed. New York: Ardent Media; 2011.
19. Trussell J. Contraceptive efficacy: global library of women's medicine; 2014 [26 September 2017]. Available from: http://www.glowm.com/section_view/heading/Contraceptive%20Efficacy/item/374.
20. Sedgh G, Ashford L, Hussain R. Unmet need for contraception in developing countries: examining Women's reasons for not using a method. New York: Guttmacher Institute; 2016.

21. Free C, Knight R, Robertson S, Whittaker R, Edwards P, Zhou W, et al. Smoking cessation support delivered via mobile phone text messaging (txt2stop): a single-blind, randomised trial. Lancet. 2011;378(9785):49–55.

22. Lester RT, Ritvo P, Mills EJ, Kariri A, Karanja S, Chung MH, et al. Effects of a mobile phone short message service on antiretroviral treatment adherence in Kenya (WelTel Kenya1): a randomised trial. Lancet. 2010;376(9755):1838–45.

23. Pop-Eleches C, Thirumurthy H, Habyarimana JP, Zivin JG, Goldstein MP, de Walque D, et al. Mobile phone technologies improve adherence to antiretroviral treatment in a resource-limited setting: a randomized controlled trial of text message reminders. AIDS. 2011;25(6):825–34.

24. Zurovac D, Sudoi RK, Akhwale WS, Ndiritu M, Hamer DH, Rowe AK, et al. The effect of mobile phone text-message reminders on Kenyan health workers' adherence to malaria treatment guidelines: a cluster randomised trial. Lancet. 2011;378(9793):795–803.

25. Orr JA, King RJ. Mobile phone SMS messages can enhance healthy behaviour: a meta-analysis of randomised controlled trials. Health Psychol Rev. 2015;9(4):397–416.

26. Hall CS, Fottrell E, Wilkinson S, Byass P. Assessing the impact of mHealth interventions in low- and middle-income countries–what has been shown to work? Glob Health Action. 2014;7:25606.

27. Aranda-Jan CB, Mohutsiwa-Dibe N, Loukanova S. Systematic review on what works, what does not work and why of implementation of mobile health (mHealth) projects in Africa. BMC Public Health. 2014;14:188.

28. Free C, Phillips G, Galli L, Watson L, Felix L, Edwards P, et al. The effectiveness of mobile-health technology-based health behaviour change or disease management interventions for health care consumers: a systematic review. PLoS Med. 2013;10(1):e1001362.

29. Head KJ, Noar SM, Iannarino NT, Grant Harrington N. Efficacy of text messaging-based interventions for health promotion: a meta-analysis. Soc Sci Med. 2013;97:41–8.

30. Hall AK, Cole-Lewis H, Bernhardt JM. Mobile text messaging for health: a systematic review of reviews. Annu Rev Public Health. 2015;36:393–415.

31. L'Engle KL, Mangone ER, Parcesepe AM, Agarwal S, Ippoliti NB. Mobile phone interventions for adolescent sexual and reproductive health: a systematic review. Pediatrics. 2016;138(3):e20160884.

32. Ippoliti NB, L'Engle KL. Meet us on the phone: mobile phone programs for adolescent sexual and reproductive health in low-to-middle income countries. Reprod Health. 2017;14(1):11.

33. Berenson AB, Rahman M. A randomized controlled study of two educational interventions on adherence with oral contraceptives and condoms. Contraception. 2012;86(6):716–24.

34. Castaño PM, Bynum JY, Andres R, Lara M, Westhoff C. Effect of daily text messages on oral contraceptive continuation: a randomized controlled trial. Obstet Gynecol. 2012;119(1):14–20.

35. Trent M, Thompson C, Tomaszewski K. Text messaging support for urban adolescents and young adults using injectable contraception: outcomes of the DepoText pilot trial. J Adolesc Health. 2015;57(1):100–6.

36. Smith C, Ngo TD, Gold J, Edwards P, Vannak U, Sokhey L, et al. Effect of a mobile phone-based intervention on post-abortion contraception: a randomized controlled trial in Cambodia. Bull World Health Organ. 2015;

37. Hall KS, Westhoff CL, Castano PM. The impact of an educational text message intervention on young urban women's knowledge of oral contraception. Contraception. 2013;87(4):449–54.

38. Rokicki S, Cohen J, Salomon JA, Fink G. Impact of a text-messaging program on adolescent reproductive health: a cluster-randomized trial in Ghana. Am J Public Health. 2017;107(2):298–305.

39. Johnson D, Juras R, Riley P, Chatterji M, Sloane P, Choi SK, et al. A randomized controlled trial of the impact of a family planning mHealth service on knowledge and use of contraception. Contraception. 2017;95(1):90–7.

40. Tsur L, Kozer E, Berkovitch M. The effect of drug consultation center guidance on contraceptive use among women using isotretinoin: a randomized, controlled study. J Womens Health (Larchmt). 2008;17(4):579–84.

41. Hou MY, Hurwitz S, Kavanagh E, Fortin J, Goldberg AB. Using daily text-message reminders to improve adherence with oral contraceptives: a randomized controlled trial.[erratum appears in Obstet Gynecol. 2010 Nov; 116(5):1224]. Obstet Gynecol. 2010;116(3):633–40.

42. Kirby D, Raine T, Thrush G, Yuen C, Sokoloff A, Potter SC. Impact of an intervention to improve contraceptive use through follow-up phone calls to female adolescent clinic patients. Perspect Sex Reprod Health. 2010;42(4):251–7.

43. Bull S, Devine S, Schmiege SJ, Pickard L, Campbell J, Shlay JC. Text messaging, teen outreach program, and sexual health behavior: a cluster randomized trial. Am J Public Health. 2016;106(S1):S117–S24.

44. McCarthy OL, Leurent B, Edwards P, Tokhirov R, Free C. A randomised controlled trial of an intervention delivered by app instant messaging to increase the acceptability of effective contraception among young people in Tajikistan: study protocol. BMJ Open. 2017;7(9):e017606.

45. McCarthy OL. A randomised controlled trial of an intervention delivered by app instant messaging to increase the acceptability of effective contraception among young people in Tajikistan: statistical analysis plan. Figshare. https://doi.org/10.6084/m9.figshare.5314714.v2.

46. Bartholomew Eldredge LK, Markham C, Ruiter R, Fernandez M, Kok G, Parcel G. Planning health promotion programs: an intervention mapping approach. 4th ed. San Francisco: Jossey-Bass; 2016.

47. Montaño D, Kasprzyk D. Theory of reasoned action, theory of planned behavior, and the integrated behavioral model. In: Glanz K, Rimer BK, Viswanath K, editors. Health behaviour: theory, research and practice. 5th ed. San Francisco: Jossey-Bass; 2015. p. 168–222.

48. Kok G, Gottlieb N, Peters G, Mullen P, Parcel G, Ruiter R, et al. A Taxonomy of Behavior Change Methods; an Intervention Mapping Approach. Health Psychol Rev. 2016;10(3):297–12.

49. Francis JJ, Eccles MP, Johnston M, Walker A, Grimshaw J, Foy R, et al. Constructing questionnaires based on the theory of planned behaviour. A manual for health services researchers 2004; 2010. p. 2–12.

50. Montano DE, Kasprzyk D, Hamilton DT, Tshimanga M, Gorn G. Evidence-based identification of key beliefs explaining adult male circumcision motivation in Zimbabwe: targets for behavior change messaging. AIDS Behav. 2014;18(5):885–904.

51. Pocock SJ, Assmann SE, Enos LE, Kasten LE. Subgroup analysis, covariate adjustment and baseline comparisons in clinical trial reporting: current practice and problems. Stat Med. 2002;21(19):2917–30.

52. Kasenda B, Schandelmaier S, Sun X, von Elm E, You J, Blumle A, et al. Subgroup analyses in randomised controlled trials: cohort study on trial protocols and journal publications. BMJ. 2014;349:g4539.

53. Gabler NB, Duan N, Liao D, Elmore JG, Ganiats TG, Kravitz RL. Dealing with heterogeneity of treatment effects: is the literature up to the challenge? Trials. 2009;10:43.

54. Kent DM, Rothwell PM, Ioannidis JPA, Altman DG, Hayward RA. Assessing and reporting heterogeneity in treatment effects in clinical trials: a proposal. Trials. 2010;11:85.

55. Brookes ST, Whitely E, Egger M, Smith GD, Mulheran PA, Peters TJ. Subgroup analyses in randomised trials: risks of subgroup-specific analyses; power and sample size for the interaction test. J Clin Epidemiol. 2004;57(3):229–36.

56. McCarthy OL, Wazwaz O, Jado I, Leurent B, Edwards P, Adada S, et al. An intervention delivered by text message to increase the acceptability of effective contraception among young women in Palestine: study protocol for a randomised controlled trial. Trials. 2017;18(1):454.

57. McCarthy OL, Osorio Calderon V, Makleff S, Huaynoca S, Leurent B, Edwards P, et al. An intervention delivered by app instant messaging to increase acceptability and use of effective contraception among young women in Bolivia: protocol of a randomized controlled trial. JMIR Res Protoc. 2017;6(12):e252.

58. Smith C, Gold J, Ngo TD, Sumpter C, Free C. Mobile phone-based interventions for improving contraception use. Cochrane Database Syst Rev. 2015;(6):CD011159.

59. Reiss K, Andersen K, Barnard S, Ngo TD, Biswas K, Smith C, et al. Using automated voice messages linked to telephone counselling to increase post-menstrual regulation contraceptive uptake and continuation in Bangladesh: study protocol for a randomised controlled trial. BMC Public Health. 2017;17(1):769.

60. Bailey JV, Pavlou M, Copas A, McCarthy O, Carswell K, Rait G, et al. The sexunzipped trial: optimizing the design of online randomized controlled trials. J Med Internet Res. 2013;15(12):e278.

61. Carswell K, McCarthy O, Murray E, Bailey JV. Integrating psychological theory into the design of an online intervention for sexual health: the sexunzipped website. JMIR Res Protoc. 2012;1(2):e16.

17

Evaluation of a family-oriented antenatal group educational program in rural Tanzania: a pre-test/post-test study

Yoko Shimpuku[1][*] , Frida E. Madeni[2], Shigeko Horiuchi[1], Kazumi Kubota[3] and Sebalda C. Leshabari[4]

Abstract

Background: To increase births attended by skilled birth attendants in Tanzania, studies have identified the need for involvement of the whole family in pregnancy and childbirth education. This study aimed to develop, implement, and evaluate a *family-oriented antenatal group educational program* to promote healthy pregnancy and family involvement in rural Tanzania.

Methods: This was a quasi-experimental 1 group pre-test/post-test study with antenatal education provided to pregnant women and their families in rural Tanzania. Before and after the educational program, the pre-test/post-test study was conducted using a 34-item Birth Preparedness Questionnaire. Acceptability of the educational program was qualitatively assessed.

Results: One-hundred and thirty-eight participants (42 pregnant women, 96 family members) attended the educational program, answered the questionnaire, and participated in the feasibility inquiry. The mean knowledge scores significantly increased between the pre-test and the post-test, 7.92 and 8.33, respectively ($p = 0.001$). For both pregnant women and family members, the educational program improved *Family Support* ($p = 0.001$ and $p = 0.000$) and *Preparation of Money and Food* ($p = 0.000$ and $p = 0.000$). For family members, *the scores for Birth Preparedness* ($p = 0.006$) and *Avoidance of Medical Intervention* (reversed item) ($p = 0.002$) significantly increased. Despite the educational program, the score for *Home-based Value* (reversed item) ($p = 0.022$) and *References of SBA* ($p = 0.049$) decreased in pregnant women. Through group discussions, favorable comments about the program and materials were received. The comments of the husbands reflected their better understanding and appreciation of their role in supporting their wives during the antenatal period.

Conclusions: The *family-oriented antenatal group educational program* has potential to increase knowledge, birth preparedness, and awareness of the need for family support among pregnant women and their families in rural Tanzania. As the contents of the program can be taught easily by reading the picture drama, lay personnel, such as community health workers or traditional birth attendants, can use it in villages. Further development of the Birth Preparedness Questionnaire is necessary to strengthen the involved factors. A larger scale study with a more robust Birth Preparedness Questionnaire and documentation of skilled care use is needed for the next step.

Keywords: Pregnancy, Childbirth, Family support, Birth preparedness, Antenatal education, Africa

* Correspondence: shimpuku.yoko.5n@kyoto-u.ac.jp
[1]Human Health Sciences, Graduate School of Medicine, Kyoto University, 53 Shogoin-kawahara-cho, Sakyo-ku, Kyoto 606-8507, Japan
Full list of author information is available at the end of the article

Plain English summary

One of the biggest challenges facing Tanzania is the large number of women who die from pregnancy and childbirth, reflecting the need for better antenatal education. In response to this need, our group of Japanese and Tanzanian midwives developed an antenatal group educational program for teaching the importance of birth preparedness and family involvement in pregnancy in rural Tanzania. For the educational material, we developed a picture drama which compared the stories of two women who had different birth preparations and family involvement. We provided the program to pregnant women and their families in Kiswahili, and asked them to fill questionnaires before and after the program and to join the discussion regarding their thoughts about the program. There were 138 participants who attended the program, answered the questionnaires, and participated in the discussion. Their knowledge of danger signs of pregnancy increased. Moreover, their perceptions toward family support and preparation of money and food improved. Family members showed better preparedness for birth and less avoidance of medical intervention. The comments about the program and materials were favorable. The husbands' comments reflected better understanding and appreciation of their role in supporting their wives during the antenatal period. Taken together, the antenatal group educational program increased knowledge, birth preparedness, and awareness of the need for family involvement and support among pregnant women and their families in rural Tanzania. Educational programs using picture dramas could add an acceptable component for increasing birth preparedness among pregnant women and their families especially in rural areas.

Background

In 2015, the Sustainable Development Goals of the United Nations were published on the basis of the achievement of the Millennium Development Goals (MDGs) [1–3]. According to the MDGs Report, greater effort is needed to reduce the global burden of maternal mortality [1]. Although a 45% reduction of maternal mortality in developing countries is a significant achievement, still about 289,000 women died in 2013 from causes related to pregnancy and childbirth [1]. World Health Organization (WHO), ICM (International Confederations of Midwives), and FIGO (International Federation of Gynecology and Obstetrics) have suggested that to reduce maternal mortality, skilled birth attendants (SBAs), namely, midwives, nurses, or doctors, should assist all births [4]. In rural areas of Tanzania, however, only 54% of all deliveries were reportedly conducted by SBAs [5]. Thus, nearly half of rural women still either chose not to use SBAs or had no access to SBAs while giving birth.

Researchers have indicated that Birth Preparedness and Complication Readiness (BP/CR) could be a key factor in influencing the choice of birthplace with SBAs [6–8]. In the WHO publication of *Birth and Emergency Preparedness in Antenatal Care* [9], 9 birth preparation components were identified: (1) the desired place of birth; (2) the preferred birth attendant; (3) the location of the closest appropriate care facility; (4) money for birth-related and emergency expenses; (5) a birth companion; (6) support in looking after the home and children while the woman is away; (7) transport to a health facility for the birth; (8) transport in the case of an obstetric emergency; and (9) identification of compatible blood donors in case of emergency. Despite the importance of BP/CR to promote SBAs, several reports have suggested a low level of BP/CR among women in African settings [10–13].

To increase BP/CR, 2 review studies have shown the accumulated findings of interventions. One study reviewed 58 articles and identified that community-based information, education, and communication interventions, which taught women when to reach out for assistance, increased awareness and knowledge of the danger signs of pregnancy complications [14]. This increase of women's awareness and knowledge has resulted in an increase in the utilization of health facility delivery services [14]. Another study using systematic review and meta-analysis found that exposure to BP/CR interventions was associated with a significant reduction of 18% in neonatal mortality risk (12 studies, RR = 0.82; 95% CI: 0.74, 0.91) and a nonsignificant reduction of 28% in maternal mortality risk (7 studies, RR = 0.76; 95% CI: 0.69, 0.85) [15]. Both home visits and community-based women's group sessions have been reported to potentially reduce the risk of neonatal mortality; however, their effects on maternal health have not been fully clarified. Moreover, home-based individual counseling has been found to be more personalized and appropriate for developing mothers' personal knowledge and skills [15]. However, other studies have revealed the lack of decision-making power of women within their family with regard to the referral and place of birth [16–18].

Intra-family or extended family decision-making also influences women's choices for childbirth [19]. The values and opinions of the husband, mother-in-law, mother, traditional birth attendant, other family members, and community members have been shown to have more influence in decisions regarding the birth place than the pregnant woman's input [19]. Implementation of the 9 BP/CR components requires family support. This implies that the decision-maker of the household, mostly the husband, must agree to provide the financial support for transportation and funds for emergency support, and the family or extended family should provide for child care, arrange for possible transport, be prepared to donate blood if necessary, and come to an agreement regarding the location for childbirth [20]. Even though husbands were typically the decision-makers regarding the place of delivery, they were rarely encouraged to attend antenatal sessions [21, 22]. August et al. [20] specifically interviewed husbands regarding their understanding of BP/CR and found them lacking particularly in the area of identifying an SBA. Therefore, community-based activities were still needed to promote family involvement because in these traditional settings the locus of decision-making was more community-based than individual-based [15]. WHO [16] recommended using BP/CR education and discussion with community participation, particularly the involvement of the male partner and other householder decision-makers.

It was found in Uganda that women who prepared for birth in consultation with their family members were more likely to give birth with the help of SBAs than women who prepared for birth by themselves [7]. A previous study investigating the partners' influence on women delivering at a health facility in Tanzania found that the agreements of partners on the importance of delivering in a health facility and on doctors having better skills than traditional birth attendants were associated with delivery in a health facility [21].

For over a decade, studies conducted in Tanzania have identified the need for involvement of the whole family in pregnancy and childbirth education [23–26]. Shimpuku et al. [26] emphasized the importance of family involvement in pregnancy and childbirth because it improved the quality of care and women's birth experiences.

Therefore, the role of the family in decision-making is a crucial issue for reducing maternal mortality, with the place of birth being an important component. However, there are only few studies that have examined family-based education. We therefore performed the present study to evaluate our recently developed *family-oriented antenatal group educational program* for pregnant women and their family members in rural Tanzania.

Methods
Study design
This was a quasi-experimental, 1 group pre-test/post--test study that included a qualitative component addressing feasibility. The *family-oriented antenatal group educational program* was provided to increase birth preparedness.

Setting
We conducted this study in Korogwe district, which is located in the center of the Tanga Region of North Eastern Tanzania. Korogwe has a total area of 3756 sq. km with 132 villages [27]. The main economic activities include agriculture and horticulture involving the natural resources of forests and game parks. The Korogwe district is predominately rural with a large population of 175,339 in reference to an urban area of 43,510. The Korogwe district has 1 public hospital and 2 private hospitals, 3 health centers, and 59 dispensaries. According to Demographic Health Survey 2 (DHS2) in 2016, delivery at health facilities 6969, deliveries with Traditional Birth Attendant (TBA) 259, home deliveries without TBA 151, birth before arrival 118 [28].

Sampling method and sample size
With the support of a local collaborator, we purposefully selected 3 mountain villages where the nearest health center was located at least 5 km away, and the majority of women deliver at home. As the villages were located in the mountain, women in these villages must walk unpaved mountain roads to reach the nearest health center. The roads become completely dark after sunset; therefore, preparation of transportation and financial support was necessary to reach skilled care because contractions could start unpredictably, even at night.

We aimed to recruit a total sample size of 100 participants (50 pregnant women and 50 family members) to meet the assumption of a normal distribution [29]. Hence, 100 participants were expected to attend the program and pre-test/post-test. The inclusion criteria for women were as follows: currently pregnant with no severe physical or psychological illness. We did not exclude women based on gestational weeks or number of pregnancies. The criteria for family members were as follows: 16 years old or older, living with or near the pregnant woman, and defined as "family" by the pregnant woman (regardless of their blood or marital relationship). Participants need to be able to read Kiswahili to complete the self-administered questionnaire. If they need assistance in answering the questionnaire, a research assistant helped for reading and marking the answer.

Recruitment and data collection process
We requested the village leaders to inform their constituents about our research activities and to ask pregnant women and their families to gather in a school or a church on a specified date and time. When we arrived in the village, pregnant women and their families gathered at the specified place. After explaining the details of our research, they were asked if they agreed to participate in the study. Because of the interest of those who gathered in the study, all agreed to participate and stayed to receive the educational program and pre-test/post-test. This data collection process was repeated in 2 more villages.

Educational program

We developed the *family-oriented antenatal group educational program* to be culturally relevant. The program lasted for approximately 2 hours and included a pre-test/post-test, picture drama, and discussion. In the educational program, pregnant women and their families were taught the importance of birth preparation to increase the safety of childbirth, namely, survival of pregnant women and their babies. The program aimed to inculcate the following ideas: (1) preparation for childbirth is important to enable women to receive health care when necessary, (2) families are encouraged to support the women's choice when deciding their birth place, and (3) women are advised to give birth with an SBA. We created a story of women's birth experiences based on a qualitative study at a rural hospital in Tanzania [26]. The story included health promotion concepts such as family decision-making processes, and family support according to the *Integrated Management of Pregnancy and Childbirth* [9].

At the beginning of our *family-oriented antenatal group educational program*, the participants were asked to answer the Birth Preparedness Questionnaire (BPQ) pre-test. The second author (FM), a female Tanzanian researcher, who has a master's degree with knowledge of local customs, shared a story using a picture drama. The picture drama depicted 2 women who had very different birth experiences, one with and one without proper birth preparation. The first woman had a very supportive family. She attended antenatal visits regularly. At the visits, a midwife provided information about nutrition, danger signs during pregnancy, risks of some traditional herbs, potential problems of the mother and baby, and necessary preparations including money, transportation, birth companions, and blood donors in case of emergency. As a result, this first woman who had properly prepared for birth with her family had a normal delivery of a healthy baby. The second woman had a family who strongly believed in home birth and did not allow her to go to antenatal visits. Because the family did not prepare anything, when the woman's labor become obstructed, they delayed leaving for the hospital and consequently, the family lost both the mother and the baby. The pictures clearly depicted the story and illustrated Tanzanian housing and clothes (*kanga*) to enable the participants to easily identify with the story.

In community settings, utilization of picture drama was found to be educationally effective. An increase in knowledge was found when providing reproductive health education using picture dramas to adolescent boys and girls in Tanzania [30]. The pictures made it easier for those who were not strong in health literacy to understand the contents. All important information was written on the backside of the pictures. This enabled the presenter to be consistent and provide comprehensive information. After the picture drama and the presenter's explanation, the participants were asked to answer the same BPQ for the post-test and then to evaluate the contents and effectiveness of the *antenatal group educational program*.

Measurements

Demographic items included age, marital status, education, occupation, daily monetary use, household assets, ethnic group, distance from health care facility, experience in losing a family member owing to pregnancy problems, and obstetric history (only pregnant women).

Birth preparedness questionnaire

The BPQ is a 34-item self-administered questionnaire consisting of a knowledge test and a BP/CR assessment that was used for both the pre-test ad the post-test. In the development of the questionnaire, the authors utilized Ajzen's theory [31] as a guide. The theory explains that intentions to perform various behaviors can be predicted from the following 3 perceptional components: 1) perceived behavioral control, 2) attitudes toward the behavior, and 3) subjective norms. The authors chose this theory to frame items related to those 3 psychological factors that may influence intention to have an SBA.

Knowledge items were added to the questionnaire because previous studies have indicated that adequate knowledge of danger signs was associated with more SBA-attended births [32, 33]. We developed a self-administered 10-item knowledge test about safe pregnancy and danger signs based on the 9 components of *Integrated Management of Pregnancy and Childbirth* [9]. The items are presented as binary *yes/no* responses. Another 24-item BP/CR assessment test was developed to assess BP/CR and the items were related to psychological values and beliefs. These 24 items were rated using a 3-point Likert scale indicating (1) *disagree*, (2) *neither disagree nor agree*, or (3) *agree*.

The questionnaire was first developed in English and then translated into Kiswahili, which is a more familiar language to most Tanzanians. The questionnaire was translated by the second author (FM) who is bilingual in Kiswahili and English, from the same district, and experienced in communicating with rural Tanzanian women. Initially, to increase face validity, 10 rural women were interviewed regarding their answers for the knowledge test and BP/CR assessment. They were asked to provide their opinions regarding any unclear or confusing questions. Thereafter, the knowledge test and BP/CR assessment were revised according to the opinions of the interviewed women and finalized for this study.

As it was the first time to introduce the program to Tanzania, a feasibility inquiry was conducted in the form of a group discussion that included all the women and their family members attending the program, followed by completion of a post-test questionnaire. This feasibility inquiry was conducted to initially determine if the delivery of the program was acceptable to the participants. The participants responded to open-ended questions to assess the feasibility of the study. The following questions were included: 1) "How did you feel about the contents of the picture drama? Did you understand it well? If not, what was difficult to understand?" 2) "Are the contents of the picture drama appropriate for educating rural women and their family members?" 3) "How can we improve the contents of the picture drama?". While observing the discussions, field notes were taken and data were transcribed in Kiswahili and then translated into English. Thematic content analysis [34] was used based on the predetermined concepts of acceptability, demand, implementation, practicality, and limited efficacy [35]. The field notes were carefully read and similar ideas were extracted, then the major ideas were discussed. Thus, the major findings were organized into 5 categories.

Ethics approval and consent to participate
The study was conducted based on the principles of ethics such as harmlessness, being voluntarily, anonymity, and protection of privacy and personal information. We explained these principles during recruitment along with the purpose, methods, and ethical considerations. We asked each participant if they agreed to participate in the study and only those who agreed were included in the study. We obtained verbal consent because the information gathered was unidentifiable and the risk from this study was minimal. Ethical clearance and permissions were obtained from the 1) Research Ethics Committee of St. Luke's International University (14–040); 2) Director of the Korogwe District Council, 3) National Institute for Medical Research, Tanzania (NIMR/HQ/R.8/Vol.IX/1604), and 4) Tanzania Commission for Science and Technology (No. 2013–273-NA-2013-101).

Data analysis
SPSS ver. 22.0 was used for descriptive analysis, correlations, exploratory factor analysis using the maximum likelihood method and promax rotation to validate the factor structure. Exploratory factor analysis was conducted using the 28 original BP/CR items to determine whether measures of the construct were consistent with authors' understanding of the nature of that construct. Before the analysis, the answers for all the reverse items were inversed (from 1 to 3 and from 3 to 1). Four items were excluded during the analysis because of low correlations. The final factor analysis included the remaining 24 items. As a result, 7 factors were identified:

Home-based Value (Factor I, 7 items, Cronbach's alpha = 0.846), *Birth Preparedness* (Factor II, 5 items, Cronbach's alpha = 0.691), *Family Support* (Factor III, 4 items, Cronbach's alpha = 0.646), *Avoidance of Medical Intervention* (Factor IV, 2 items, Cronbach's alpha = 0.548), *Preparation of Money and Food* (Factor V, 2 items, Cronbach's alpha = 0.615), *Preference of SBA* (Factor VI, 2 items, Cronbach's alpha = 0.472), *Pregnant Women's Workload* (Factor VII, 2 items, Cronbach's alpha = 0.337). Table 1 shows the results of factor analysis. Wilcoxon signed-rank test was used to determine any significant difference in the BP/CR scores before and after the educational program. For the feasibility inquiry, the qualitative data were analyzed using thematic content analysis.

Results
Demographic and obstetric characteristics
There were a total of 139 prospective participants from 3 villages (42 pregnant women and 97 family members). One participant did not complete the questionnaire and was therefore excluded. Hence, 138 participants (42 pregnant women and 96 family members) were included for the analysis. Table 2 shows a summary of the participants' characteristics. Although the group included both pregnant women and their family members, there was no significant difference in education, occupation, daily expenses, or household assets. There was a significant difference in the mean age ($p < 0.001$). Among the 42 pregnant women, 8 (19%) were primipara and 34 were multipara ($M = 1.45$, SD 1.194, range 0–5). For antenatal visits, 17 (40.5%) attended once and 23 (54.8%) attended twice (2 had missing data). There were 24 multiparas who had given birth at a health facility, one of whom had caesarean section. None had lost a baby during pregnancy or childbirth. All the participants attended the *antenatal group educational program* and the *feasibility inquiry*.

Pre-test and post-test differences in knowledge
Figure 1 shows that the mean knowledge score of all the participants significantly increased between pre-test and post-test ($p = 0.001$). After the education, both pregnant women and family members showed significantly higher means in knowledge scores ($p = 0.011$ and $p = 0.020$, respectively).

Pre-test/post-test differences in BPQ
There were significant differences between pre-test and post-test both in pregnant women and family members in *Family Support* ($p = 0.001$ and $p = 0.000$, respectively) and *Preparation of Money and Food* ($p = 0.000$ and $p = 0.000$, respectively). Table 3 shows the mean score and standard deviation of the 7 factors between pregnant

Table 1 Exploratory factor analysis Birth Preparedness Questionnaire using maximum likelihood method and promax rotation among 138 rural adults in Tanzania

Item#	Items	I	II	III	IV	V	VI	VII
Factor 1: Home-based value								
Q36	I plan to give birth at home. (reverse item)	**.839**	-.026	.029	.058	-.019	-.051	.091
Q25	I want (I want her) to give birth at home with family because we do not know people in health care facilities (reverse item)	**.799**	.025	.040	.049	.158	-.299	-.058
Q38	God will help me, so I don't plan anything for childbirth. (reverse item)	**.755**	.153	.122	.201	-.211	-.183	-.165
Q29	A pregnant woman should stay at home to give birth if no one else takes care of the children in the family. (reverse item)	**.621**	-.179	-.160	.030	.104	.087	.284
Q28	A woman should give birth at home if her husband does not allow her to go to a health center. (reverse item)	**.593**	-.095	-.295	-.067	.071	.341	-.038
Q24	I like to give birth with traditional birth attendants because they are kinder than nurses at the hospital. (reverse item)	**.554**	.050	.129	.434	.012	-.048	.156
Q31	A baby belongs to the family, so woman should follow their family's wishes about where to give birth. (reverse item)	**.474**	-.004	-.517	-.139	.000	.152	-.131
Factor 2: Birth preparedness								
Q18	My family members think it is okay for me to access health care.	.060	**.754**	.121	.113	-.050	.040	-.130
Q13	I have someone who can go with me when going to a health care facility for birth	-.083	**.667**	.021	.206	.034	.223	.155
Q12	I have someone who can take over my family responsibilities when I need to go to a health center.	-.083	**.625**	-.123	.028	.353	-.042	.142
Q15	I know where to find a health care facility for delivery and emergencies.	.154	**.607**	-.128	-.361	.100	-.183	.134
Q14	I can identify where a trained health care provider is to help me.	-.153	**.574**	-.205	-.330	-.173	.088	-.053
Factor 3: Family support								
Q34	I will prepare for childbirth with my family	.056	-.139	**.770**	-.056	.280	-.107	-.078
Q30	A woman should discuss her birth with her husband and other family members.	-.081	-.047	**.746**	-.029	.089	.003	.158
Q22	It is better to go to a health center for deliveries with family members because of their support.	.138	.058	**.507**	-.411	-.314	.333	.101
Q35	I am going to give birth at a health care facility	.051	.150	**.461**	.155	.074	.287	-.247
Factor 4: Avoidance of medical intervention								
Q23	I would not go to a health center because I do not want a C-section or a vaginal cut. (reverse item)	.180	.113	-.020	**.771**	-.096	-.084	-.114
Q20	It is okay to give birth at home when a pregnant women and her baby have no problems. (reverse item)	.138	-.122	-.027	**.507**	-.095	.277	.073
Factor 5: Provision of money and food								
Q11	I have saved enough money to reach a health facility for birth.	.115	.073	.111	-.157	**.791**	.091	-.309
Q32	I plan to eat healthy during my pregnancy.	-.052	-.014	.267	.010	**.688**	.278	.076
Factor 6: Preference of SBA								
Q37	I will visit a health centre if there is a problem for my baby or me after delivery.	-.171	.020	-.026	.003	.187	**.815**	-.165
Q26	I want to be with doctors and nurses during childbirth because they are the experts.	.108	.276	.022	.089	.281	**.409**	.121
Factor 7: Pregnant women's workload								
Q21	Women should rest and should not work hard during their pregnancy.	.082	.084	.215	-.413	.033	-.153	**.746**
Q27	A woman should work hard for her family during pregnancy. (reverse item)	-.002	.054	-.125	.245	-.290	-.074	**.723**

Component values are captured in bold

Table 2 Comparison of the sociodemographic characteristics of the participants

	Pregnant women (N = 42)		Family (N = 96)		p-value
	Mean (SD)	n (%)	Mean (SD)	n (%)	
Age	27.67		35.29		< 0.001
Educational level					0.148
Lower than secondary level		34 (82.9)		62 (73.8)	
Secondary level and above		7 (17.1)		22 (26.2)	
Missing data		1 (2.4)		12 (12.5)	
Occupation					0.203
Farmer		33 (80.5)		63 (73.3)	
Housewife/student		8 (19.5)		23 (26.7)	
Missing data		1 (2.4)		10 (10.4)	
Daily expense					0.662
< 1000 TSH		18 (42.9)		39 (47.0)	
1000–5000 TSH		21 (50.0)		32 (38.6)	
≥ 5000 TSH		3 (7.1)		12 (14.4)	
Missing data		0		13 (13.5)	
Household assets ownership					0.83
Low (0–1)		38 (90.5)		70 (75.3)	
High (2+)		4 (9.5)		23 (24.7)	
Missing data		0		3 (3.1)	

women and family members for the pre-test and post-test. There was a significant decrease in two reversed items of *Home-based Value* and *Preference of SBA* ($p = 0.022$ and $p = 0.049$, respectively) among only pregnant women. There were significant differences in *Birth Preparedness* and *Avoidance of Medical Intervention* ($p = 0.006$ and $p = 0.002$, respectively) among only family members.

Correlation among BPQ factors

Among the 7 factors, *Home-based Value* was positively associated with *Avoidance of Medical Intervention* ($r = 0.55$, $p = 0.000$) and *Pregnant Women's Workload* ($r = 0.22$, $p = 0.011$) and negatively associated with *Family Support* ($r = -0.34$, $p = 0.000$) and *Preparation of Money and Food* ($r = -0.26$, $p = 0.000$). *Birth Preparedness* was positively associated with *Family Support* ($r = 0.26$, $p =$

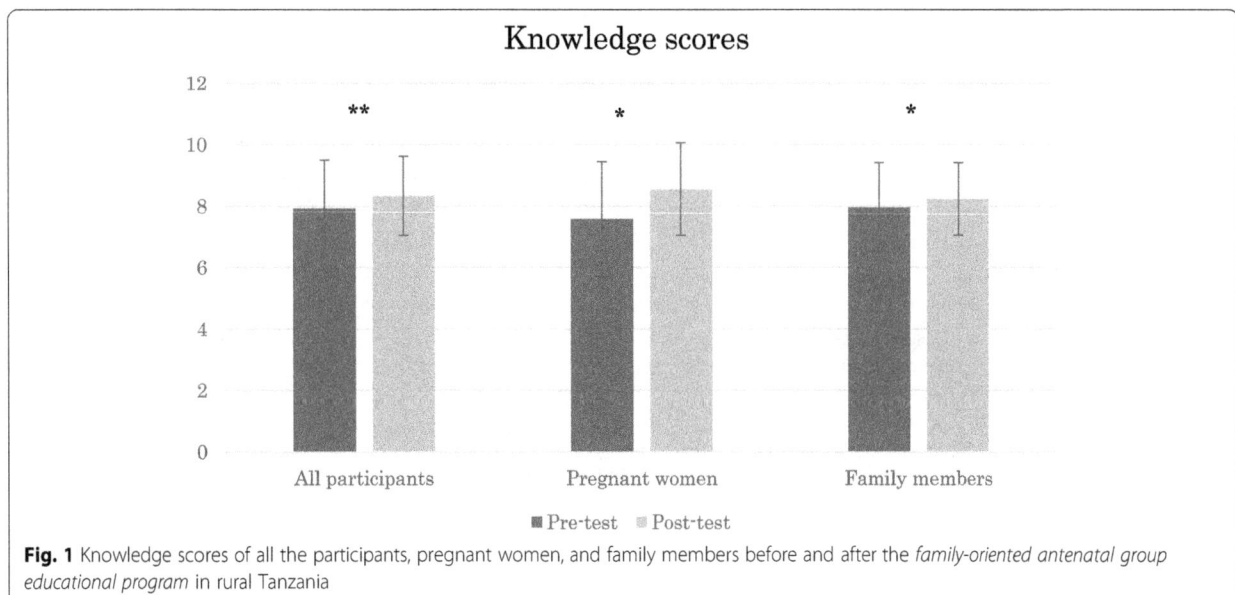

Fig. 1 Knowledge scores of all the participants, pregnant women, and family members before and after the *family-oriented antenatal group educational program* in rural Tanzania

Table 3 Comparison of pre-test/post-test Birth Preparedness Questionnaire scores among pregnant women and family members

	Pregnant women (n = 42)			Family members (n = 96)		
	Pre	Post	p	Pre	Post	p
1) Home-based Value	17.32 (3.49)	16.33 (3.88)	0.022*	16.33 (3.88)	16.24 (3.51)	0.312
2) Birth Preparedness	14.13 (1.07)	14.38 (1.01)	0.135	14.38 (1.01)	13.99 (1.76)	0.006**
3) Family Support	10.02 (1.76)	11.18 (1.58)	0.001**	11.18 (1.58)	10.95 (1.52)	0.000**
4) Avoidance of Medical Intervention	3.92 (1.61)	4.25 (1.56)	0.078	4.25 (1.56)	4.26 (1.37)	0.002**
5) Preparation of Money and Food	4.77 (1.28)	5.68 (0.75)	0.000**	5.68 (0.75)	5.71 (0.66)	0.000**
6) Preference of SBA	5.78 (0.70)	5.51 (0.93)	0.049*	5.51 (0.93)	5.53 (0.77)	0.105
7) Pregnant Women's Workload	4.80 (1.31)	5.08 (1.11)	0.108	5.08 (1.11)	4.64 (1.10)	0.215

*$p < 0.05$, **$p < 0.01$
Note: The Wilcoxon signed-rank test. The p-value is asymptotic significance (two-tailed)

0.002), *Preparation of Money and Food* ($r = -0.28$, $p = 0.001$), and *Preference of SBA* ($r = 0.24$, $p = 0.05$), and negatively associated with *Avoidance of Medical Intervention* ($r = -0.29$, $p = 0.001$). *Family Support* was positively associated with *Preparation of Money and Food* ($r = 0.41$, $p = 0.000$) and *Preference of SBA* ($r = 0.26$, $p = 0.003$) and negatively associated with *Avoidance of Medical Intervention* ($r = -0.27$, $p = 0.002$). *Avoidance of Medical Intervention* was negatively associated with *Preparation of Money and Food* ($r = -0.25$, $p = 0.003$). *Preparation of Money and Food* was positively associated with *Preference of SBA* ($r = 0.31$, $p = 0.000$).

Feasibility inquiry

Bowen et al. [35] suggested 8 general areas of focus for a feasibility study: *acceptability, demand, implementation, practicality, adaptation, integration, expansion,* and *limited efficacy*. Within these areas, this study focused on acceptability, demand, implementation, practicality, and limited efficacy, which fit with the preliminary stage of this study. The details and outcomes are described in Table 4.

Acceptability indicates how the intended participants and program staff react to the intervention [35]. Regarding the educational materials in this study, a woman shared, "The picture is good and makes it easy for us to understand." Another woman mentioned, "We are very happy to learn many things, no one feels bad. Everybody is happy." After the education, a woman said, "Husbands should change their behaviors. For example, giving the women heavy loads." One man stated, "We learned how to make a good relationship between pregnant women and their families." Another man expressed, "We learned to increase love to unborn baby and his/her mother."

Demand indicates the estimated or actual use of the intervention. As an example of demand, a man stated, "We need to tell the government to add more health centers to the villages near people's houses." Another man mentioned, "This type of education should be given to all Tanzanian people, pregnant women, and their families."

Implementation indicates the extent, likelihood, and manner in which an intervention is fully implemented. In this study, more time was needed to complete the self-administered questionnaire than as planned.

Table 4 Observations and qualitative data for the feasibility inquiry

Focus areas	Questions in feasibility inquiry[a]	Study outcomes
Acceptability	To what extent is a new idea, program, process or measure judged as suitable, satisfying, or attractive to program deliverers? To program recipients?	"The picture is good and enables us to easily understand." "We are very happy to learn many things, no one feels bad. Everybody is happy."
Demand	To what extent is a new idea, program, process, or measure likely to be used (i.e., how much demand is likely to exist?)	"This type of education should be given to all Tanzanian people, pregnant women and their families."
Implementation	To what extent can a new idea, program, process, or measure be successfully delivered to intended participants in some defined, but not fully controlled, context?	It takes more time to complete the self-administered questionnaire than what was planned by the researchers.
Practicality	To what extent can an idea, program, process, or measure be carried out with intended participants using existing means, resources, and circumstances and without outside intervention?	The collaborator can conduct the intervention, but more local nurses or community health workers need to be educated to implement the intervention and expand the research.
Limited efficacy	Does the new idea, program, process, or measure show promise of being successful with the intended population, even in a highly controlled setting?	The scores of the measure showed some significant differences before and after the intervention with the limited convenient sample. More changes are expected.

[a]Referred from Bowen et al. [35], p. 8

Practicality indicates the extent to which an intervention can be delivered depending on the available resources, time, commitment, or a combination of factors. We identified that a local collaborator can conduct the research; however, training is required to be able to extend the research.

Limited efficacy indicates whether the study was successful even at a limited extent such as the evaluation of a convenient sample. We conducted this study using a convenient sample and we found several statistically significant findings. If we conduct this study using a larger sample with possible randomization, it is expected that more significant differences will be found after the intervention.

Discussion

The *family-oriented antenatal group educational program* in rural Tanzania succeeded in providing information about the importance of birth preparation and how to strengthen family involvement. The program specifically improved the scores of *Knowledge, Family Support,* and *Preparation of Money and Food* among all the participants. As *Knowledge* increased among all the participants, the educational program utilizing a picture drama and discussion was effective and culturally compatible with the participants.

It was an important finding that *Family Support* changed significantly. This variable includes the items about discussion on birthplace among family members. The increase of discussion among family members including women may improve women's decision-making power within the family. Household equity indeed has also been shown to increase women's facility delivery in Nepal [36]. Notably, when Nepalese women were actually communicating with their husbands, they were more likely to discuss health issues during pregnancy and birth preparedness with their husbands, and the husbands had a higher likelihood of being present during health facility delivery [37]. When women in Guatemala [38] and Uganda [39] made a birth plan with their husbands or other family members, they were more likely to seek the care of SBAs. Thus, although we did not increase SBA-assisted deliveries this time, the educational program contributed to increasing the participation of women in decision-making and birth preparation, which could increase facility delivery with a larger sample size.

Similarly, the increase of monetary preparation from the program shows that the program had the potential to increase SBA-assisted deliveries. Other studies also showed that monetary preparation was found to be one of the key factors for achieving deliveries with SBAs [8, 33, 40].

The next step is the necessity to improve education on *Preference of SBA*. Among pregnant women, the score

was significantly decreased; this change was not our intent. This factor included perceptions toward health care providers. We deduced that the participants from this rural area might have had perceptions toward health care providers that the educational program did not address. For example, disrespect and abuse of birthing women by health care providers have been reported in Tanzania [41–43]. As suggested by WHO [3], education for health care providers might also be needed. Another possible area for study is a follow-up of community volunteers for women to utilize skilled care at delivery as recommended by a *community-based safe motherhood program* in Tanzania [44]. As the present study provided only 1 session of education, continuous education or follow-up might be a more effective method for increasing readiness to use a health facility for an emergency.

Regarding the changes in the scores between family members and pregnant women, family members showed an increase in the scores for more variables than pregnant women. For example, the scores for *Birth Preparedness* and *Avoidance of Medical Intervention* increased significantly among only the family members. Some possible explanations why the scores of pregnant women did not significantly increase were the higher pre-test scores and the smaller sample size of the pregnant women. On the other hand, the scores for the *Home-based Value* of women decreased significantly, which was not our intended change. As the factor was composed of reverse items, the participants might not have answered carefully and instead answered in a response set, which is the opposite course. Reverse items could be reduced so that participants answer the questionnaires as researchers intended.

The study was significant in terms of obtaining preliminary data from pregnant women and their families who were difficult to reach in rural Tanzania. The study can be further improved in terms of more efficient implementation and greater community involvement in a subsequent larger scale study. At this stage of the educational program development, the study limitations of a small sample size, less rigorous sampling methods, and no-comparison group restrict the demonstration of the robust effects of the educational program, and therefore the generalizability is limited. Due to the small sample size, normality was not confirmed, and therefore only non-parametric analysis was used. With a larger sample size, the BPQ could benefit from additional psychometric testing to clarify and strengthen the concepts. In addition, this study would benefit more if it were conducted in districts with higher home birth rate. Although this study focused on increasing the knowledge and psychological aspects of BP/CR immediately after education, it did not evaluate outcome behaviors, such as delivery at a health facility. Further study is needed to investigate whether the participants who received education delivered with SBAs at a health facility, and to clarify the neonatal and maternal outcomes. Ultimately, a longitudinal randomized controlled study that replicates the educational intervention and includes outcome data in rural settings of Tanzania will provide more generalizable data.

Conclusions

The *family-oriented antenatal group educational program* has potential to increase knowledge, birth preparedness, and awareness of the need for family support among pregnant women and their families in rural Tanzania. As the contents of the program can be taught easily by reading the picture drama, lay personnel, such as community health workers or traditional birth attendants, can use it in villages. Further development of the Birth Preparedness Questionnaire is necessary to strengthen the involved factors. A larger scale study with a more robust BPQ and documentation of skilled care use is needed for the next step.

Abbreviations
BP/CR: Birth Preparedness and Complication Readiness; BPQ: Birth Preparedness Questionnaire; MDGs: Millennium Development Goals; SBAs: Skilled Birth Attendants; WHO: World Health Organization

Acknowledgements
The authors appreciate the contribution of all study participants. The following student assistants played a crucial role in developing the education materials: Kana Shimoda, Nao Tanaka, Ritsuko Yamada, Aiko Itokawa, Takae Kurahashi, and Mariko Komada. Our sincere gratitude goes to Dr. Maimbo Mndolwa, the Bishop of Korogwe who supported us in arranging data collection in the villages. Dr. Sarah E. Porter provided editing on behalf of St. Luke's International University. We thank Dr. Edward Barroga (http://orcid.org/0000-0002-8920-2607) for the editorial review of the manuscript.

Funding
The study was funded by the Japan Society for the Promotion of Science, Grants-in-Aid for Scientific Research: Research Activity Start-up (No. 248902460001).

Authors' contributions
YS conceptualized and designed of the study. YS, FM, and SL contributed to the acquisition of data. YS and KK participated in data analysis and/or interpretation. YS drafted the first manuscript. SH reviewed and suggested revisions. All authors reviewed and approved the final manuscript.

Authors' information
YS is a Japanese midwifery researcher who obtained her PhD from the University of Illinois at Chicago, USA. She has been conducting research on maternal child health and midwifery in Tanzania since 2008. She speaks fluent English and Swahili which were necessary for conducting this study. FM and SL are Tanzanian midwifery researchers who provided cultural understanding of the data. KK is a nurse and statistician who provided analytical expertise into the study. SH is a Japanese midwifery professor who has conducted, supervised, and published numerous midwifery research studies across the world, and who currently spearheads many on-going studies in this field.

Competing interests
The authors declare that they have no competing interests.

Author details
[1]Human Health Sciences, Graduate School of Medicine, Kyoto University, 53 Shogoin-kawahara-cho, Sakyo-ku, Kyoto 606-8507, Japan. [2]Magunga District Hospital, P. O. Box 430, Old-Korogwe, Tanga, Tanzania. [3]Department of Biostatistics, Yokohama City University School of Medicine, 3-9 Fukuura, Kanazawa-ku, Yokohama 236-0004, Japan. [4]School of Nursing, Muhimbili University of Health and Allied Sciences, P. O. Box 65169, Dar es Salaam, Tanzania.

References
1. United Nations. The millennium development goals report. New York: United Nations; 2015.
2. United Nations Development Group. 2014. Delivering the post-2015 development agenda: opportunities at the national and local levels. Available from: [cited 2016 April 30] Available at: http://www.worldwewant2015.org/file/459043/download/499855. Accessed 20 July 2017.
3. World Health Organization. 2015. WHO recommendations on health promotion interventions for maternal and newborn health. Available at: [cited 2017 January 14] http://apps.who.int/iris/bitstream/10665/172427/1/9789241508742_report_eng.pdf. Accessed 20 July 2017.
4. World Health Organization. 2004. Making pregnancy safer: the critical role of the skilled attendant. Available at: [cited 2016 April 30] http://www.who.int/maternal_child_adolescent/documents/9241591692/en/. Accessed 20 July 2017.
5. Ministry of Health, Community Development, Gender, Elderly and Children (MoHCDGEC) [Tanzania Mainland], Ministry of Health (MoH) [Zanzibar], National Bureau of Statistics (NBS), Office of the Chief Government Statistician (OCGS), and ICF. Tanzania Demographic and Health Survey and Malaria Indicator Survey (TDHS-MIS) 2015–16. Dar es Salaam, Tanzania, and Rockville, Maryland, USA: MoHCDGEC, MoH, NBS, OCGS, and ICF; 2016.
6. Hailu M, Gebremariam A, Alemseged F, Deribe K. Birth preparedness and complication readiness among pregnant women in southern Ethiopia. PLoS One. 2011;6:e21432.
7. Kabakyenga JK, Östergren PO, Turyakira E, Pettersson KO. Influence of birth preparedness, decision-making on location of birth and assistance by skilled birth attendants among women in south-western Uganda. PLoS One. 2012;7:e35747.
8. Moran AC, Sangli G, Dineen R, Rawlins B, Yameogo M, Baya B. Birth-preparedness for maternal health: findings from Koupela district, Burkina Faso. J Health Popul Nutr. 2006;24:489–97.
9. World Health Organization 2006. Birth and emergency preparedness in antenatal care. Available at: http://www.who.int/reproductivehealth/publications/maternal_perinatal_health/emergency_preparedness_antenatal_care.pdf. Accessed 20 July 2017.
10. Kaso M, Addisse M. Birth preparedness and complication readiness in Robe Woreda, Arsi zone, Oromia region, Central Ethiopia: a cross-sectional study. Reprod Health. 2014;11:55.
11. Markos D, Bogale D. Birth preparedness and complication readiness among women of child bearing age group in Goba Woreda, Oromia region, Ethiopia. BMC Pregnancy Childbirth. 2014;14:282. https://doi.org/10.1186/1471-2393-14-282.
12. Mbalinda SN, Nakimuli A, Kakaire O, Osinde MO, Kakande N, Kaye DK. Does knowledge of danger signs of pregnancy predict birth preparedness? A critique of the evidence from women admitted with pregnancy complications. BMC Health Res Policy Syst. 2014;12:60. Available at: http://www.health-policy-systems.com/content/12/1/60. Accessed 20 July 2017.

Evaluation of a family-oriented antenatal group educational program in rural...

201

13. Tura G, Afework MF, Yalew AW. The effect of birth preparedness and complication readiness on skilled care use: a prospective follow-up study in Southwest Ethiopia. Reprod Health. 2014;11:60. https://doi.org/10.1186/1742-4755-11-60.

14. Nyamtema AS, Urassa DP, van Roosmalen J. Maternal health interventions in resource limited countries: a systematic review of packages, impacts and factors for change. BMC Pregnancy Childbirth. 2011;11:30. https://doi.org/10.1186/1471-2393-11-30.

15. Soubeiga D, Gauvin L, Hatem MA, Johri M. Birth preparedness and complication readiness (BPCR) interventions to reduce maternal and neonatal mortality in developing countries: systematic review and meta-analysis. BMC Pregnancy Childbirth. 2014;14:129. https://doi.org/10.1186/1471-2393-14-129.

16. Mrisho M, Schellenberg JA, Mushi AK, Obrist B, Mshinda H, Tanner M, Schellenberg D. Factors affecting home delivery in rural Tanzania. Trop Med Int Health. 2007;12:862–72.

17. Pembe AB, Urassa DP, Darj E, Carlsted A, Olsson P. Qualitative study on maternal referrals in rural Tanzania: decision making and acceptance of referral advice. Afr J Reprod Health. 2008;12:120–31.

18. Pembe AB, Carlstedt A, Urassa DP, Lindmark G, Nyström L, Darj E. Effectiveness of maternal referral system in a rural setting: a case study from Rufiji district, Tanzania. BMC Health Serv Res. 2010;10:326.

19. Ganle, JK, Obeng B, Segbefia AY, Mwinyuri V, Yeboah JY, Baatiema L. How intra-familial decision-making affects women's access to, and use of maternal healthcare services in Ghana: a qualitative study. BMC Pregnancy Childbirth 2015;15:173. Available at: http://doi.org/10.1186/s12884-015-0590-4. Accessed 20 July 2017.

20. August F, Pembe A, Mpembeni R, Aximo P, Darj E. Men's knowledge of obstetric danger signs, birth preparedness and complication readiness in rural Tanzania. PLoS One 2015. Available at: http://dx.doi.org/10.1371/journal.pone.0125978. Accessed 20 July 2017.

21. Danforth EJ, Kruk ME, Rockers PC, Mbaruku G, Galea S. Household decision-making about delivery in health facilities: evidence from Tanzania. J Health Popul Nutr. 2009;27:696–703.

22. Magoma M, Requejo J, Campbell OM, Cousens S, Filippi V. High ANC coverage and low skilled attendance in a rural Tanzanian district: a case for implementing a birth plan intervention. BMC Pregnancy Childbirth. 2010;10(13) https://doi.org/10.1186/1471-239.

23. Kruk ME, Paczkowski M, Mbaruku G, de Pinho H, Galea S. Women's preferences for place of delivery in rural Tanzania: a population-based discrete choice experiment. Am J Public Health. 2008;99(9):1666–72.

24. Lugina HI, Lindmark G, Johansson E, Christensson K. Tanzanian midwives' views on becoming a good resource and support person for postpartum women. Midwifery. 2001;17(4):267–78.

25. Mbekenga CK, Lugina HI, Christensson K, Olsson P. Postpartum experiences of first-time fathers in a Tanzanian suburb: a qualitative interview study. Midwifery. 2011;27(2):174–80.

26. Shimpuku Y, Patil CL, Norr KF, Hill PD. Women's perceptions of childbirth experience at a hospital in rural Tanzania. Health Care Women Int. 2013;34:461–81.

27. The Planning Commission Dar es Salaam & Regional Commissioner's Office Tanga Tanga Region Socio-Economic Profile 1997. Available at: http://www.tzonline.org/pdf/Tanga.pdf. Accessed 20 July 2017.

28. Korogwe District. Demographic health survey 2. 2016.

29. Ueda T. Statistics: approval and estimation. Tokyo Japan: Ohmsha.

30. Madeni F, Horiuchi S, Iida M. Evaluation of a reproductive health awareness program for adolescence in urban Tanzania-a quasi-experimental pre-test post-test research. Reprod Health. 2011;8:21.

31. Ajzen I. Theory of planned behavior. Organ Behav Hum Decis Process. 1991;50:179–211.

32. Pembe AB, Urassa DP, Carlstedt A, Lindmark G, Nystrom L, Darj E. Rural Tanzanian women's awareness of danger signs of obstetric complications. BMC Pregnancy Childbirth. 2009;9:12.

33. Urassa PD, Pembe BA, Mganga F. Birth preparedness and complication readiness among women in Mpwapwa district, Tanzania. Tanzanian J Health Res. 2012;14:1–7.

34. Sandelowski M. Focus on research methods: whatever happened to qualitative description? Res Nurs Health. 2000;23:334–40.

35. Bowen DJ, Kreuter M, Spring B, Cofta-Woerpel L, Linnan L, Weiner D, Bakken S, Kaplan CC, Squiers L, Fabrizio C, Fernandez M. How we design feasibility studies. Am J Prev Med. 2009;36(5):452–7. https://doi.org/10.1016/j.amepre.2009.02.002.

36. Nonyane BA, KC A, Callaghan-Koru JA, Guenther T, Sitrin D, Syed U, et al. Equity improvements in maternal and newborn care indicators: results from the Bardiya district of Nepal. Health Policy Plan. 2016;31(4):405–14. https://doi.org/10.1093/heapol/czv077.

37. Thapa DK, Niehof A. Women's autonomy and husbands' involvement in maternal health care in Nepal. Soc Sci Med. 2013;93:1–10.

38. Becker S, Fonseca-Becker F, Schenck-Yglesias C. Husbands' and wives' reports of women's decision-making power in western Guatemala and their effects on preventive health behaviors. Soc Sci Med. 2006;62(9):2313–26.

39. Njuki R, Kimani J, Obare F, Warren C. Using verbal and social autopsies to explore health-seeking behavior among HIV-positive women in Kenya: a retrospective study. BMC Womens Health. 2014;14:77. https://doi.org/10.1186/1472-6874-14-77.

40. Kalisa R, Malande CO. Birth preparedness, complication readiness and male partner involvement for obstetric emergencies in rural Rwanda. Pan Afr Med J. 2016;17(25):91. https://doi.org/10.11604/pamj.2016.25.91.9710.

41. Kujawski S, Mbaruku G, Freedman LP, Ramsey K, Moyo W, Kruk ME. Association between disrespect and abuse during childbirth and women's confidence in health facilities in Tanzania. Matern Child Health J. 2015;19(10):2243–50. https://doi.org/10.1007/s10995-015-1743-9.

42. Larson E, Hermosilla S, Kimweri A, Mbaruku GM, Kruk ME. Determinants of perceived quality of obstetric care in rural Tanzania: a cross-sectional study. BMC Health Serv Res. 2014;14:483. https://doi.org/10.1186/1472-6963-14-483.

43. Sando D, Kendall T, Lyatuu G, Ratcliffe H, McDonald K, Mwanyika-Sando M, et al. Disrespect and abuse during childbirth in Tanzania: are women living with HIV more vulnerable? J Acquir Immune Defic Syndr. 2014;67(Suppl 4):S228–34. https://doi.org/10.1097/QAI.0000000000000378.

44. Mushi D, Mpembeni R, Jahn A. Effectiveness of community based safe motherhood promoters in improving the utilization of obstetric care. The case of Mtwara rural district in Tanzania. BMC Pregnancy Childbirth. 2010;10(14) https://doi.org/10.1186/1471-2393-10-1.

18

Values clarification workshops to improve abortion knowledge, attitudes and intentions: a pre-post assessment in 12 countries

Katherine L. Turner[1,2], Erin Pearson[4], Allison George[3] and Kathryn L. Andersen[4*] ⓘ

Abstract

Background: Women's access to abortion care is often denied or hampered due to a range of barriers, many of which are rooted in abortion stigma. Abortion values clarification and attitude transformation (VCAT) workshops are conducted with abortion providers, trainers, and policymakers and other stakeholders to mitigate the effects of abortion stigma and increase provision of and access to abortion care. This study assesses changes in knowledge, attitudes, and behavioral intentions of VCAT workshop participants.

Methods: Pre- and post-workshop surveys from 43 VCAT workshops conducted in 12 countries in Asia, Africa, and Latin America between 2006 and 2011 were analyzed to assess changes in three domains: knowledge, attitudes and behavioral intentions related to abortion care. A score was created for each domain (range: 0-100), and paired t-tests or Wilcoxon matched-pairs signed-ranks tests were used to test for significant differences between the pre- and post-workshop scores overall and by region and participant type (providers, trainers, and policymakers/other stakeholders). We also assessed changes in pre- and post-workshop scores for participants with the lowest knowledge and negative attitudes on the pre-workshop survey.

Results: Overall, the mean knowledge score increased significantly from 49.0 to 67.1 ($p < 0.001$) out of a total possible score of 100. Attitudes and behavioral intentions showed more modest, but still statistically significant improvements between the pre- and post-workshop surveys. The mean attitudes score increased from 78.2 to 80.9 ($p < 0.001$), and the mean behavioral intentions score rose from 82.2 to 85.4 ($p = 0.03$). Among participants with negative attitudes pre-workshop, most shifted to positive attitudes on the post-workshop survey, ranging from 35.2% who switched to supporting unrestricted access to second-trimester abortion to 90.9% who switched to feeling comfortable working to increase access to contraceptive services in their country. Participants who began the workshop with the lowest level of knowledge experienced the greatest increase in mean knowledge score from 20.0 to 55.0 between pre- and post-workshop surveys ($p < 0.001$).

Conclusions: VCAT workshop participants demonstrated improvements in knowledge, attitudes, and behavioral intentions related to abortion care. Participants who entered the workshops with the lowest levels of knowledge and negative attitudes had the greatest gains in these domains.

Keywords: Values clarification, Attitude transformation, Abortion, Stigma

* Correspondence: andersenk@ipas.org
[4]Technical Innovation and Evidence, Ipas, P.O. Box 9990, Chapel Hill 27515, NC, USA
Full list of author information is available at the end of the article

Plain English summary

Women are often unable to access safe abortion services due to abortion stigma, which prevents potential abortion providers from offering abortion services and prevents other decision-makers such as policymakers or community leaders from supporting abortion service provision. This study found that abortion values clarification and attitude transformation (VCAT) workshops improve participants' knowledge and attitudes about abortion as well as their intentions to support abortion care, especially among those who come to the workshops with the least knowledge and most negative attitudes.

Background

Globally, an estimated 22 million unsafe abortions occur each year, resulting in the preventable deaths of 47,000 women annually [1]. Nearly all unsafe abortions occur among women in developing countries [2]. The determinants of safety for an induced abortion, such as method used and gestational age, are greatly influenced by underlying social factors, including the legal context, the availability services, levels of stigma, women's access to information and women's age and socioeconomic status [3]. Young, poor, rural and indigenous women often have the least access to high-quality abortion care and suffer the most negative consequences; 41% of unsafe abortions in developing regions are among young women aged 15–24 years [4].

Stigma is a learned behavior that impacts provision of and access to abortion care and the social environment surrounding it. Research suggests that abortion care providers in sub-Saharan Africa and Southeast Asia face personal conflicts, stigmatization and victimization with regards to delivering abortion care because of negative attitudes belonging to family, community and policymakers as well as their colleagues [5]. The World Health Organization recommends use of values clarification interventions as an integral part of training for abortion providers [6] to address abortion stigma as a root cause of barriers to abortion service delivery. A range of other stakeholders, influenced by their values, beliefs, attitudes and biases, may also impede women's right to access abortion care. Policymakers and law enforcement impact abortion availability and accessibility through the language, passage, interpretation and enforcement of laws and policies. Ministry of health officials develop service delivery standards and guidelines that outline how and by whom services will be delivered at each level of the health system and the roles, responsibilities and limitations of health system administrators, providers and other health workers. These standards and guidelines may include restrictions that are not required by law or medically necessary that impede women's access to care. All of these stakeholders possess and act upon values

and attitudes which may be guided by misinformation and unexamined, internalized social norms and mores against abortion rather than factually-correct information and a belief in women's right to abortion or an understanding of how restricting access to abortion increases women's risk of death and disability.

Values clarification

Values clarification (VC) is the process of examining one's basic moral reasoning [7] to identify the values that one finds most meaningful and important [8]. The process can help an individual (1) identify when these core values conflict with assumptions or actions that may be informed by social norms and other external influences and (2) examine alternate values and their consequences. Although there is little published literature evaluating strategies for changing attitudes and behaviors of health care providers or other stakeholders [9–13], evidence supports the use of VC principles to improve attitudes and behaviors for social and health issues [14, 15]. In the field of sexual and reproductive health, VC has been employed to reduce HIV stigma [16], aid the integration of medical abortion into health care facilities [17, 18] and increase support for abortion care [19–23].

Use of VC to increase support for abortion services has yielded success in South Africa as shown in a study by Dickson-Tetteh & Reese. An evaluation of over 4000 providers who participated in such workshops demonstrated that close to 70% said that the workshop was helpful in strengthening their ability to work with abortion clients compared to before the workshop [24]. Interviews with a variety of stakeholders who participated in 3-day VC workshops in Limpopo, South Africa indicated that 93.2% of participants expressed increased compassion for women seeking abortions and the clinicians providing services [19]. Another study examining a three-part VC exercise used with 34 nursing students in South Africa found that the number of participants who were against abortion at the start of the training decreased by almost half; additionally, three of the five participants who were originally in favor of abortion only under specific circumstances decided they were not in a position to judge those seeking services upon completion of the exercise [23].

Abortion values clarification and attitude transformation (VCAT)

Abortion values clarification and attitude transformation (VCAT) is an intervention that is grounded in values theory [7] and the Transtheoretical Model [25–27] and builds on similar interventions in other fields [28]. Abortion VC was first implemented in South Africa [19] and then developed by Turner into a global VCAT toolkit and strategy [28]. In VCAT interventions, trained facilitators lead diverse stakeholders through a process conducted in an emotionally safe environment in which they examine their personal values, attitudes and actions related to abortion; engage in honest, open-minded and critical reflection and evaluation of personally-relevant abortion information and situations and fully comprehend the harmful consequences of stigmatizing abortion and restricting service delivery and access to care. In abortion VCAT workshops, participants:

- Challenge deeply-held assumptions and myths
- Clarify and affirm their values and potentially resolve values conflicts
- Potentially transform their beliefs and attitudes that impact behaviors
- State their intentions to act in accordance with their affirmed values

Through this process, VCAT addresses some of the root causes of stigma-related barriers to abortion service delivery, access and quality.

The VCAT theoretical framework developed by Turner and Chapman Page [28] posits that values play a critical role in determining how people make decisions and ultimately act (Fig. 1). The abortion VCAT process takes place within existing cultural and social structures and norms, which are extremely influential in shaping people's attitudes and values. As Dewey states [29], "Valuing occurs when the head and the heart...unite under the direction of action." Values tend to have persistence, assume a pattern in our lives and impact our *attitudes* and behaviors. This framework places the

process of VC within a larger context of attitude transformation, behavioral intentions and, ultimately, behavior or performance. This is unlike traditional VC, in which the end goal is clarified values.

The framework begins with the willingness to change; people must be open to examining their values and potentially changing their attitudes and practices. Participants who effectively engage in the abortion VCAT process: gain new knowledge, deepen their understanding of existing or new knowledge, experience empathy for people who seek, provide or are affected by abortion, clarify current values on abortion, explore alternative values, recognize barriers to change, and remain open to change. Turner and Chapman Page [28] modified the three main stages of values clarification: making an informed value choice, affirming that choice, and acting on the chosen value, which reflects the process and cognitions an individual would go through when thoughtfully choosing among competing alternatives and deciding on a particular course of action. The framework hypothesizes that, after undergoing the values clarification process, participants' attitudes are expected to be consistent with their clarified, affirmed values. Attitudes and beliefs influence behavioral intentions, which in turn predict behaviors [25–27]. These constructs of personal attitude and behavioral intention have been successful in predicting health workers' behaviors in several studies [30, 31].

The VCAT strategy and activities
Strategies based on the abortion VCAT framework focus on the real consequences of abortion stigma: unsafe abortion, which can result in women's injury or death. Faced with these potentially dire consequences, participants in

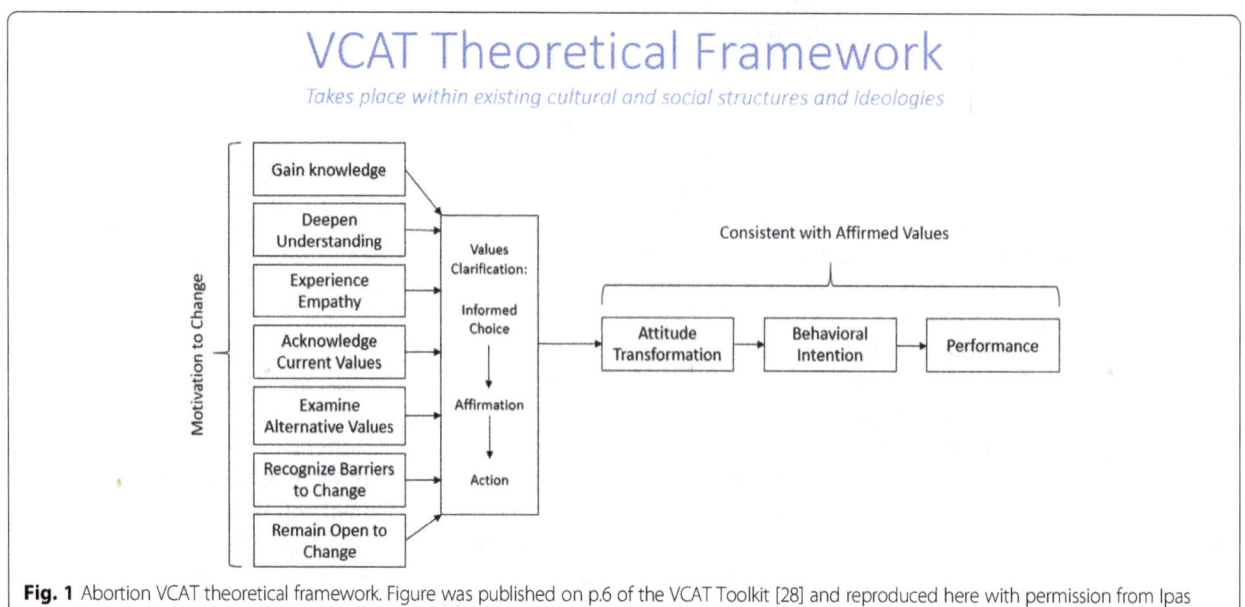

Fig. 1 Abortion VCAT theoretical framework. Figure was published on p.6 of the VCAT Toolkit [28] and reproduced here with permission from Ipas

the VCAT process often move along a progressive continuum from obstruction to tolerance to acceptance to provision or support, and for some, to advocacy for high-quality, comprehensive abortion care for all women. The VCAT intervention consists of participatory presentations and activities (14 total activities in the Toolkit) that engage participants with accurate abortion information, realistic scenarios, critical self-reflection, empathy-evoking experiences and meaningful dialogue on abortion beliefs, values and professional ethics and responsibilities. Each activity includes specific, timely, measureable and detailed learning objectives for participants. Activities are intended to cultivate attitudes that are supportive of women's right to safe abortion care. Participants are given vignettes to discuss and asked to consider the health and social implications when policymakers, providers and other stakeholders restrict access to safe abortion services for certain women. VCAT workshops employ adult learning principles and methodologies, including large and small group discussion, expressive activities, case studies, individual and group work, personal journals and interviews, and self-analysis worksheets. VCAT workshops were designed for use with diverse audiences. Additional versions of the VCAT toolkit activities have been developed to specifically address second trimester abortion, medical abortion, young women's needs and perspectives on abortion care, and sex selective abortion as well as other health areas, including contraceptive services and respectful maternity care.

The present study sought to assess whether VCAT workshops implemented by Ipas, an international NGO seeking to reduce unsafe abortion and increase women's access to comprehensive abortion care, improved participants' knowledge, attitudes and behavioral intentions pertaining to abortion care.

Methods
Study design
This study used matched pre- and post-workshop surveys to assess changes in three domains: knowledge, attitudes and behavioral intentions related to abortion care. During the study period of 2006 to 2011, 118 VCAT workshops were reported, but only 46 of those workshops (39%) conducted matched pre- and post-surveys with participants. The other workshops either did not conduct the pre- and post-workshop surveys, or no code was used to link the pre-workshop survey to a participant's post-workshop survey. In addition, data from three workshops were excluded due to excessive missing data. This analysis presents findings for the convenience sample of 43 workshops in Africa ($n = 22$), Asia ($n = 18$), and Latin America ($n = 3$), which included a total of 641 participants with matched pre- and post-workshop surveys. The participants in workshops

included in this study comprise three main groups: 1) stakeholders, including elected and ministry of health officials, lawyers, journalists, and other political and community leaders; 2) trainers attending training-of-trainer (TOT) events to become trainers on abortion clinical skills; and 3) health care providers, including physicians and mid-level providers such as midwives and nurses. Workshop participants were typically self-nominated or selected based on a perceived or assessed willingness to support, provide or advocate for abortion care, reflecting the reality of conducting interventions such as VCAT.

Data
Standardized pre- and post- workshop surveys were administered to all participants in each of the workshops included in this analysis. Questions were developed in conjunction with the VCAT curriculum to ensure that the measures matched the content of the workshops. The questionnaires were developed in English, then translated and back-translated into both Spanish and French to ensure consistency across country settings. Overall, the survey aimed to measure changes in participants' knowledge, attitudes and behavioral intentions related to abortion care.

Facilitators were able to modify the standard questionnaires to better reflect their country setting. As a result, not all workshops' surveys included all of the standardized components. In particular, all (43 workshops, 641 participants) included the attitude component, 39 workshops (564 participants) included the knowledge component, and 32 workshops (471 participants) included the behavioral intentions component. The pre-workshop survey was completed at the beginning of each workshop, and the post-workshop survey was completed at the end. Data were entered using EpiData software.

Measures
Three domains were assessed by the survey: knowledge, attitudes, and behavioral intentions. The number of items assessing each domain varied somewhat across workshops, and to account for this, scores on a scale of 1 to 100 were created for each of the three domains. Knowledge questions evaluated the participants' knowledge about abortion laws in their country, safe abortion methods, consequences of unsafe abortion, and statistics on unsafe abortion in their country. Knowledge scores were calculated by dividing the number of correct responses by the total number of items (20 on the standard survey), and multiplying by 100. Attitude questions were asked on a five-point Likert scale and evaluated the participants' comfort with the topic of abortion, including their willingness to discuss abortion with colleagues, family and friends, attitudes toward the legality and provision of abortion in their setting. Attitude scores were

calculated by summing the five-point responses, dividing by five times the total number of items (18 on the standard survey), and multiplying by 100. Behavioral intention questions evaluated the participants' intent to participate in activities such as information sharing and advocacy for abortion and, among clinical providers, intentions to perform or assist with abortion procedures in the next six months. Behavioral intention scores were calculated by dividing the number of positive responses by the total number of items (7 on the standard survey), and multiplying by 100.

Missing data

Missing data were handled in two ways. For the knowledge and behavioral intentions components, items that were left unanswered were conservatively coded as "incorrect" or "no, does not intend", respectively. On the knowledge section it was assumed that a participant did not know the correct answer to the question if she or he left the question unanswered. Similarly, on the behavioral intentions section it was assumed that the participant did not intend to participate in the activity or was unsure of whether they would participate in the activity if she or he did not answer the question.

Missing data in the attitudes section could not be easily recoded because attitudes were measured using scales. Missing data were considered to be "not missing at random" since leaving an item blank, such as agreement with second trimester abortion, was expected to be related to the unobserved value. Multivariate multiple imputation was used to assign values for each missing item under the attitude domain using the iterative Markov chain Monte Carlo (MCMC) method [32].

Analysis

Data are presented for each domain overall and by workshop participant type (stakeholder, trainer or provider) and by region (Africa, Asia or Latin America). The mean score and associated standard deviation (SD) are presented for the knowledge and behavior scores, while the mean and standard error (SE) are presented from the

multiple imputation sample for attitude scores. Paired t-tests were used to test for significant differences between the pre- and post-workshop scores where the sample size was sufficient to assume a normal distribution. For analyses with small sample sizes, such as for Latin America, the non-parametric Wilcoxon matched-pairs signed-ranks test was used to test for significant differences between the pre- and post-workshop scores.

We also assessed whether changes in the pre- and post-workshop knowledge scores varied based on participants' knowledge levels at the beginning of the workshop. The pre-workshop scores were divided into quartiles, and within each quartile of the pre-workshop score, the mean pre- and post-workshop scores were calculated. Differences between the pre- and post-workshop scores within each quartile of the pre-workshop score were assessed using the paired t-test.

Finally, we present an analysis of changes in attitudes between the pre- and post-workshop surveys among participants with negative pre-workshop attitudes. This analysis presents data by question and was restricted to the 317 participants who received the 18 standard attitudes questions. For each question, participants' attitudes were classified in three categories: 1) negative, "strongly disagree" or "disagree"; 2) neutral, "neither disagree nor agree"; or 3) positive, "agree" or "strongly agree." Among those who were classified as negative on the pre-workshop survey, we present the proportion classified as negative, neutral and positive on the post-workshop survey. The Kruskal-Wallis one-way analysis of variance test, the non-parametric version of the one-way analysis of variance (ANOVA), was used to test for differences between the pre- and post-workshop surveys. Statistical significance was assessed at an alpha level of 0.05 for all analyses. Statistical analyses were conducted using Stata version 11.2.

Results

Table 1 presents the mean scores for each domain overall and by workshop participant type. Overall, the mean

Table 1 Mean pre- and post-workshop knowledge, attitude and behavioral intention scores, overall and by type of participants

	Knowledge						Attitudes						Behavioral Intentions					
		Pre-workshop		Post-workshop				Pre-workshop		Post-workshop				Pre-workshop		Post-workshop		
	n	Mean	(SD)	Mean	(SD)	p-value	n	Mean	(SE)[1]	Mean	(SE)[1]	p-value	n	Mean	(SD)	Mean	(SD)	p-value
Providers	300	36.7	(19.4)	60.9	(20.2)	<0.001	332	77.9	(0.71)	81.6	(0.62)	<0.001	162	81.6	(27.0)	88.1	(22.1)	0.007
Trainers	167	68.1	(17.9)	77.8	(13.7)	<0.001	167	80.1	(0.93)	83.1	(0.76)	0.001	167	86.3	(26.4)	91.5	(17.7)	0.007
Stakeholders	97	54.3	(19.4)	68.1	(17.4)	<0.001	142	77.4	(0.71)	76.7	(0.82)	0.177	142	77.9	(30.3)	75.0	(36.0)	0.374
Total	564	49.0	(23.5)	67.1	(19.4)	<0.001	641	78.2	(0.47)	80.9	(0.43)	<0.001	471	82.2	(28.0)	85.4	(26.8)	0.027

[1]Standard error (SE) is presented for the attitudes scores rather than the standard deviation (SD) because the mean for this score was derived from the multiple imputation sample

[2]P-values associated with paired t-tests

knowledge score increased from 49.0 (SD = 23.5) on the pre-workshop survey to 67.1 (SD = 19.4) on the post-workshop survey (p < 0.001) (Table 1). Trainers had the highest mean pre-workshop knowledge score (mean = 68.1; SD = 17.9), which increased by almost 10 points on the post-workshop survey (p < 0.001). Among stakeholders, the mean score increased from 54.3 (SD = 19.4) on the pre-workshop survey to 68.1 (SD = 17.4) on the post-workshop survey (p < 0.001). Though providers had the lowest mean pre-workshop knowledge score (36.7), they also had the largest increase between the pre- and post-workshop surveys; the mean score increased by almost 25 points between the pre- and post-workshop surveys (p < 0.001).

Overall, attitudes showed modest but statistically significant improvement between the pre- and post-workshop surveys from 78.2 (SE = 0.47) on the pre-workshop survey to 80.9 (SE = 0.43) on the post-workshop survey (p < 0.001). The largest increases were observed for providers whose mean attitude score increased by 4 points from 77.9 (SE = 0.71) on the pre-workshop survey to 81.6 (SE = 0.62) on the post-workshop survey (p < 0.001) (Table 1). A statistically significant increase in the attitudes score was also observed for trainers, from a mean of 80.1 (SE = 0.93) on the pre-workshop survey to 83.1 (SE = 0.76) on the post-workshop survey (p = 0.001). Statistically significant changes were not observed for stakeholders.

Similarly, behavioral intentions showed modest gains between the pre- and post-workshop surveys from 82.2 (SD = 28.0) on the pre-workshop survey to 85.4 (SD = 26.8) on the post-workshop survey (p = 0.027). Providers' mean behavioral intentions score increased by almost 7 points from a mean of 81.6 (SD = 27.0) on the pre-workshop survey to 88.1 (SD = 22.1) on the post-workshop survey (p = 0.007) (Table 1). Among trainers, mean behavioral intention scores increased by 4 points from 86.3 (SD = 26.4) on the pre-workshop survey to 91.5 (SD = 17.7) on the post-workshop survey (p = 0.007). Again, no statistically significant changes were observed for stakeholders.

Table 2 presents the mean scores for each domain by region. Statistically significant improvements were observed in knowledge, attitudes and behavioral intentions for the participants in Africa. The mean knowledge score increased by almost 17 points between the pre- and post-workshop surveys (p < 0.001), and the mean attitudes score increased by 3 points (p < 0.001). The mean behavioral intentions score increased from 83.0 (SD = 28.6) on the pre-workshop survey to 86.8 (SD = 26.5) on the post-workshop survey (p = 0.030). In Asia there were significant increases in knowledge and attitude scores, but not in the behavioral intentions score. The mean knowledge score increased by 20 points, from 43.7 (SD = 24.3) on the pre-workshop survey to 63.7 (SD = 21.2) on the post-workshop survey (p < 0.001). The mean attitude score showed a more modest increase from 78.3 (SE = 0.72) on the pre-workshop survey to 81.0 (SE = 0.66) on the post-workshop survey (p = 0.001). In Latin America, statistically significant changes were not observed in any of the domains.

Figure 2 presents a comparison of the mean pre- and post-workshop knowledge scores by quartile of the pre-workshop knowledge score. Increases in the mean knowledge score were observed between the pre- and post-workshop surveys for all participants, regardless of pre-workshop knowledge. However, the participants who began the workshop with the lowest level of knowledge, those in the 25th percentile, experienced the greatest increase in mean knowledge score (35 points) between the pre- and post-workshop surveys (p < 0.001). Participants in the 50th and 75th percentiles of the pre-workshop knowledge score saw similar increases in mean score of 18 points (p < 0.001) and 13 points (p < 0.001), respectively. A smaller increase in mean score was observed for participants in the highest quartile of the pre-workshop knowledge score (2 points; p = 0.04). Similar, statistically-significant results were found for attitudes and behavioral intentions; those who reported more negative attitudes and behavioral intentions on the pre-workshop survey showed the largest gains in mean score on the post-workshop survey (data not shown).

Table 2 Mean pre- and post-workshop knowledge, attitude and behavioral intention scores, overall and by region

	Knowledge						Attitudes						Behavioral Intentions					
		Pre-workshop		Post-workshop				Pre-workshop		Post-workshop				Pre-workshop		Post-workshop		
	n	Mean	(SD)	Mean	(SD)	p-value[2]	n	Mean	(SE)[1]	Mean	(SE)[1]	p-value[2]	n	Mean	(SD)	Mean	(SD)	p-value[2]
Africa	275	54.0	(21.7)	70.9	(17.0)	< 0.001	320	78.3	(0.67)	81.5	(0.59)	< 0.001	320	83.0	(28.6)	86.8	(26.5)	0.030
Asia	279	43.7	(24.3)	63.7	(21.2)	< 0.001	279	78.3	(0.72)	81.0	(0.66)	0.001	109	80.2	(28.4)	81.8	(28.3)	0.636
Latin America	10	60.5	(11.4)	61.0	(12.6)	0.907	42	77.0	(1.48)	76.7	(1.62)	0.882	42	80.9	(22.0)	84.1	(24.1)	0.147
Total	564	49.0	(23.5)	67.1	(19.4)	< 0.001	641	78.2	(0.47)	80.9	(0.43)	< 0.001	471	82.2	(28.0)	85.4	(26.8)	0.027

[1]Standard error (SE) is presented for the attitudes scores rather than the standard deviation (SD) because the mean for this score was derived from the multiple imputation sample
[2]P-values associated with paired t-tests or Wilcoxon matched-pairs signed-ranks test, as appropriate

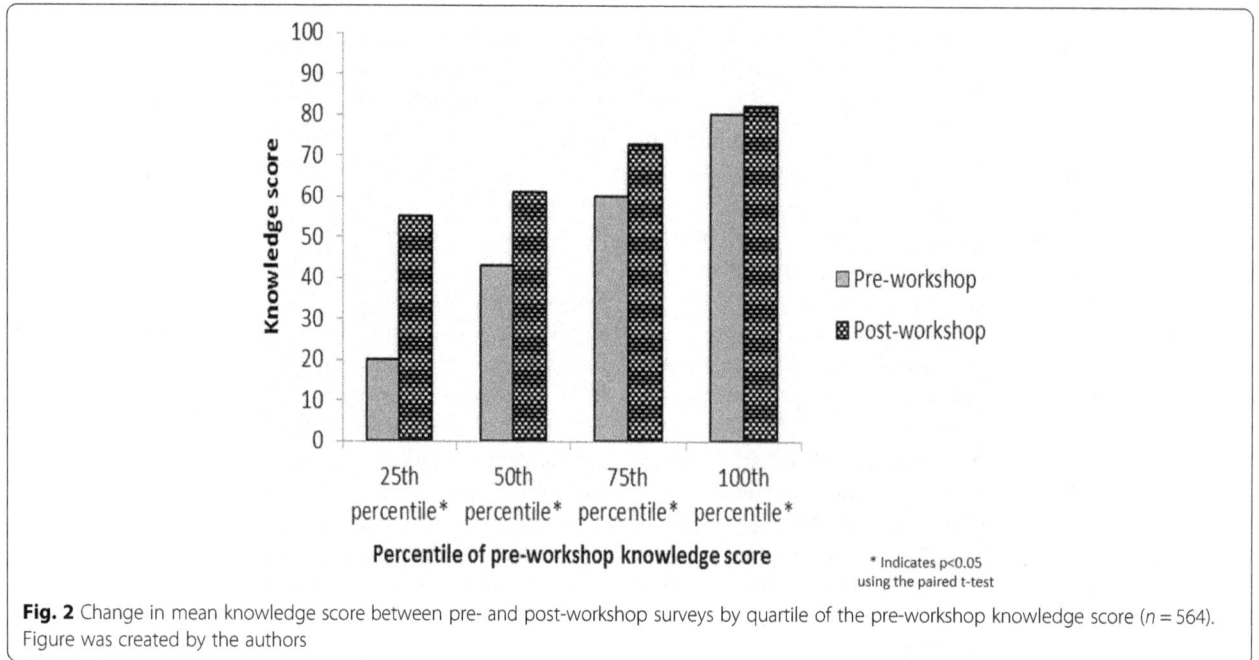

Fig. 2 Change in mean knowledge score between pre- and post-workshop surveys by quartile of the pre-workshop knowledge score (n = 564). Figure was created by the authors

Table 3 presents an analysis of the post-workshop attitudes among those who had negative attitudes on the pre-workshop survey. Among the 317 participants who completed the standardized attitudes questions, the number who had negative attitudes pre-workshop ranged from 9 (2.8%) who did not support provision of family planning in their country to 156 (49.2%) who felt that access to second trimester abortion services should be restricted to certain circumstances. Most participants who had negative attitudes pre-workshop reported a shift to positive attitudes on the post-workshop survey. Of particular interest were attitudes about support for abortion services as permitted by law; of the 47 participants who were unsupportive pre-workshop, 31 (66.0%) reported positive attitudes, 8 (17.0%) reported neutral attitudes, and 8 (17.0%) maintained their negative attitudes on the post-workshop survey ($p = 0.010$). Similarly, 41 participants reported that they were uncomfortable with working to increase access to abortion services pre-workshop, and the majority (63.4%) reported positive attitudes on the post-workshop survey ($p < 0.001$). Comfort with performing or assisting with an abortion procedure showed a smaller improvement; of the 41 who reported being uncomfortable pre-workshop, 17 (41.5%) reported positive attitudes, 8 (19.5%) reported neutral attitudes, and 16 (39.0%) maintained their negative attitudes on the post-workshop survey ($p < 0.001$). Support for access to safe, comprehensive abortion care increased for both the first and second trimester, but 36.4% of participants maintained their negative attitudes about second trimester care, compared to only 10.5% for first trimester care.

Discussion

This study documents the results of abortion VCAT workshops to improve knowledge, attitudes and intentions to provide support, assist or advocate for abortion care. Across workshop types and locations, the greatest improvements were observed in knowledge. Mean knowledge scores were low pre-workshop, especially among providers and participants from Asia, but these scores increased by up to 24 points between the pre- and post-workshop surveys. Participants who entered the workshops with the lowest levels of knowledge experienced the greatest gains. However, participants with the lowest pre-workshop knowledge did not catch up to their more knowledgeable peers; their post-workshop scores were still lower than those of participants who had high pre-workshop scores. Previous work has demonstrated a dose-response relationship between exposure to abortion messages and abortion knowledge, suggesting that multiple exposures to messages about abortion may be needed over time to increase knowledge in a meaningful way [33]. A question that could be further explored is whether the post-survey mean knowledge scores were sufficiently high, and given the relationship between knowledge and attitudes in the VCAT theoretical framework, whether higher knowledge gains might result in more positive attitudes.

More modest increases in the attitudes scores were observed, which was expected because attitudes may be less pliable than knowledge and is in line with other studies [34]. The VCAT workshops' effect on participants' attitudes varied by question. VCAT workshops were more successful in shifting those with negative

Table 3 Post-workshop attitudes among 317 participants with negative attitudes at pre-workshop survey

Attitude question	Negative attitude at pre-test	Post-workshop attitudes among those who had negative attitudes at pre-test						
		Negative		Neutral		Positive		
	n	n	(%)	n	(%)	n	(%)	p-value[1]
The issue of abortion is important to me	41	13	(31.7)	2	(4.9)	26	(63.4)	0.002
I support the provision of FP and contraceptive services in my country	9	1	(11.1)	0	(0)	8	(88.9)	0.909
I feel comfortable working to increase access to FP and contraceptive services in my country	11	1	(9.1)	0	(0)	10	(90.9)	0.419
I support the provision of abortion services as permitted by law in my country	47	8	(17.0)	8	(17.0)	31	(66.0)	0.010
I feel comfortable working to increase access to abortion services as permitted by law in my country	41	4	(9.8)	11	(26.8)	26	(63.4)	< 0.001
I feel comfortable talking with my closest friends about my involvement with abortion care	30	6	(20.0)	4	(13.3)	20	(66.7)	0.007
I feel comfortable talking with my closest family members about my involvement with abortion care	47	13	(27.7)	9	(19.1)	25	(53.2)	< 0.001
I would feel comfortable observing an abortion procedure[2]	41	13	(31.7)	9	(22.0)	19	(46.3)	< 0.001
I would feel comfortable performing or assisting an abortion procedure[2]	41	16	(39.0)	8	(19.5)	17	(41.5)	< 0.001
I am clear about my personal values concerning abortion	18	1	(5.6)	1	(5.6)	16	(88.8)	0.534
I do not feel conflicted about abortion	67	17	(25.4)	13	(19.4)	37	(55.2)	0.013
I can clearly explain my personal values concerning abortion	19	3	(15.8)	3	(15.8)	13	(68.4)	0.106
I can respectfully explain values concerning abortion that conflict with mine	22	3	(13.6)	2	(9.1)	17	(77.3)	0.276
I feel empathy for women who have experienced abortion	25	9	(36.0)	6	(24.0)	10	(40.0)	< 0.001
All women should have access to safe, comprehensive abortion care in the first trimester	38	4	(10.5)	12	(31.6)	22	(57.9)	0.002
Access to first-trimester abortion should not be restricted to certain circumstances	111	47	(42.3)	14	(12.6)	50	(45.1)	< 0.001
All women should have access to safe, comprehensive abortion care in the second trimester	88	32	(36.4)	16	(18.2)	40	(45.4)	< 0.001
Access to second-trimester abortion should not be restricted to certain circumstances	156	77	(49.4)	24	(15.4)	55	(35.2)	< 0.001

[1]P-value associated with the Kruskal-Wallis one-way analysis of variance test
[2]Excludes attendees of stakeholder workshops since most were non-clinical (n = 198)

attitudes pre-workshop to neutral or positive attitudes for questions that were less controversial, such as support for family planning. Meanwhile, attitudes about more stigmatized issues, such as second trimester abortion care, were not as readily improved, which is in line with other studies that have shown challenges in improving provider attitudes about reasons for abortion that may be considered more controversial in some settings [34]. At the community level, studies have shown that exposure to abortion messages is associated with positive attitudes about abortion [35], but more research is needed to understand what is required to achieve the tipping point from negative to positive attitudes about abortion. Though the increase in the mean attitude score was small, it is important that the majority of participants who had negative attitudes pre-workshop showed improved attitudes on the post-workshop survey. A goal

of the VCAT workshops is to shift individuals along the continuum from obstructionist to tolerant to supportive attitudes. Those whose attitudes shift from negative to neutral may be less likely to obstruct and may even support or facilitate women's access to care and colleagues' service provision. In addition, individuals who leave VCAT workshops with positive attitudes may be the most likely to provide, support and advocate for abortion.

The smallest increases were observed in the behavioral intentions scores, which are partially explained by the very high scores on the pre-workshop survey. It is likely that the pre-workshop behavioral intentions scores were high because participants were either selected by NGO staff and colleagues due to past support for or work in abortion or because they meet other screening criteria for abortion VCAT workshops. Thus, many of the participants likely intended to support or provide abortion services prior to the VCAT workshop. This affects how much change is likely or possible between pre- and post-test. The data suggest that those who enter the workshops with the lowest levels of knowledge and more negative attitudes and behavioral intentions are the participants who experience the greatest gains in these domains. However, it is possible that even modest improvements in attitudes and behavioral intentions could affect workshop participants' willingness to support or provide abortion services or improve the quality of care they provide, based on an improved understanding of women's right to abortion and consequences of poor access to or quality of care. VCAT workshops and post-test scores can help organizations decide which participants are committed to abortion service provision and thus merit the significant investment of clinical training and follow-up support at their facilities.

Statistically significant increases were observed in all three domains for provider and trainer workshops, but stakeholder workshops only resulted in a statistically significant increase in knowledge. Abortion VCAT workshops were originally designed for use with abortion providers, but the stakeholder workshops were conducted with a diverse group of people, including politicians, journalists and community leaders. Results suggest that new VCAT toolkit modules may be needed to improve attitudes and behavioral intentions for non-clinician participants such as those who participate in stakeholder workshops.

Regional variation was observed in the results with statistically significant improvement across all three domains in Africa, in knowledge and attitudes in Asia, and in none of the domains in Latin America. In Asia, we did not observe statistically significant changes in behavioral intentions, which may be due to the smaller sample size for this domain compared to the knowledge and attitudes domains. Approximately 60% of the participants in Asia did not receive the behavioral intentions component of the pre- and post-workshop surveys, which resulted in a much smaller sample size for analysis of this domain (109 participants) compared to the knowledge and attitudes domains (279 participants). In Latin America, significant changes were not observed in any of the domains. The VCAT organizers and facilitators in this region attribute this to the survey instrument and maintain that a context-specific pre- and post-test is needed. More contextual analysis is needed to better understand the results of abortion VCAT workshops in Latin America.

Limitations

This study had several limitations. The primary limitation of this study was that surveys were only conducted before and immediately following each workshop, and as a result, it was not possible to measure lasting change. Because identifiers were not recorded on the participants' pre- and post-workshop surveys, the changes in the three domains assessed by the surveys could not be linked to behavioral outcomes such as abortion procedures performed or advocacy efforts. It is possible that better attitudes and behavioral intentions on the post-workshop survey reflect social desirability bias rather than a true improvement in attitudes and intentions, and though the results of this study suggest positive change, behavior change cannot be assessed. Future research could link changes in knowledge, attitudes and behavioral intentions with actual behaviors and practices.

Another limitation is selection bias. As previously mentioned, it is likely that pre-workshop behavioral intention scores were high because participants self-selected or were selected by workshop organizers to participate in the VCAT workshops because they had demonstrated support for abortion service provision and access in their previous work. Though selection bias should be recognized, it also represents a reality of implementing an intervention such as VCAT in that workshops would usually be conducted with willing participants. In addition, this study only reflects findings from a small convenience sample of all VCAT workshops. It is possible that the workshops for which data were available had more conscientious organizers and facilitators, which could be associated with more positive workshop outcomes. As a result, results may not be representative of all VCAT workshop participants.

Finally, missing data was a limitation. A conservative approach was taken, and missing data for the knowledge and behavioral intentions was coded as "incorrect" or "no". As a result, the calculated scores may be an underestimate of the true knowledge and behavioral intentions scores.

Conclusions

This study demonstrated that abortion VCAT workshops led to improvements in participant knowledge, attitudes, and behavioral intentions regarding abortion. Findings suggest that participants who enter the workshops with the lowest levels of knowledge and more negative attitudes are the participants who experience the greatest improvements in those domains. Additional research is needed to understand long-term gains in knowledge and attitudes resulting from VCAT as well as actual behavior change in support for or provision of abortion services.

Abbreviations

ANOVA: Analysis of variance; NGO: Non-governmental organization; SD: Standard deviation; SE: Standard error; TOT: Training of the trainer; VC: Values clarification; VCAT: Values clarification and attitude transformation

Acknowledgements

The authors would like to thank Kimberly Chapman Page, co-author of the Toolkit, Joan Healy for her review and inputs, Kyle Pennisi for her research and inputs and the many Ipas staff, colleagues and workshop facilitators and participants around the world who contributed to abortion VCAT implementation and evaluation.

Funding

This study was internally funded by Ipas as data were collected as a part of routine data collection for monitoring and evaluation purposes.

Authors' contributions

KT developed the VCAT Toolkit, theoretical framework, strategy and workshop curricula, and KT and AG supported implementation of the VCAT workshops, design and interpretation of study results, and wrote portions of the manuscript. KA and EP led the design, analysis and interpretation of study results and wrote portions of the manuscript. All authors reviewed and approved the final version of the manuscript.

Competing interests

The authors declare that they have no competing interests.

Author details

[1]Global Citizen, LLC Consulting, 732 Ninth St., No. 521, Durham 27705, NC, USA. [2]UNC-Chapel Hill Gillings School of Global Public Health, Chapel Hill, USA. [3]Public Health Solutions, 40 Worth Street, 5th Floor, New York 10013, NY, USA. [4]Technical Innovation and Evidence, Ipas, P.O. Box 9990, Chapel Hill 27515, NC, USA.

References

1. Ahman E, Shah IH. New estimates and trends regarding unsafe abortion mortality. Int J Gynecol Obstet. 2011;115(2):121–6.
2. World Health Organization (WHO): Unafe abortion: Global and regional estimates of the incidence of unsafe abortion and associated mortality in 2008: Sixth ed. Italy: WHO; 2011.
3. Ganatra B, Tunçalp Ö, Johnston HB, Johnson BR, Gülmezoglu AM, Temmerman M. From concept to measurement: operationalizing WHO's definition of unsafe abortion. Bull World Health Organ. 2014;92(3):155.
4. Shah I, Åhman E. Unsafe abortion differentials in 2008 by age and developing country region: high burden among young women. Reprod Health Matters. 2012;20(39):169–73.
5. Loi UR, Gemzell-Danielsson K, Faxelid E, Klingberg-Allvin M: Health care providers' perceptions of and attitudes towards induced abortions in sub-Saharan Africa and Southeast Asia: a systematic literature review of qualitative and quantitative data. BMC Public Health. 2015;15(139):1 13. https://bmcpublichealth.biomedcentral.com/track/pdf/10.1186/s12889-015-1502-2?site=bmcpublichealth.biomedcentral.com.
6. World Health Organization (WHO). Safe abortion: technical and policy guidance for health systems. 2nd ed. Geneva: WHO; 2012.
7. Rokeach M. The nature of human values. New York: Free Press; 1973.
8. Steele S. Values clarification in nursing. New York: Appleton-Century-Crofts; 1979.
9. Harris LH, Debbink M, Martin L, Hassinger J. Dynamics of stigma in abortion work: findings from a pilot study of the providers share workshop. Soc Sci Med. 2011;73(7):1062–70.
10. Bingham A, Drake JK, Goodyear L, Gopinath CY, Kaufman A, Bhattarai S. The role of interpersonal communication in preventing unsafe abortion in communities: the dialogues for life project in Nepal. J Health Commun. 2011;16(3):245–63.
11. Banerjee SK, Andersen KL, Warvadekar J, Pearson E. Effectiveness of a behavior change communication intervention to improve knowledge and perceptions about abortion in Bihar and Jharkhand, India. Int Perspect Sexual Reprod Health. 2013;39(3):142–51.
12. Rowe A, de Savigny D, Lanata C, Victora CG. How can we achieve and maintain high-quality performance of health workers in low-resource settings? Lancet. 2005;366(9490):1026–35.
13. World Health Organization (WHO): Strategies for assisting health workers to modify and improve skills: developing quality health care – a process of change. 2000,
14. Karel M, Powell J, Cantor M. Using a values clarification guide to facilitate communication in advance care planning. Patient Educ Couns. 2004;55:22–31.
15. Mosconi J, Emmett J. Effects of a values clarification curriculum on high school students' definitions of success. ASCA Prof Sch Couns. 2003;7(2):68–78.
16. Kidd R, Clay S, Chiiya C: Understanding and challenging HIV stigma: toolkit for action. 2007,
17. Leeman L, Espey E. "You Can't do that 'round here": a case study of the introduction of medical abortion care at a university medical center. Contraception. 2005;71(2):84–8.
18. Prine L, Lesnewski F, Bregman R. Integrating abortion into a residency practice. Fam Med. 2003;35(7):469–71.
19. Mitchell E, Trueman K, Gabriel M, Bickers Bock L. Building alliances from ambivalence: evaluation of abortion values clarification workshops with stakeholders in South Africa. Afr J Reprod Health. 2005;9(3):89–99.
20. Turner KL, Hyman A, Gabriel M. Clarifying values and transforming attitudes to improve access to second trimester abortion. Reprod Health Matters. 2008;16(31, Suppl. 1):108–16.
21. Gómez Ponce de León R, Turner KL. Clarificación de valores para la transformación de actitudes : Una herramienta para el mejoramiento de la calidad de la asistencia a mujeres en situación de aborto. (Clarifying values for attitude changes: A tool for improving quality assistance to women in abortion situations). Revista Peru Ginecol Obstet. 2009;55(4):240–7.
22. Capiello J, Beal MW, Gallogly-Hudson K. Applying ethical practice competences to the prevention and management of unintended pregnancy. J Obstet Gynecol Neonatal Nurs. 2011;40(6):808–16.
23. Mpeli MR, Botma Y. Abortion-related services: value clarification through 'difficult dialogues' strategies. Educ Citizenship Social Justice. 2015;10(3):278–88.
24. Dickson-Tetteh K, Rees H. Efforts to reduce abortion-related mortality in South Africa. In: Berer M, Sundari Ravindran TK, editors. Safe motherhood initiatives: critical issues. Oxford, England: Blackwell Science; 1999. p. 198–219.
25. Ajzen I. From intentions to actions: a theory of planned behavior. In: Kuhl J, Beckman J, editors. Action-control: from cognition to behavior. Heidelberg: Springer; 1985. p. 11–39.
26. Ajzen I. Attitudes, personality, and behavior. Chicago: Dorsey Press; 1988.
27. Ajzen I. The theory of planned behavior. Organ Behav Hum Decis Process. 1991;50:179–211.
28. Turner KL, Chapman Page K: Abortion attitude transformation: a values clarification toolkit for global audiences. 2008,
29. Dewey J. Theory of valuation. Chicago: University of Chicago Press; 1939.
30. Millstein SG. Utility of the theories of reasoned action and planned behavior for predicting physician behavior: a prospective analysis. Health Psychol. 1996;15(5):398–402.
31. Armitage CJ, Christian J. Planned behavior: The relationship between human thought and action. New Brunswick, New Jersey: Transaction Publishers; 2004.
32. Rubin D. Multiple Imputation for Nonresponse in Surveys. New York, NY: John Wiley & Sons; 2009.
33. Banerjee S, Andersen KL, Pearson E, Warvadekar J, Khan D, Batra S. Evaluating the relative effectiveness of high-intensity and low-intensity models of behavior change communication interventions for abortion care-seeking in Bihar and Jharkhand, India: a cross-sectional study. BMJ Open. 2017;7(2):e012198.
34. Pace L, Sandahl Y, Backus L, Silveira M, Steinauer J. Medical students for Choice's reproductive health externships: impact on medical students' knowledge, attitudes and intention to provide abortions. Contraception. 2008;78(1):31–5.
35. Banerjee SK, Andersen KL, Buchanan RM, Warvadekar J: Woman-centered research on access to safe abortion services and implications for behavioral change communication interventions: a cross-sectional study of women in Bihar and Jharkhand, India. BMC Public Health 2012; 12(175):1–13. https://bmcpublichealth.biomedcentral.com/track/pdf/10.1186/1471-2458-12-175?site=bmcpublichealth.biomedcentral.com.

19

Childbirth experiences and their derived meaning: a qualitative study among postnatal mothers in Mbale regional referral hospital, Uganda

Josephine Namujju[1]*[ID], Richard Muhindo[1], Lilian T. Mselle[2], Peter Waiswa[3,4], Joyce Nankumbi[1] and Patience Muwanguzi[1]

Abstract

Background: Evidence shows that negative childbirth experiences may lead to undesirable effects including failure to breastfeed, reduced love for the baby, emotional upsets, post-traumatic disorders and depression among mothers. Understanding childbirth experiences and their meaning could be important in planning individualized care for mothers. The purpose of this study was to explore childbirth experiences and their meaning among postnatal mothers.

Methods: A phenomenological qualitative study was conducted at Mbale Regional Referral Hospital among 25 postnatal mothers within two months after birth using semi-structured interviews and focus group discussions and data was thematically analyzed.

Results: The severity, duration and patterns of labour pains were a major concern by almost all women. Women had divergent feelings of yes and no need of biomedical pain relief administration during childbirth. Mothers were socially orientated to regard labour pains as a normal phenomenon regardless of their nature. The health providers' attitudes, care and support gave positive and negative birth experiences. The Physical and psychosocial support provided comfort, consolation and encouragement to the mothers while inappropriate care, poor communication and compromised privacy contributed to the mothers' negative childbirth experiences. The type of birth affected the interpretations of the birth experiences. Women who gave birth vaginally, thought they were strong and brave, determined and self-confident; and were respected by members of their communities. On the contrary, the women who gave birth by operation were culturally considered bewitched, weak and failures.

Conclusion: Childbirth experiences were unique; elicited unique feelings, responses and challenges to individual mothers. The findings may be useful in designing interventions that focus on individualized care to meet individual needs and expectations of mothers during childbirth.

Keywords: Childbirth, Experiences, Meaning, Postnatal mothers, Uganda

* Correspondence: mwanjejose@yahoo.com
[1]Department of Nursing, Makerere University, College of Health Sciences, P.O Box 7072, Kampala, Uganda
Full list of author information is available at the end of the article

Plain ENGLISH summary

Childbirth experiences are the women's personal feelings and interpretations of birth processes. Birth experiences to some women have meant hard work, exciting lovely event and to others it is a stressful, exhausting and unpredictable experience. Negative experiences have been associated with poor support and care, fear, excessive pain, discomfort and undesirable outcomes. Participating in making decisions regarding childbirth care and being supported by healthcare providers gives a positive memory and increases the woman's confidence and love for the baby and better adjustment to motherhood. Understanding the women's childbirth experiences and their meaning is important in providing socially acceptable individualized care during and after birth. In Uganda, few studies on childbirth experiences of mothers and their meanings have been done. This study explored childbirth experiences and their meanings among women within two months after giving birth. Twelve women were interviewed one on one and thirteen women in two groups of seven and six in Mbale Regional Referral Hospital, in the Eastern part of Uganda. The women reported unique experiences of labour pains, they had social orientation on labour and gave different views on pain management during birth. Negative and positive attitudes and care by service providers were described and the social support from the significant others was noted as a source of comfort and encouragement. The personal women's and society's interpretations of birth experiences focused on the type of birth undergone. The vaginal birth meant braveness to some mothers and caesarean birth was associated with witchcraft and weakness of a woman. In conclusion, the individual mothers had unique childbirth experiences that required service provider's understanding and personalized care.

Background

Childbirth is a significant event in a woman's life and a transition to motherhood. Childbirth experiences are the subjective psychological and physiological processes, influenced by the social and environmental factors [1]. Birth experiences elicit uncertainties of the next destination with feelings of inabilities [2]. Labour pain has been regarded as a "well kept – secret" whose true reality cannot be explained until you go through it causing fear and emotional upsets [3]. Childbirth is perceived as a paradox of moments of sadness and disappointment initially and joy crowns its end if a baby is alive [3]. The interpretations of birth experiences further include hard work, exciting intimate event and a stressful, exhausting and unpredictable phenomenon [4]. To some women, giving birth is life itself, a fulfillment of God's plan and the law of procreation and a turning point between death and life for the woman and her baby [5].

Childbirth experiences could be both positive and negative. Negative experiences are characterized by fear, excessive pain, poor support and care, discomfort and undesirable outcomes [6–8]. The negative experiences of medical interventions like epidural analgesia, induction of labor and instrumental vaginal delivery have been found to be associated with post-traumatic stress, fear of childbirth, reduced child care and emotional upsets among women [7, 9]. The positive memories of being in control over the situational happenings and the decisions on care coupled with the healthcare providers' support are said to enhance self-confidence with feelings of accomplishment and better adjustment to motherhood [9–11]. The positive birth experiences are thus said to improve the bonding between the mother and the baby [12–14].

Understanding the women's childbirth experiences and their meaning is crucial in the provision of individualized and culturally sensitive care during and after childbirth [15–17]. A number of studies have described women's childbirth experiences and their meaning but these studies were done in the developed world. In Uganda, studies on childbirth experiences of mothers and the perceived meanings are scarce. This study therefore, describes the childbirth experiences and the perceived meanings among postnatal mothers seeking postnatal services at Mbale Regional Referral Hospital in Eastern Uganda to broaden the information base for appropriate intervention development and individualized care during childbirth.

Methods

Study design and setting

A phenomenological qualitative research design was used. Phenomenological qualitative research is an approach that describes life experiences and gives them meaning [18]. The design allows exploration of participants' experiences, perspectives and feelings, in depth, through a holistic framework. Childbirth is a lived experience to women whose truth and reality is deeply embedded in the lives of those that have experienced it [19, 20]. In this study, it was specifically used to explore experiences, feelings and perspectives of women who had given birth. The study was conducted at Mbale Regional Referral Hospital (MRRH) located in Mbale Municipality, Northeast of Kampala, Uganda. MRRH is a public hospital with 500 bed capacity. The hospital serves 13 districts (with about 4 million people in the region) and about 800 women give birth per month in this hospital. Specifically, the study was carried out at the Young Child Clinic (YCC), one of the clinics run by the Department of Obstetrics and Gynaecology in MRRH. The clinic had four certified health care providers including 3 midwives and 1 public health nurse. It offers immunization, health education, monitoring growth and development to children under 5 years;

postnatal care services, HIV counseling and testing, and referral services for example HIV positive mothers and babies were being referred to the HIV clinic for care. On average, 35 mothers and babies were attended to at this clinic per day.

Participants and recruitment

Purposive sampling was used to recruit participants. Purposive sampling allows a researcher to get rich information to a particular research question [21]. The researcher oriented the staff of the YCC on the study and worked with the midwife in charge of the clinic to identify potential participants. The inclusion criteria were the postnatal mothers who gave birth within two months with live babies and those that were able to communicate in English, Luganda or Lumasaba. Luganda however, which all participants understood and spoke fluently was preferred in the two discussions. After receiving the services they had come for, all the potential participants were requested to meet with the researcher. She explained to them the study, its aim and how it was going to be conducted including their rights and the principles of confidentiality. Those who agreed to take part in the study gave written consent and a suitable place (with privacy) at hospital was arranged for an interview or discussion.

Data collection

To build the credibility and better understanding of the childbirth experiences two methods of data collection were used; the semi-structured interviews (SSI) and the focus group discussions (FGDs).

Semi-structured interviews

Twelve (12) semi-structured interviews with postnatal mothers were conducted in Luganda and English by the first author at YCC in a quiet room adjacent to the clinic. The saturation was reached with 12 interviews where the answers from mothers seemed to repeat information gained earlier with little new information [22]. A semi-structured interview guide with open ended questions and probes were used to explore and understand better the issues as they emerged [23] and elicited broader and deeper views from participants. All the interviews were audio recorded and lasted within 30 min.

Focus group discussions

Two FGDs with postnatal mothers were conducted. The discussion groups included 6 and 7 postnatal mothers. The first author moderated the discussions and notes and non-verbal clues were taken by the assistant, the clinic midwife who was not involved during the participants' recruitment process. The FGD guide used centered on the mothers' childbirth experiences and their

meanings. The discussions were held in Luganda, the local language of instruction in schools, spoken and preferred by all participants and all the discussions were audio recorded with permission from participants. The discussions lasted between 60 and 80 min.

Data analysis

Thematic analysis guided the analysis of data. All the audio recorded interviews and discussions were transcribed verbatim and were translated from Luganda to English. The English translated transcripts were reviewed and edited to ensure correct interpretation of the mothers' accounts. The analysis procedure included familiarization with the material through careful reading of sentence by sentence for many times, identification of the codes, searching for subcategories, formulation, revision and interpretation of themes. Phrases and sentences related to the mothers' experiences of childbirth were coded in the margin of the transcript sheets. The coding was predominantly close to the text using mothers' own descriptions. The codes with similar content were then brought together into sub-categories and themes. The authors discussed and reflected on the interpretations of the mothers' descriptions of their childbirth experiences and agreed on the themes. Anonymous quotes were used to illustrate the facts.

Methodological considerations

Qualitative researchers suggest the use of credibility, transferability, dependability and conformability as methods to ensure trustworthiness in qualitative studies [24, 25]. The researcher ensured credibility through use of multiple data collection methods (focus group discussions and in depth-interviews) which allowed triangulation of findings. Also the researcher established good rapport through having prolonged engagement in the field, used Luganda language (during FGDs) to build trust with participants. Bracketing was done through the researcher's honest self-examination of the values, beliefs, interests and prior experiences. These were noted down and kept at the back of the mind right from proposal development through data collection, analysis and report writing to ensure that the findings were the views of the participants and not the researcher's imaginations.Dependability and conformability were promoted through inquiry audit where by the researchers reviewed and examined the research process and the data analysis in order to ensure that the findings were consistent. Further, the thick description of the phenomenon under study, the purposive sampling used, the data collection methods that were employed and using participant's own words during analysis and write up enhance the understanding of childbirth experiences and will allow for others to determine its transferability to other contexts [26].

Results

The 25 women who were interviewed about their childbirth experiences described themselves as housewives (*n* = 7), teachers (*n* = 6), business women (n = 6), students (*n* = 2), a journalist, an administrator, a peasant and health information assistant (*n* = 1). They were between 18 and 33 years of age, 88% (*n* = 22) were married; 88% (n = 22)gave birth in the health facilities and 12% delivered at their homes or from the traditional birth attendant. Their parity ranged from one to five and the majority were Christians (Born again (32%), Protestants (24%), Catholics (12%), the rest were Moslems (32%).

From the 12 semi-structured interviews and 2 focus group discussions, five (5) themes emerged. These included the Childbirth experiences (Labour pains and management, Institutional care and support, Childbirth fears and Social support) and the Meaning attached to childbirth experiences (Individual and Cultural interpretations). The Women reported diverse trends in their birth experiences that provided the differences and the basis for emphasis. Numbers were used to identify participants during group discussions instead of names for privacy purposes and fictive names are used in the presentation of quotes.

Childbirth experiences
Labour pains and management
The memory of labour pains remained in the minds of almost all women and formed the basis for their stories. The women's birth pain experiences were viewed and expressed in terms of intensity, duration and patterns. The severe labour pains to some women were characterized by the temporary moments of confusion and loss of understanding as one mother expressed:

This is the 4th born, other children never pained me like this one,...contractions were very strong and I reached a point when I did not understand well, they just lifted me up on to the bed. ....I just found myself delivered. After delivering, my senses came back (Zaifa, 27 years, a mother of 4)

Rose who experienced abnormal labour patterns also said:

Labour for my last born was hard, because the pains were much and later the contractions stopped. .....later the midwives put on a drip for contractions (Rose, 30 years, a mother of 4).

Some womenexperienced labour for a long duration and its effects were reported with dismay, frustration and loss of hope as one mother explained:

*...the contractions pained me for 3 days... I went back, they examined me ... I was still not ready. I walked and walked .... I went back at 6.00pm (second day, I was still not ready. I went back at 10.00 p.m, they told me I was not ready. I went back at midnight, the midwife told me, aaaah we are fed up with you, you go and walk so that the baby can move down, ...the body was feeling like a metal, I said this time I am dead (*Eseza, 23years, a mother of one).

The labour pain aspect of childbirth is one dimension that is given attention in various ways. In this study, the women were socially oriented to view labour pains as a normal phenomenon regardless of intensity, duration and varying patterns. This psychological care in preparation for birth provided consolation, hope and encouragement as narratives below indicate:

"My attendants told me, contractions pain but you must be strong, and when time comes for the baby to come out, the baby itself will force you" (Shifa, a 28 year old mother of 2).

"Getting much pain happens and is human and normal to a woman, but it is God who gives you the life and energy" (Rehema, a 33 year old mother of five).

Labour pain management elicited mixed feelings from participants. Some women believed childbirth is natural and therefore should be left to take the natural course, while others felt it was necessary to reduce on the birth pains through medication if it was possible. According to the women's descriptions, none of them received biomedical painkillers during birth and one mother explained:

Next time I deliver, I would not want to have too much labour pains like the ones I went through. If that medicine was there, I would feel like having such a drug to reduce the pain (Christine, 25 years, a first time mother).

Some women doubted as to whether medicine could have an effect on a natural process like labour pains as they had no prior knowledge to the intervention

"I think no need of medicine, because it is natural. I think even if they give you some medicine for pain, contractions would still come because the baby has to come out. I think the drugs cannot reduce those pains...every other woman goes through that" (Irene, 26 years, a primepara).

Institutional care and support

The experiences of women regarding care and support received in the health facilities varied from positive by some mothers to negative and non-satisfying by others. Regarding institutional **births,** majority of women had **given birth** from the Regional Referral Hospital apart from one woman who had delivered from a private maternity centre. The women's comments generally centred on the attitude of service providers, the interpersonal communication, the physical and psychological support and how the labour complications were managed. For those who felt good about their labour experiences described them in form of the good reception and attention given to them, the physical and psychological support through counseling; being listened to and having been given appropriate management to the complications as some mothers narrated:

*The midwives were good.... even when they were attending to other people, when I would also call her (musawo) meaning a health care provider, also come and help me, She would not shout at me, would say let me come, I am hearing. I used to hear that they shout at people but for me they never shouted at me. (*Christine, a 25 year old mother of one).

Another one said:

*The midwives welcomed me well, examined me ... delivery time had not reached. I told them, basawo, I am sick, (HIV positive) they said you have done a good thing to tell us..., they said don't fear. Some hide and do not tell us. ....when the time reaches you will push well and in case something wrong happens, we will help you. When time came, the midwife helped me to climb the bed. After delivery, I bled a lot ... quickly they ran and gave me an injection and blood stopped. ... weighed the baby, wrote treatment and gave the syrup for the baby (*Rehema, a 33year mother of 5*).*

As some mothers expressed their birth experiences with confidence and trust in service providers, to others it was a moment of reflection on the sadness, suffering and agony they went through. The women described experiences of non- caring attitude, limited technical care and support; quarreling and being rough to them. Rose,one of the mothers that was cared for by the morning and evening ward staff described her experience with the midwife of the 2nd shift:

.... I called her that I feel like something pushing me, she never bothered. She said, "Keep quiet, for you, you are making yourself tired for nothing, you are not going to deliver now". I forced to deliver myself, what can I

do? *(Voice tone lowered) I said that if I relax I would lose my baby.... When the midwife reached, the baby was out and a lot of water (liquor) had poured on the baby. She (midwife) got annoyed, quarreled.... She cut the baby's cord from that water yet I normally see midwives cut the cord from the mother's abdomen. I felt too bad.*

The practices reflected by some health care providers were unethical and violated the rights of the clients as one mother who was slapped during the time she pushed her baby narrated:

... the midwife told me to push. I tried to push and push, she was even slapping me telling me to push. The old woman (attendant) had given the midwife some money, now she was on my "bamper" (on my neck). "I have told you to push the baby with slaps"

(Ruth, a 20 year old mother of 2)

Giving birth by caesarean was a hurdle. One mother who was taken to the theatre for the caesarean birth experienced delay to be operated as theatre was unready causing her stress and anxiety. This was heighted by being left exposed naked, a factor that compromised her privacy as she lamented:

....now you are under stress and you feel like... they have to do it (operation) immediately. "They take you in the theatre room, you again spend some good time there when they are still organizing. It was too bad, ...now even you feel stress is coming back again , you try to console yourself , you control...As you wait, you are naked, you are exposed there... (laughed while shaking her head)... you know how funny it is. ..you are nude. It was not good, privacy was not enough". (Caroline, a 30 year old mother of 3 children).

Many women were giving birth for the first time and as such needed more information regarding labour and its proceedings. Women noted limited effective communication and sharing of information by the service providers. The non-involvement of a mother in decision-making regarding her care resulted in a number of unanswered questions as one woman explained:

..... the doctor told me, Irene, with you, you are just going for an operation. ...I had to break down... because I was like what has gone wrong? ... why not me to deliver like other women? ....they are telling me I am going for an operation but they are not telling me the cause! Doctor Just told me, the baby was big. He then used some medical language that I did not

understand. She did not convince me as to why I should have an operation... they were talking alone! (Irene, a first time mother).

Social support

The mothers according to their narratives appreciated the presence, proximity, the physical and psychological support from their birth companions that were basically family members (the mums, sisters, mothers-in law, aunties, husbands) and friends. Physically, the women were supported by giving them food and drinks like tea, they were supported to walk around before reaching second stage of labour and their backs were rubbed to provide relief during contractions by their birth companions.

Eseza a 23 year old mother of 3 recounted:

Attendants (birth companions) helped me to get tea to drink, they kept around, and during that time when I could get the contractions, they could support me at the back, rub it, I could get some relief of about one minute.

Irene, a 26 year old primipara, who was supported through counselling by a relative before a caesarean birth recalled:

"At that time when I broke down,... my sister in law and mother in law were there for me. They tried to counsel and consoled me but still it wasn't an easy moment"

The male partners were involved in intrapartum care of their spouses at different times and in various ways. Although their (male partners') physical presence was registered at the hospital, their participation in real care was minimal. One mother whose husband was in hospital but at a distance from the maternity unit commented:

My husband was not near, had feared and moved away. I never wanted him to be near because when you are in labour the face changes, you may say that it is this one who brought the problems and get annoyed with him (laughed) (Shifa, a mother of 2).

Another mother whose husband fully participated in the processes of the birth of their baby by being present at the side of his partner and providing physical and psychological support during the pushing time gave her story:

When I came back to the labour ward they told me "the baby has reached you push", I was not feeling any energy. ....my husband helped me, held me and he

never feared. When the baby was coming out, he told me that "bambi" (meaning my friend) push more, the head is coming, add in more effort. ... I felt good, I liked it so much because he gave me support, and he was there (Faith, a mother of one).

Childbirth fears

Childbirth is a moment of unpredictable "next" in terms of the outcome of the baby and mother both to those who give birth normally and by caesarean birth. In this study, these experiences were worsened by giving birth by a caesarean resulting into mothers' fear, anxiety and loss of hope for survival as one woman recalled:

It is hard when you are going for a cesarean birth, you are always worried. ...... you are not sure of what is going to happen there..... in such situation the mother is not sure of the baby's survival and her own wellbeing; or she might come out with complications. Yah...it is like you are going for trouble when you are seeing (mother laughed) (Catherine, a 30-year mother of 3, with 3 previous scars).

The situation can be more terrifying to those who are giving birth for the first time. Irene, a first time mother had refused a caesarean birth for fear of losing her life in theatre until all hope of delivering normally was lost.

The doctor told me, "Irene, with you, you are just going for an operation at 10am". ....I had to break down, I did not know ... "if others can push normally, why not me?" At 10 a.m I refused the operation. I told them I don't want, give me time ......I had feared the theatre because with me I knew whoever goes to theatre, does not come back. They just die like that. I imagined very many things

Multidimensional sources of fear were reported in this study. One mother who experienced excessive bleeding and a retained placenta regretted the decision she had made of delivering at home: "being with aunt alone I feared, I felt my life was going and regretted not having been in hospital". The mistreatment of women by health care providers was so frightening that one mother vowed never again to deliver in that hospital as she expressed it:

"... I forced to deliver myself"....in that difficulty situation I went through, I got scared, I feared the midwives of the main hospital (government). I feared too much, I said next time when I deliver, at least I go to private but not go back to main hospital. (Rose, a mother of 4 children).

The negative stories (the past experiences by other mothers) about the institutional care were noted to be far reaching and a source of childbirth fears regarding the place of delivery. One mother who presumed and perceived hospital care negatively resorted to practices that undermine the quality of birth outcomes as she gave birth at the TBA's home and gave her account:

"I refused going to hospital. I had no appetite of going there. What I hear threatened me. I hear in the hospital they don't care about you, you care for yourself. ....You are seeing this one is complaining, that one grumbling, another one is dying, I avoided such things. I said at least, for me let me die from here (TBA's) and those other ones die there in hospital" (Amina, an 18-year-old primipara).

Meaning attached to childbirth experiences: The individual woman's and societal interpretations
The individuals' childbirth experience meaning

The individual women interviewed had varying personal interpretations of their birth experiences. The sense made out of it was determined by what preoccupied the woman at that time of labour, the transpirations of the day and the outcomes. The supremacy of God in the event of childbirth was strongly expressed by many women but in union with self-belief and determination of an individual. The women were convinced that God had to be in control for a successful birth. One woman said; *....things to do with childbirth, it is God's grace* and others affirmed:

You must believe in yourself and believe in God. ....for me during birth, I said yes I will do it... I became firm and pushed the baby. Believing in yourself helps you to push the baby (Zaharah, 24 years, mother of one).

"It's not an easy thing but when you are determined, God can be by your side, yah then you will get a child" (Irene, a 26-year-old first time mother).

As some women believed childbirth had a strong bearing on one's personal effort put in during labour, to others birthing without complications was perceived and directly associated with "being strong and brave" as accounts below indicated:

.... people used to consider me as a weak person and thought I would not manage to give birth by myself... but I demonstrated that I am strong, (She stressed the point very happily, entire group went into laughter)...I pushed the baby without any problem (Amina, an 18 year old, primipara)

Anna, a 28-year-old first time mother also added:

"..... others when they start to push, they push and even die. I had to push and I saw the baby; then what I concluded is that i am brave because it is not easy there"

Societal and cultural interpretation of childbirth experiences
When women were asked to comment on how society perceived the different birth experiences they had gone through, the responses were cross cutting despite mothers being from different tribal and cultural backgrounds. The socio- cultural interpretations were mainly bent on the type of birth a woman went through. A mother was considered a strong woman if she gave birth well (vaginally) and the operated were regarded bewitched, failures or weak women.

Caroline, who had 3 consecutive operations said:

The Gisu's themselves think that when you go for an operation, ... you are bewitched. ...you are unable to have children, unable to be a real housewife; ... not a good house woman to make a child for somebody.

Irene, a first- time mother who delivered by caesarean birth was insulted by the community members as she explained:

Culturally, to the illiterate, they assume whoever goes for an operation failed to push. You are a weak woman. So, they were insulting me "eeeh she had just fattened, but you see, she failed to push the baby".

Discussion
The study explored and presents the childbirth experiences among postnatal mothers and the meaning attributed to such experiences. The themes that emerged majorly focused on childbirth pains and management, institutional care and support, social support, childbirth fears and the meaning attributed to their childbirth experiences.

Childbirth pains and management
The intensity of labour pains, the duration and patterns gave women different birth experiences and responses. The varied experiences were a reflection that each labour and birth a woman goes through is a unique experience even to women who have given birth before [27].This calls for proper assessment and understanding of the individual intrapartum needs of a woman by the health care providers and emotional support by the birth companion for a positive childbirth experience [28]. It

was noted that people in the communities orient women to consider labour pains natural and normal regardless of their nature and this is intended to build courage and self-confidence of women during birth. Similarly, in a study done in Ghana, a first time mother was told in advance by her mother that labour was painful but should harden and remain strong [29]. Although women experienced prolonged and exhaustive labour pains with moments of confusion, inability to move, backs being felt in pieces and feelings of despair, divergent feelings of yes and no need regarding biomedical pain relief administration during childbirth were elicited. The women that were not in favour of the administration of drugs for pain relief simply felt birth pains were natural and medicine could not stop them. These expressions were of no surprise given that use of drugs to control pain during childbirth is still a rare occurrence in the country's health care system like it is reported in other settings [29]. The evidence that none of the mothers received medication for pain relief despite a few of them expressing desire to have it, was a clear indication of limited access to such interventions. The women posited that without pain a baby could not come out, an indication of a knowledge gap on use of drugs for pain relief during labour. This calls for orientation of women on pain management options to empower them demand for their right of a pain free labourexperience as also recommended by the WHO intrapartum care model of 2018 [28].

Institutional care and support

The women's experiences of care and support varied from positive to negative and non-satisfying. The majority of women had given birth from the Regional Referral Hospital apart from one woman who had given birth from a private maternity centre. The needs and expectations of mothers in labour may seem to be many, however from this study it became apparent that giving attention and listening to women; good interpersonal communication and involving them in their care plans were key; the provision of physical and psychological support and competence in the management of complications were all paramount. The extent to which care met the individual expectations of mothers influenced the individual comments which were either reflective of a positive or negative birth experience. The women who received attention, good care and support expressed comfort and contentment of the hospital services and built high degree of confidence in the service providers and themselves. In a study done in Australia, women who were under supportive midwives felt contented with their childbirth experiences as opposed to those who were not and felt frustrated [27]. Similar findings have been reported in studies done in Iceland and India,

where kindness and supportiveness to women in labour were strongly emphasized and closely related to a satisfying childbirth experience [30, 31]. On the contrary, in this study, women who received little attention, minimal technical, physical and psychological support had their birth experiences non-notable. And as such women lost self-confidence, distanced themselves from the care providers and some built bitterness against them. It was also noted that lack of provision of adequate information about labour processes and progression, poor communication and low involvement of mothers in their plans of care deprived them of full situational control and increased anxiety, stress and other emotional tendencies. Such findings are strongly backed by studies [27, 32], in which involvement of mothers in decision making during childbirth increased self-confidence, self-esteem, feelings of being in control and felt they had accomplished a task. These aspects of care are far reaching [28] that a mother, who misses them, will register a gap and a negative childbirth experience. This therefore calls for a positive attitude of a service provider to enhance and promote these indispensable needs during childbirth.

Social support

Support from family members (mums, sisters, mothers in-law, aunties, husbands) and friends was strongly noted during this study. Escorting women to the birth places, provision of food and other requirements; rubbing the back, helping the mother to move to and forth were among the physical support given. Psychologically, they were supported through consolation and counseling and orientation on labour pains before or during labour. Social support in this study was strongly noted as a source of comfort, encouragement and hope to the mothers as strongly supported in other studies [33].

The presence of the male partner in the labour ward and his proximity to the spouse was appreciated by some women while others felt comfortable when their spouses were at a distance for fear of shifting blame to their male partners as trouble causers. Such divergent views and feelings about the men's availability in labour wards have been cited in [34] in which some women expressed fear of their partners being impolite and non-loving to them while others were comfortable and in agreement with the practice. In Uganda, the practice of a female partner being with her spouse in a labour suite is just starting (mainly in private hospitals) and thus it is new to most women and men contrary to the developed world where the culture is deeply embedded in their care [35]. In a Swedish study [36] men from other countries appreciated the Swedish culture that transformed them from being "men at a distance" and women at "close proxy" to "a family" at the centre of every family member's health concerns including childbirth. In this study, most participants had given birth from a government hospital and like most other government health facilities in this country, it had a general labour ward whose admission capacity was up to six mothers at a single moment. This minimized the space for a single laboring woman whose privacy was fragile and only protected by a curtain in between the beds. This further explains the low number of male partners and their low levels of involvement in labour processes for their female partners especially in the labour wards. Similar findings of a non-supportive environment for male involvement, have been reported in a study done in Mulago hospital [37].The findings of the study clearly indicated that mothers in labour currently have two schools of thought regarding the presence of male partners in labour suites. This calls for more research in this area to fully understand the factors that influence male partner involvement in labour and birth processes.

Childbirth fears

The fears of childbirth reported in this study were majorly associated with the uncertainties of birth outcomes especially women who underwent an operation for they were not sure of the lives of the baby and self; or whether it would result in complications. Similarly, Corbett and Callister [30] found out that the Tamil Nadu women had fear of "the unknown" as they could not imagine the birth pains, and also feared caesarean birth leading to anxiety. In a Taiwan study [38] the caesarean births augmented more the risk of stress compared to women who gave birth vaginally and it was thought to be associated with hormonal differences or lack of self-confidence. In a Turkish study, the complications greatly contributed to birth fears [39]. These fears are further justified by Harrison and Goldenberg [40] who found out that complications like heamorrhage, embolism, hypovolemic shock, pre-eclampsia and eclampsia contributed to poor or severe maternal outcomes especially in resource limited geographies among caesarean births.

The non-satisfying childbirth experience due to the negative attitudes and practices of the health care providers frightened women and as such they vowed never again to give birth in the public hospitals. Furthermore, the stories the mothers heard from other women about the care and the practices of health care providers in hospital, caused some women to resist moving to hospital with the eventual decision to give birth with the TBA. This puts a woman further at risk and undermines the quality of the outcomes of labour given the limited level of knowledge and skills of the traditional birth attendant [41].Although labour pains were significantly noted by almost all women, to a lesser extent they were reported to be a source of fear possibly due to the social orientation of women about labour. These findings are

contrary to what was found out in a Turkish study where labour pains was the most feared component of childbirth [42].Generally,fear caused stress and anxieties to mothers, both of which are factors that have been found to distort contractions and prolong labour and render one's birth experience negative [33]. Overall, it is important to note, that creating a conducive birthing environment, free of fear, is key in promoting a sense of trust and confidence both in the health care providers and in theservices they offer for a positive childbirth experience.

Meaning attached to childbirth experiences

The meaning of the childbirth experiences captured was two folded. The first one was – the mother's personal interpretation of her own birth experience and two was how other people in the community interpreted the birth experience she went through. The women drew personal meanings and lessons of their birth experiences mainly from the nature of labour pains they had, the treatment by the service providers, the complications experienced and the labour outcomes. According to their accounts, women felt it was important and safer to deliver in a hospital especially those who had given birth at home and those who got complications like severe bleeding.Such lessons learnt could be helpful to a woman to subsequently make rational decisions regarding the birthing place. On the contrary, in a study done among Hmong women of Vietnam, majority of participants preferred a home birth for fear of loss of control over birth care decisions, limited comfort and loss of the placenta for cultural rituals [30].Findings also revealed that self-determination, self-confidence, self-belief and perseverance contributed to their successful childbirth. Although these ideologies may sound non- objective, they are important to note for they provide a basis for further assessment of their underlying causes from which objective interventions can be designed to improve childbirth. Self-belief and self-confidence have been found to promote and were closely related to positive childbirth experiences [43]. The women associated a normal vaginal birth (a birth free of complications) to braveness and being strong as they withstood and tolerated the birth hardships especially contractions. Such beliefs are important to understand by a health care provider so as to provide appropriate counseling to those who may experience complications during childbirth and those who undergo cesarean birth to prevent frustration, loss of self-esteem and feelings of inadequacy.

The cultural and social interpretations of childbirth experiences were the perceived meanings of childbirth by other people. Given the fact that these mothers were living in the same communities, it was speculated that the participants knew or had heard what people say about their birth experiences. According to the accounts of mothers, the majority of meanings were drawn from the type of birth one underwent. Culturally, every woman is expected to be strong, endure with pain and give birth vaginally. So, if a woman gave birth by caesarean, she would be considered bewitched, failed to push (a failure), weak and a woman not good to make a housewife. These findings might be so because in many African cultures, what goes wrong is thought to be an influence of evil spirits. They also believe in big number of children yet a mother, who is operated right from the first child, can safely produce four. Such interpretations may cause loss of self-esteem leading to poor adjustment to motherhood [43]. Understanding the cultural interpretations of childbirth experiences helps a health care provider to provide emotional support to the sufferers and their families and generally for the decision makers to design interventions that can address knowledge gaps regarding birthing options.

Limitations

Childbirth experiences were got from mothers of parity five and below despite trying hard to look for those ones with parity above five. These possibly would have given different stories regarding childbirth. Literature from Africa on childbirth experiences and their meaning to mothers was limited giving a narrow point of reference when discussing the results in regard to the African context. Therefore, we recommend that subsequent similar or related studies look at settings like Latin America for a broader and closer contextual comparison. The socio cultural interpretations of the childbirth experiences may not fully reflect the views of all the other people in the studied community given the narrow source of the views.

Conclusion

Childbirth experiences were unique and elicited unique feelings, responses and challenges to individual mothers, thus the need for the proper assessment and understanding of women for personalized care. It is important to note that pain management during labour is a necessity and a right of a woman to experience a pain free labour and birth for a positive childbirth outcome for those who embrace it. Creating a good birthing environment with the health care providers that are competent, compassionate and supportive to their clients, builds a sense of trust, and confidence in them and their services and the institution at large which promotes the general wellbeing of a woman at birth. Understanding the societal perceptions of childbirth experiences provides a basis for identifying and designing interventions to support the victimized mothers and the communities to understand childbirth.

Operational definitions

Childbirth experiences: Is an individual woman's life event that incorporates interrelated subjective psychological and physiological processes, influenced by social, environmental, organizational and policy contexts [1].

Childbirth: In this study, childbirth referred to labour and birth.

Experiences: the personal lived through encounter of the phenomenon.

Mothers: women who had been pregnant and delivered.

Meaning: were the individual and subjective interpretations of a situation or a happening (her childbirth experiences) by the mother.

Postpartum period: Is the period from one hour following the delivery of the placenta up to six weeks (WHO, 1998). However, in this study the postpartum period referred to the period from one hour after the birth of the placenta up to eight weeks or two months.

Abbreviations

DHO: District Health Officer; FGD: Focus Group Discussion; M. o. H: Ministry of Health; SSI: Semi Structured Interviews; WHO: World Health Organization; YCC: Young Child Clinic

Acknowledgments

The authors would like to thank the Centre of Excellence for Maternal, Newborn and Child Health Research, Makerere University, School of Public Health for the funds that supported the research. Thanks are also due to the administration and staff of Mbale Regional Referral Hospital for their cooperation and support during data collection and the dear mothers for accepting to participate in the study.

Funding

The Centre of Excellence for Maternal, Newborn and Child Health supported the study from data collection, analysis, interpretation of data and writing the report. The grant further covered the dissemination / sharing of results at the study site and in scientific conferences within the country.

Authors' contributions

JN conceived the research idea and participated in the design, coordination of data collection, and drafting of the manuscript. RM participated in refining the research idea and drafting of the manuscript. LTM performed the analysis and participated in refining the presentation of results and their discussion. PW, JN did critical revision of the research work and provided additional inputs and comments for further improvement of the manuscript. PM participated in the refining the research idea and design. All authors read and approved the final manuscript.

Competing interests

The authors declare that they have no competing interests in this section.

Author details
[1]Department of Nursing, Makerere University, College of Health Sciences, P.O Box 7072, Kampala, Uganda. [2]Department of Clinical Nursing, Muhimbili University of Health and Allied Sciences, Nursing and Midwifery Services Muhimbili Academic Medical Centre, P.O. Box 65427, Dar es Salaam, Tanzania. [3]Department of Health, Policy, Planning and Management, Makerere University, College of Health Sciences, School of Public Health, Kampala, Uganda. [4]Global Health Division Karolinska Institutet, Sweden and Leader Makerere University Maternal and Newborn Centre of Excellence and the INDEPTH Network Maternal and Newborn Health Research, Stockholm, Sweden.

References

1. Larkin P, Begley CM, Devane D. Women's experiences of labour and birth: an evolutionary concept analysis. Midwifery. 2009;25(2):e49–59.

2. Mensah R, Mogale R, Richter M. Birthing experiences of Ghanaian women in 37th military hospital, Accra, Ghana. International Journal of Africa Nursing Sciences. 2014;1:29–34.

3. Semenic SE, Callister LC, Feldman P. Giving birth: the voices of orthodox Jewish women living in Canada. J Obstet Gynecol Neonatal Nurs. 2004;33(1):80–7.

4. Winter C, et al. Depression, pregnancy-related anxiety and parental-antenatal attachment in couples using preimplantation genetic diagnosis. Hum Reprod. 2016;31(6):1288–99.

5. Wilkinson SE, Callister LC. Giving birth: the voices of Ghanaian women. Health Care Women Int. 2010;31(3):201–20.

6. Leeners B, et al. Birth experiences in adult women with a history of childhood sexual abuse. J Psychosom Res. 2016;83:27–32.

7. Nilsson C. The delivery room: is it a safe place? A hermeneutic analysis of women's negative birth experiences. Sex Reprod Healthc. 2014;5(4):199–204.

8. Waldenström U, et al. A negative birth experience: prevalence and risk factors in a national sample. Birth. 2004;31(1):17–27.

9. Størksen HT, et al. The impact of previous birth experiences on maternal fear of childbirth. Acta Obstet Gynecol Scand. 2013;92(3):318–24.

10. Karlström A, Nystedt A, Hildingsson I. The meaning of a very positive birth experience: focus groups discussions with women. BMC pregnancy childbirth. 2015;15(1):251.

11. Stoll K, Hall W. Vicarious birth experiences and childbirth fear: does it matter how young Canadian women learn about birth? J Perinat Educ. 2013;22(4):226.

12. Elvander C, Cnattingius S, Kjerulff KH. Birth experience in women with low, intermediate or high levels of fear: findings from the first baby study. Birth. 2013;40(4):289–96.

13. Muzik M, et al. Mother–infant bonding impairment across the first 6 months postpartum: the primacy of psychopathology in women with childhood abuse and neglect histories. Arch Womens Ment Health. 2013;16(1):29–38.

14. O'Higgins M, et al. Mother-child bonding at 1 year; associations with symptoms of postnatal depression and bonding in the first few weeks. Arch Womens Ment Health. 2013;16(5):381–9.

15. Hodnett ED, et al. Continuous support for women during childbirth. Cochrane Database Syst Rev. 2012;10:1–77.

16. Renfrew MJ, et al. Midwifery and quality care: findings from a new evidence-informed framework for maternal and newborn care. Lancet. 2014; 384(9948):1129–45.

17. Shiferaw S, et al. Why do women prefer home births in Ethiopia? BMC pregnancy childbirth. 2013;13(1):5.

18. Burns N, Grove SK. The practice of nursing research. Philadelphia: WB. Saunders Company; 1997.

19. Callister LC. Making meaning: Women's birth narratives. J Obstet Gynecol Neonatal Nurs. 2004;33(4):508–18.

20. Smith JA. Qualitative psychology: A practical guide to research methods. London: Sage; 2015.

21. Tongco MDC. Purposive sampling as a tool for informant selection. Ethnobot Res Appl. 2007;5:147–58.

22. Morse JM. Data were saturated. Los Angeles: Sage publications Sage CA; 2015.

23. Browne J, Minichiello V. The social meanings behind male sex work: Implications for sexual interactions. Br J Sociol. 1995;46:598–622.

24. Elo S, et al. Qualitative content analysis: a focus on trustworthiness. SAGE Open. 2014;4(1):2158244014522633.

25. Houghton C, et al. Rigour in qualitative case-study research. Nurse researcher. 2013;20(4):12–7.

26. Yazan B. Three approaches to case study methods in education: yin, Merriam, and stake. Qual Rep. 2015;20(2):134–52.

27. Murray L, et al. The experiences of African women giving birth in Brisbane. Australia Health Care for Women International. 2010;31(5):458–72.

28. Oladapo O, et al. WHO model of intrapartum care for a positive childbirth experience: transforming care of women and babies for improved health and wellbeing. BJOG: An International Journal of Obstetrics & Gynaecology; 2018.

29. Wilkinson S. and Callister L., Perceptions of childbearing among women in the Ashanti region of Ghana. , 2010. 31(3): p. 201–220

30. Corbett CA, et al. The meaning of giving birth: voices of Hmong women living in Vietnam. Perinat Neonatal Nurs. 2017;31(3):207–15.

31. Halldorsdottir S, Karlsdottir SI. Journeying through labour and delivery: perceptions of women who have given birth. Midwifery. 1996;12(2):48–61.

32. Simkin P. Just another day in a woman's life? Women's long-term perceptions of their first birth experience. Part I Birth. 1991;18(4):203–10.

33. Iliadou M. Supporting women in labour. Health Sci J. 2012;6(3):385.

34. Singh D, Lample M, Earnest J. The involvement of men in maternal health care: cross-sectional, pilot case studies from Maligita and Kibibi, Uganda. Reprod Health. 2014;11(1):68.

35. Redshaw M, Henderson J. Fathers' engagement in pregnancy and childbirth: evidence from a national survey. BMC pregnancy childbirth. 2013;13(1):70.

36. Ny P, et al. The experience of middle eastern men living in Sweden of maternal and child health care and fatherhood: focus-group discussions and content analysis. Midwifery. 2008;24(3):281–90.

37. Kaye DK, et al. Male involvement during pregnancy and childbirth: men's perceptions, practices and experiences during the care for women who developed childbirth complications in Mulago hospital, Uganda. BMC pregnancy childbirth. 2014;14(1):54.

38. Chen HH, et al. Understanding the relationship between cesarean birth and stress, anxiety, and depression after childbirth: a nationwide cohort study. Birth. 2017;44(4):369–76.

39. JamshidiManesh M, et al. The process of women's decision making for selection of cesarean delivery. Iran J Nurs. 2009;21(56):55–67.

40. Harrison MS, Goldenberg RL. Cesarean section in sub-Saharan Africa. Maternal health, neonatology and perinatology. 2016;2(1):6.

41. Turinawe EB, et al. Traditional birth attendants (TBAs) as potential agents in promoting male involvement in maternity preparedness: insights from a rural community in Uganda. Reprod Health. 2016;13(1):24.

42. روند ت   میم گـیری زنان در انتـخاب زایـمان بـه روش سـزارین. et al ,منش, ج نـشریه بـر. سـتأری ایـران. 2009;21(56):55–67

43. Fenwick J, et al. Study protocol for reducing childbirth fear: a midwife-led psycho-education intervention. BMC Pregnancy childbirth. 2013; 13(1):190.

Permissions

List of Contributors

Mamakiri Mulaudzi, Busisiwe Nkala Dlamini, Jenny Coetzee and Janan Janine Dietrich
Perinatal HIV Research Unit (PHRU), Faculty of Health Sciences, University of the Witwatersrand, Chris Hani Road, Diepkloof, Soweto, Johannesburg 1864, South Africa

Kathleen Sikkema
Duke University, Department of Psychology and Neuroscience, Durham, USA

Glenda Gray
Perinatal HIV Research Unit (PHRU), Faculty of Health Sciences, University of the Witwatersrand, Chris Hani Road, Diepkloof, Soweto, Johannesburg 1864, South Africa
South African Medical Research Council, Cape Town, South Africa

Wakgari Binu
Department of Midwifery, Arba Minch College of Health Sciences, Arba Minch, Ethiopia

Taklu Marama
Department of Midwifery, College of Health Sciences and Medicine, Wolaita Sodo University, Wolaita Sodo, Ethiopia

Mulusew Gerbaba and Melese Sinaga
Department of Population and Family Health, College of public Health and Medical Sciences, Jimma University, Jimma, Ethiopia

Angela Odiachi
Abuja, Nigeria

Salome Erekaha and Christopher Isah
International Research Center of Excellence, Institute of Human Virology Nigeria, Abuja, Nigeria

Llewellyn J. Cornelius
School of Social Work and College of Public Health, University of Georgia Athens, Athens, USA

Habib O. Ramadhani
Institute of Human Virology, University of Maryland School of Medicine, Baltimore, USA

Laura Rapoport
Harvard T. H. Chan School of Public Health, Boston, USA

Nadia A. Sam-Agudu
International Research Center of Excellence, Institute of Human Virology Nigeria, Abuja, Nigeria
Institute of Human Virology, University of Maryland School of Medicine, Baltimore, USA

Edward Antwi
Julius Global Health, Julius Center for Health Sciences and Primary Care, University Medical Center Utrecht, Utrecht University, Utrecht, the Netherlands
Ghana Health Service, P.M.B, Ministries, Accra, Greater Accra, Ghana

Kerstin Klipstein-Grobusch
Julius Global Health, Julius Center for Health Sciences and Primary Care, University Medical Center Utrecht, Utrecht University, Utrecht, the Netherlands
Division of Epidemiology and Biostatistics, School of Public Health, Faculty of Health Sciences, University of the Witwatersrand, Johannesburg, South Africa

Joyce L. Browne and Diederick E. Grobbee
Julius Global Health, Julius Center for Health Sciences and Primary Care, University Medical Center Utrecht, Utrecht University, Utrecht, the Netherlands

Peter C. Schielen
Center for Infectious Diseases Research, Diagnostics and Screening (IDS), National Institute for Public Health and the Environment (RIVM), Bilthoven, the Netherlands

Kwadwo A. Koram
Noguchi Memorial Institute for Medical Research, College of Health Sciences, University of Ghana, Legon, Accra, Ghana

Irene A. Agyepong
Ghana Health Service, P.M.B, Ministries, Accra, Greater Accra, Ghana

R. Rima Jolivet and Mary Nell Wegner
Maternal Health Task Force, Women and Health Initiative, Department of Global Health and Population, Harvard T.H. Chan School of Public Health, 651 Huntington Avenue, Boston, MA 02115, USA

Bella Vasant Uttekar and Kanchan Lakhwani
Centre for Operations Research and Training, 402 Woodland Apartment, Race Course Circle, Vadodara, Gujarat 390 007, India

Meaghan O'Connor
Maternal Health Task Force, Women and Health Initiative, Harvard T.H. Chan School of Public Health, 651 Huntington Avenue, Boston, MA 02115, USA

Jigyasa Sharma
Department of Global Health and Population, Harvard T. H. Chan School of Public Health, 677 Huntington Ave, Boston, MA 02115, USA

Yao-Yao Du, Na Guo, Xiang Hua, Tao-Ran Deng, Xue-Mei Teng, Yang-Cheng Yao and Yu-Feng Li
Reproductive Medicine Center, Tongji Hospital, Tongji Medical College, Huazhong University of Science and Technology, 1095 JieFang Avenue, Wuhan, Hubei, People's Republic of China

Yi-Xin Wang
Department of Occupational and Environmental Health, School of Public Health, Tongji Medical College, Huazhong University of Science and Technology, Wuhan, Hubei, People's Republic of China
Key Laboratory of Environment and Health, Ministry of Education and Ministry of Environmental Protection, and State Key Laboratory of Environmental health (incubating), School of Public Health, Tongji Medical College, Huazhong University of Science and Technology, Wuhan, Hubei, People's Republic of China

Kazuyo Machiyama and John Cleland
Faculty of Epidemiology and Population Health, London School of Hygiene and Tropical Medicine, Keppel Street, London WC1E 7HT, UK

Fauzia Akhter Huda and Faisal Ahmmed
icddr, b, Dhaka, Bangladesh

George Odwe and Francis Obare
Population Council, Nairobi, Kenya

Joyce N. Mumah and Marylene Wamukoya
African Population and Health Research Center, Nairobi, Kenya

John B. Casterline
Institute for Population Research, Ohio State University, Columbus, USA

Sumiyo Okawa and Masamine Jimba
Department of Community and Global Health, Graduate School of Medicine, The University of Tokyo, Tokyo, Japan

Sylvia Mwanza-Kabaghe
Department of Educational Psychology, Sociology, and Special Education, School of Education, University of Zambia, Lusaka, Zambia

Paediatric HIV Centre of Excellence, University Teaching Hospital, Lusaka, Zambia

Mwiya Mwiya and Chipepo Kankasa
Paediatric HIV Centre of Excellence, University Teaching Hospital, Lusaka, Zambia

Kimiyo Kikuchi
Institute of Decision Science for a Sustainable Society, Kyushu University, Fukuoka, Japan

Naoko Ishikawa
Bureau of International Health Cooperation, National Center for Global Health and Medicine, Tokyo, Japan

Upuli Amaranganie Pushpakumari Perera
Postgraduate Institute of Medicine, University of Colombo, 36/1, Naiwala, Essalla, Veyangoda, Sri Lanka

Chrishantha Abeysena
Department of Public Health, Faculty of Medicine, University of Kelaniya, Kelaniya, Sri Lanka

Javier A. Schvartzman, Hugo Krupitzki, Angel E. Fiorillo, Enrique C. Gadow, Francisco M. Vizcaino, Felicitas von Petery and Victoria Marroquin
Department of Obstetrics and Gynecology, Centro de Educación Médica e Investigaciones Clínicas "Norberto Quirno" (CEMIC-IUC - CONICET), University Hospital, Av. Galván 4102 1431FWO, Buenos Aires, Argentina

Mario Merialdi
UNDP/UNFPA/UNICEF/WHO/World Bank Special Programme of Research, Development and
Research Training in Human Reproduction (HRP), Department of Reproductive Health and Research, World Health Organization, Avenue Appia 20, CH-1211 Geneva 27, Switzerland
Becton Dickinson and Company (BD), Franklin Lakes, NJ, USA

Ana Pilar Betrán, My Huong Nguyen, A Metin Gülmezoglu and Mercedes Bonet
UNDP/UNFPA/UNICEF/WHO/World Bank Special Programme of Research, Development and Research Training in Human Reproduction (HRP), Department of Reproductive Health and Research, World Health Organization, Avenue Appia 20, CH-1211 Geneva 27, Switzerland

Jennifer Requejo
Partnership for Maternal, Newborn and Child Health, World Health Organization, Avenue Appia 20, CH-1211 Geneva 27, Switzerland

Effy Vayena
Department of Health Sciences and Technology, ETH Zurich, Auf der Mauer 17, 8092 Zurich, Switzerland

María Luisa Cafferata, Agustina Mazzoni and Fernando Althabe
Instituto de Efectividad Clínica y Sanitaria (IECS - CONICET), Dr Emilio Ravignani 2024, C1414CPV Buenos Aires, Argentina

Valerie Vannevel and Robert C. Pattinson
SAMRC Maternal and Infant Health Care Strategies, Department of Obstetrics and Gynaecology, University of Pretoria, Pretoria, South Africa

Alex Müller, Sarah Spencer, Talia Meer and Kristen Daskilewicz
Gender, Health and Justice Research Unit, University of Cape Town, Observatory, Cape Town, South Africa

Rajani Shah
Nepal Public Health Foundation, Kathmandu, Nepal
Center for International Health, Ludwig-Maximilians-University, Munich, Germany

Eva A. Rehfuess
Center for International Health, Ludwig-Maximilians-University, Munich, Germany
Institute for Medical Information Processing, Biometry and Epidemiology, Pettenkofer School of Public Health, Ludwig-Maximilians-University, Munich, Germany

Deepak Paudel
Center for International Health, Ludwig-Maximilians-University, Munich, Germany
Save the Children, Kathmandu, Nepal

Mahesh K. Maskey
Nepal Public Health Foundation, Kathmandu, Nepal

Maria Delius
Center for International Health, Ludwig-Maximilians-University, Munich, Germany
Department of Obstetrics and Gynecology – Campus Grosshadern, Ludwig-Maximilians-University, Munich, Germany

M. M. Dynes, E. Twentyman, L. Kelly and F. Serbanescu
Centers for Disease Control and Prevention, Division of Reproductive Health, Atlanta, Georgia

G. Maro
Bloomberg Philanthropies Tanzania, Kigoma, Tanzania

A. A. Msuya
AMCA Inter Consult, Dar es Salaam, Tanzania

S. Dominico
Thamini Uhai, Kigoma, Tanzania

P. Chaote
Kigoma Region Ministry of Health, Kigoma, Tanzania

R. Rusibamayila
Ministry of Health Community Development Gender Elderly and Children, Dar es Salaam, Tanzania

Andrea C. Johnson, W. Douglas Evans and Nicole Barrett
Milken Institute School of Public Health, The George Washington University, 950 New Hampshire Avenue, NW, Washington, DC 20052, USA

Howida Badri, Tamador Abdalla and Cody Donahue
UNICEF, Kassala, Sudan

Tina Khanna, Murari Chandra, Ajay Singh and Sunil Mehra
MAMTA Health Institute for Mother and Child, B-5, Greater Kailash Enclave-II, New Delhi 110048, India

Ona McCarthy, Irrfan Ahamed, Phil Edwards, Melissa Palmer and Caroline Free
Department of Population Health, Faculty of Epidemiology and Population Health, London School of Hygiene and Tropical Medicine, Keppel Street, London WC1E 7HT, UK

Firuza Kulaeva, Ravshan Tokhirov and Salokhiddin Saibov
Tajik Family Planning Association, 10 Rudaki Avenue, TC 'Sadbarg', 7th floor, Dushanbe, Tajikistan

Marieka Vandewiele and Sarah Standaert
International Planned Parenthood Federation European Network, Rue Royale 146, 1000 Brussels, Belgium

Baptiste Leurent
Department of Medical Statistics, Faculty of Epidemiology and Population Health, London School of Hygiene and Tropical Medicine, Keppel Street, London WC1E 7HT, UK

Yoko Shimpuku and Shigeko Horiuchi
Human Health Sciences, Graduate School of Medicine, Kyoto University, 53 Shogoin-kawahara-cho, Sakyo-ku, Kyoto 606-8507, Japan

Frida E. Madeni
Magunga District Hospital, Old-Korogwe, Tanga, Tanzania

Kazumi Kubota
Department of Biostatistics, Yokohama City University School of Medicine, 3-9 Fukuura, Kanazawa-ku, Yokohama 236-0004, Japan

Sebalda C. Leshabari
School of Nursing, Muhimbili University of Health and Allied Sciences, Dar es Salaam, Tanzania

Katherine L. Turner
Global Citizen, LLC Consulting, 732 Ninth St., No. 521, Durham 27705, NC, USA
UNC-Chapel Hill Gillings School of Global Public Health, Chapel Hill, USA

Erin Pearson and Kathryn L. Andersen
Technical Innovation and Evidence, Ipas, Chapel Hill 27515, NC, USA

Allison George
Public Health Solutions, 40 Worth Street, 5th Floor, New York 10013, NY, USA

Josephine Namujju, Richard Muhindo, Joyce Nankumbi and Patience Muwanguzi
Department of Nursing, Makerere University, College of Health Sciences, Kampala, Uganda

Lilian T. Mselle
Department of Clinical Nursing, Muhimbili University of Health and Allied Sciences, Nursing and Midwifery Services Muhimbili Academic Medical Centre, Dar es Salaam, Tanzania

Peter Waiswa
Department of Health, Policy, Planning and Management, Makerere University, College of Health Sciences, School of Public Health, Kampala, Uganda
Global Health Division Karolinska Institutet, Sweden and Leader Makerere University Maternal and Newborn Centre of Excellence and the INDEPTH Network Maternal and Newborn Health Research, Stockholm, Sweden

Index